Paediatric neurosurgery for nurses

Paediatric Neurosurgery for Nurses provides accessible and up-to-date information for nurses working in paediatric neurosurgery. Referring throughout to the evidence-base for care and interventions, this complex area is described and explained in a meaningful and easily understandable way.

The text includes chapters on the underpinning knowledge and principles for the care of children who need neurosurgery as well as the following common neurological problems:

- hydrocephalus
- traumatic brain injury
- craniosynostosis
- brain tumours
- surgical management of epilepsy in children
- cerebrovascular disorders
- neural tube defects.

The complexity of the nervous system and principles of care are presented logically with points to consider and essential care clearly highlighted. Where available, evidence-based practice is presented, complete with a range of pedagogical features, such as chapter overviews and summaries, diagrams, sample care plans, text boxes and a glossary.

This book is essential reading for pre-registration nursing students and newly qualified nurses but will also be of use to allied healthcare professionals working with children and young people requiring neurosurgery.

Joanna Smith is Lecturer in Child Health Nursing at the University of Leeds, UK.

Catherine Martin is a staff nurse on the Regional Paediatric and Adolescent Oncology Unit at St James's Hospital, Leeds, UK.

Paediatric neurosurgery for nurses

Evidence-based care for children and their families

Joanna Smith and Catherine Martin

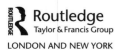

Routledge
Taylor & Francis Group

LONDON AND NEW YORK

First published 2009
by Routledge
2 Park Square, Milton Park, Abingdon, Oxon OX14 4RN

Simultaneously published in the USA and Canada
by Routledge
270 Madison Ave, New York, NY 10016

Routledge is an imprint of the Taylor & Francis Group, an informa business

Typeset in Garamond by
HWA Text and Data Management, London
Printed and bound in Great Britain by
CPI Antony Rowe, Chippenham, Wiltshire

British Library Cataloguing in Publication Data
A catalogue record for this book is available from the British Library

Library of Congress Cataloging-in-Publication Data
Smith, Joanna, 1963–
    Paediatric neurosurgery for nurses : evidence-based care for children and their
    families / Joanna Smith & Catherine Martin.
        p. ; cm.
    Includes bibliographical references.
    1. Pediatric neurology. 2. Pediatric nursing. 3. Neurological nursing. 4. Nervous
    system – Surgery. I. Martin, Catherine, 1976– II. Title.
    [DNLM: 1. Neurosurgical Procedures – nursing. 2. Child. 3. Evidence-Based
    Medicine – methods. 4. Nervous System Diseases – physiopathology. 5. Nervous
    System Diseases – surgery. 6. Pediatric Nursing – methods.
    0415446198 (hbk) / WY 160.5 S651p 2008]
    RJ486.S628 2008
    618.92′8--dc22   2007051018

ISBN10: 0–415–44619–8 (hbk)
ISBN10: 0–415–44620–1 (pbk)
ISBN10: 0–203–89511–8 (ebk)

ISBN13: 978–0–415–44619–8 (hbk)
ISBN13: 978–0–415–44620–4 (pbk)
ISBN13: 978–0–203–89511–5 (ebk)

Contents

Figures

Tables

Foreword

Neurosurgery in children is not new. Much of the work of the early pioneers of neurosurgery, such as Cushing or Dandy, involved surgery in children. However, the recognition of the need for a subspecialty of paediatric neurosurgery, or indeed paediatric neuroscience, is a much more recent phenomenon. That children are not small adults has become something of a cliché used by those promoting and developing paediatric services. Nonetheless, this point is at the root of why paediatric neurosurgery has emerged as a subspecialty. Not only are the conditions affecting children, and the clinical skills necessary to manage them, different from their counterparts in adults, but also for an optimal outcome (short term and long term), this treatment must be delivered in a way that understands the emotional and social needs of the child in relation to their age or cognitive abilities and, of course, the central role of parents and carers in the child's life.

This is, of course, why delivering optimal treatment requires a multi-professional team approach where each team member understands each other's roles and is prepared to learn from others within the team. It has been a privilege for me to have been part of such a team and to have watched our nursing colleagues develop paediatric neuroscience nursing from a niche interest to a fully fledged subspecialty with university recognition.

This book by Joanna Smith and Catherine Martin represents a coming of age for paediatric neuroscience nursing. The authors are to be congratulated for rising to the challenge of presenting an ever-growing body of clinical knowledge in the context of the pragmatic needs of the child and family who are undergoing neurosurgery. The authors have observed, listened to and learnt from their patients and in this book they are passing on a wealth of knowledge, expertise and opinion that will be invaluable to those who are embarking on the challenge of nursing children undergoing neurosurgery.

John Livingston
Consultant Paediatric Neurologist,
The General Infirmary at Leeds

Preface

The twenty-first century has, rightly so, placed an unprecedented emphasis on child health issues. Within the United Kingdom (UK) the emphasis on the health and well-being of children is underpinning the government's Every Child Matters agenda (DfES 2004). A commitment to the National Service Framework for Children, Young People and Maternity Services: Change for Children – Every Child Matters (DH 2004) requires healthcare professionals to place the child and family at the centre of care and respond appropriately to their needs. This is linked to ensuring that the people working with children are valued, rewarded and trained. In addition to the National Service Framework there is a range of guidance documents aimed at meeting the needs of people with neurological disorders such as:

- Head injury: triage, assessment, investigation and early management of head injury in infants, children and adults, 2nd edition (National Institute for Health and Clinical Excellence 2007).
- The epilepsies: the diagnosis and management of epilepsy in children and adults in primary and secondary care (National Institute for Clinical Excellence 2004).
- Stroke in childhood: clinical guidelines for diagnosis management and rehabilitation (Royal College of Physicians 2004).

The increase in guidance relating to the care and management of children with neurological disorders is excellent news for healthcare professionals working with these children and their families because there has, until recently, been a paucity of evidence on which to base care and service provision has been inconsistent.

Disorders of the nervous system are an important group of childhood conditions; central nervous system malformations account for approximately 75 per cent of fetal deaths and 40 per cent of deaths within the first year of life (Padgett 2002). Furthermore, it has been estimated that 15–20 per cent of hospitalised children have a neurological problem, either as the sole or associated complaint (Aicardi 1998). Diseases of the neurological system in infancy and childhood have a profound effect on the lives of the child and family and are probably the most disruptive of all ailments. As a group of conditions they provoke extreme anxiety, not only for the child and family, but also for healthcare professionals caring for these children. These anxieties are complex and include:

- The uncertain outcome and the potential to cause dramatic changes in function, both cognitively and physically.

- Although collectively common, many healthcare professionals do not have experience of caring for children with specific, rare neurological problems.
- Families often have expert knowledge of their child's condition and needs and although this should be viewed positively, can lead to frustration for parents and feelings of inadequacy for healthcare professionals involved in the care of the child.

Healthcare professionals may have a potential knowledge deficit because pre-registration curricula pressures have resulted in limited opportunity to include issues relating to the field of children's neurosciences into programmes of study. Furthermore, there is a dearth of post-registration courses, across healthcare professions, specifically focusing on children's neurosciences. In reality staff will be learning through experience. There is recognition that paediatric neurosurgery forms a significant neurosurgical workload and there is a drive towards the development of paediatric neurosurgery as a discrete subspecialty within neurosurgery (Chumas *et al.* 2002).

The aim of caring for a child with a neurological problem is to work within a developmental context to integrate the child into their family, school and community. Traditionally, models of care have focused on the disease (illness and dependence) and treatment; this is obviously inappropriate for a child with a neurological problem. Care must be individually designed and strongly influenced by encouraging children to reach their full potential. This can only be achieved through a structured, caring and safe environment. Care will be provided for by a variety of disciplines and the team must have common goals and programmes of care must be integrated into the child's daily routines. A detailed understanding of the role and function of the multidisciplinary team is essential. This will be a theme throughout the book.

The aim of this book is to provide accessible and up-to-date information relating to aspects of caring for a child with a neurological problem, and the family, when the child's treatment is primarily surgical. Chapter 1 will provide an overview of anatomy and physiology of the nervous system to enable readers to have a quick reference guide for subsequent chapters. This is in recognition that many neurological deficits correlate to structure or functional abnormalities (Raimondi and Hirschauer 1984). Those wishing greater depth of knowledge are advised to refer to one of the numerous texts relating specifically to anatomy and physiology of the nervous system. Chapter 2 outlines the general principles of caring for a child with a neurological problem, such as diagnostic procedures, neurological assessment, raised intracranial pressure and seizure management, of which an understanding is essential when caring for a child who has had or will have cranial surgery. There is a section specifically relating to the principles of rehabilitation programmes. This is justifiable within a book focusing upon neurosurgery because some children who have had major neurosurgery will require extensive rehabilitation programmes and these children may be cared for on a neurosurgical ward. Chapter 3 provides an overview of the general principles of care of children requiring surgery including perioperative care, pain management and wound care. The remaining chapters focus upon the management of a child with a specific disease process that requires primarily surgical treatment. Terminology relating to surgical procedures is provided in Appendix I. A glossary of terms is provided in Appendix II.

Although the book is primarily aimed at pre-registration nursing students and qualified nurses new to the children's neurosurgical environment, it is hoped that it will be a valuable resource to a range of healthcare professionals, both junior and experienced, working with children and young people requiring surgery. Policy documents cited within the book are primarily from relevant government departments in England. Many of the principles are contained within equivalent documents for Scotland, Wales and Ireland. The term child will be used to represent infants, children and young people unless otherwise stated. Well-accepted information will not be referenced. Where available, evidence-based care will be reflected upon and supported by appropriate references. In the absence of available literature to support care, descriptions will be provided based on current care delivery with rationale; however there will be an indication that there is lack of evidence in the area being described. Text boxes will be used throughout to enable key information to be highlighted and easily located.

References

Aicardi J (1998) *Diseases of the Nervous System in Childhood*, 2nd edn. Cambridge University Press, London.

Chumas P, Hardy D, Hockley A *et al.* (2002) Safe paediatric neurosurgery 2001. *British Journal of Neurosurgery* **16** (3): 208–10.

Department for Education and Skills (2004) *Every Child Matters: Change for Children*. The Stationery Office, London.

Department of Health (2004) N*ational Service Framework for Children, Young People and Maternity Services: Every Child Matters – Change for Children*. The Stationery Office, London.

National Institute for Clinical Excellence (2004) *The Epilepsies: The Diagnosis and Management of Epilepsy in Children and Adults in Primary and Secondary Care*. The Stationery Office, London.

National Institute for Health and Clinical Excellence (2007) *Head Injury. Triage, Assessment, Investigation and Early Management of Head Injury in Infants, Children and Adults*. NICE, London.

Padgett K (2002) Alterations of neurological function in children. In McCance KL, Huether SE (eds) *Pathophysiology: The Biologic Basis for Disease in Adults and Children*, 4th edn. Mosby, St Louis, MO.

Raimondi AJ, Hirschauer J (1984) Head injury in the infant and toddler. Coma scoring and outcome scale. *Child's Brain* **11**: 12–35.

Royal College of Physicians (2004) *Stroke in Childhood: Clinical Guidelines for Diagnosis, Management and Rehabilitation*. Royal College of Physicians, London.

Acknowledgements

This book is dedicated to all those working with children who require care in a neurosurgical setting.

We would like to express our thanks to our families and friends for their support and encouragement during the writing of this book.

We would particularly like to thank Sharon Peacock, Sister (Children's Neurosciences Ward) and John Livingston, Paediatric Neurologist, both based at Leeds General Infirmary for diligently reading and commenting on each chapter, and providing enthusiastic encouragement. We would like to thank all those who gave specialist advice including Julie Cooper and Andie Mulkeen, Sisters (Children's Neurosciences Ward, General Infirmary at Leeds), Angela Hughes, Sister (Children's Intensive Care, General Infirmary at Leeds), Rachel Hollis, Senior Sister (Paediatric and Adolescent Oncology and Haematology Unit at St James's University Hospital, Leeds), Anne Aspin, Nurse Consultant (Neonatal Surgery, General Infirmary at Leeds) and Bernadette Baldwin and Geraldine Binstead, Advisors for the Northern Region of the Association for Spina Bifida and Hydrocephalus.

1 Overview of anatomy and physiology of the central nervous system

The nervous system is a fascinating, complex and remarkable structure. It is one of the two major regulatory systems of the body, the other being the endocrine system. However, the nervous system not only regulates internal body functions, it facilitates the body's ability to interact with the environment. The nervous system is the body's most rapid means of maintaining homeostasis and to achieve this it must be able to constantly react and adjust to internal and external stimuli. These stimuli are detected and conveyed by nerves to the brain where they are analysed and interpreted resulting in a coordinated response. Neuroanatomy and physiology are the foundations upon which an understanding of nervous system disorders is based (Crossman and Neary 2000). The aim of this chapter is to provide a clear and concise overview of anatomy and physiology of the nervous system, with particular emphasis upon changes that occur as part of normal childhood growth and development.

At the end of reading this chapter you will be able to:

Learning outcomes

- Describe the main divisions of the nervous system
- Outline the key anatomical structures of the brain
- Describe the physiology of nerve conduction
- Appreciate embryological development of the nervous system

1.1 Introduction and overview of the organization of the nervous system

Although the nervous system functions as a whole, for descriptive purposes it is divided into the central nervous system (CNS) and the peripheral nervous system (PNS) (Sugarman 2002).

Central nervous system

The CNS consists of the brain and spinal cord which are respectively enclosed in the cranial vault and spinal column. The three main functions of the nervous system are *sensory* (detect changes), *integrative* (interpret changes) and *motor* (respond to changes initiating action). The CNS is the control centre for the entire nervous system (Figure 1.1a).

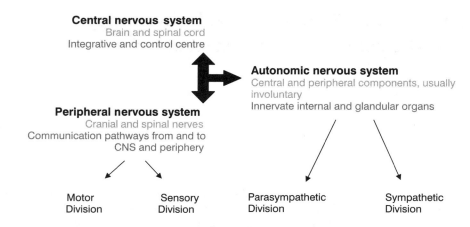

Figure 1.1a Relationship between the components of the nervous system

Peripheral nervous system

The PNS consists of all the nerve networks which link the CNS with the periphery, such as the body's receptors, muscles, glands and organs. Peripheral nerve pathways are further differentiated into ascending or afferent pathways that carry information towards the CNS, and descending or efferent pathways that carry information away from the CNS to the effector organs (Sugarman 2002). Clinically the PNS has two main subdivisions, the somatic nervous system (SNS) and autonomic nervous system (ANS) (Sugarman 2002). Actions carried out by the SNS are both voluntary and involuntary with sensations consciously perceived, while actions carried out by the ANS are involuntary and are not usually consciously perceived.

Somatic nervous system

The SNS can be divided into:

- Sensory afferent nerve receptors which are located in the skin and transmit impulses to the brain. Impulses are perceived as general senses such as touch, pressure, temperature and pain;
- Special sense organs transmit impulses to the brain. Impulses are perceived as smell, taste, vision and hearing;
- Motor efferent nerves that conduct impulses away from the CNS to the skeletal muscles;
- Mixed nerves containing both sensory and motor neurons;
- The 12 pairs of cranial nerves (Table 1.1a) and 31 pairs of spinal nerves.

Sensory spinal nerves carry information from specific areas of the body to the CNS. These regions can be graphically represented by known as a dermatome (Figure 1.1b). Similarly each group of muscles innervated by nerves from a particular spinal nerve can be represented graphically known as a myotome. A plexus is a network of nerves, for example the brachial plexuses is formed from C 5, 6, 7, 8 and T1 spinal nerves, which innervate the skin and muscles of the upper limbs and chest muscles.

Table 1.1a Summary of the cranial nerves and their functions

Cranial nerve	Function
CN I Olfactory nerve	The nerve fibre originates in the nasal olfactory bulb and transmits sensory impulses to the temporal lobes, where the stimulus is perceived as smell
CN II Optic nerve	The nerve fibre originates in the retina of the eye and transmits sensory impulses to the occipital cortex, where the stimulus is perceived as vision
CN III Oculomotor nerve	Mixed nerve
1.	The motor nerve fibre originates in the midbrain and extends to the extraocular muscles and smooth muscles of the iris. Nerve stimulation results in elevation and adduction of the eyes and constriction of the pupils
2.	The sensory nerve fibres from the extraocular muscles relay information relating to the position of the eyes to the brain
CN IV Trochlear nerve	Mixed nerve
1.	The motor nerve fibre originates in the midbrain and extends to the superior oblique muscles. Nerve stimulation results in depression of an adducted eye
2.	The sensory nerve fibres from the superior oblique muscles relay information relating to the position of the eyes to the brain
CN V Trigeminal nerve	Mixed nerve fibre originates from the pons and branches to convey motor and sensory impulses to the mouth, nose, surface of the eyes, dura mater and motor fibres which stimulate chewing
CN VI Abducens nerve	Mixed nerve
1.	The motor nerve fibre originates in the pons and extends to the lateral rectus muscles. Nerve stimulation results in abduction of the eyes
2.	The sensory nerve fibres from the lateral rectus muscles relay sensory information relating to the position of the eyes to the brain
CN VII Facial nerve	Mixed nerve
1.	The motor nerve fibre originates in the pons and extends to the facial muscles, lacrimal ducts and salivary glands
2.	The sensory nerve fibres from the facial muscles and the taste buds in the anterior two thirds of the tongue are relayed to the brain
CN VIII Vestibulocochlear nerve	The nerve fibre originates in the inner ear (cochlea and semi-circular canals) and transmits sensory impulses to the brain stem, where the stimuli are perceived as sound and body orientation (essential for balance and helps provide a sense of equilibrium)
CN IX Glossopharyngeal nerve	Mixed nerve
1.	The motor nerve fibre originates in the midbrain and extend to the throat muscles and salivary glands
2.	The sensory nerve fibres from the pharynx relay information from the throat and the taste buds of the posterior third of the tongue to the brain

continued...

Table 1.1a continued

Cranial nerve	Function
CN X Vagus nerve	Mixed nerve
1.	The motor nerve fibre originates in the medulla and extends to the neck, thorax, and abdominal region
2.	The sensory nerve fibres from the abdomen relay information relating to visceral organs to the brain
CN XI Spinal accessory nerve	Nerve fibres originating in the back and neck transmit sensory impulses to the medulla and superior spinal cord, and motor nerves from the medulla and superior spinal cord transmit impulses to the back and neck, allowing for coordinated movement of the head and neck
CN XII Hypoglossal nerve	Nerve fibre originating in the tongue transmit sensory impulses to the medulla, and motor impulse from the medulla transmit impulses to the tongue, allowing for movement and positioning of the tongue to be coordinated

Source: adapted from Sugarman 2002

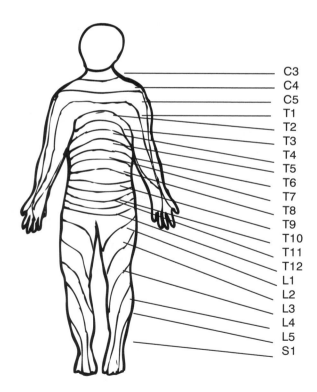

Figure 1.1b Dermatome map (anterior view) (Source: Crossman and Neary 2000)

Autonomic nervous system

The ANS has components within both the central nervous system and the peripheral nervous system (Crossman and Neary 2000). The ANS can be further divided into the sympathetic and parasympathetic divisions, and the enteric nervous system (Figure 1.1c).

The ANS is primarily concerned with the innervation and control of visceral organs, smooth muscle and secretory glands with the overall aim to maintain homeostasis in the internal environment (Crossman and Neary 2000). Sensory neurons of the ANS carry impulses to the central nervous system from the receptors of the body's organs. Motor neurons of the ANS carry impulses from the central nervous system to smooth muscle, cardiac muscle and the glands. Where organs have both sympathetic and parasympathetic nerve innovation their actions have an antagonistic effect. Table 1.1b provides examples of the opposing actions of the ANS.

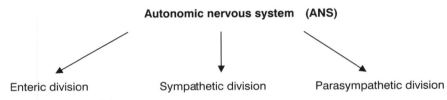

Autonomic nervous system (ANS)

Enteric division   Sympathetic division   Parasympathetic division

Figure 1.1c Divisions of the autonomic nervous system

Table 1.1b Actions of the sympathetic and para-sympathetic divisions of the ANS

Organ	Sympathetic activity	Parasympathetic activity
Heart	Increased force of muscle contraction Heart rate increases	Reduction in force of muscle contraction Heart rate decreases
Lungs	Smooth muscle of the bronchial tree relaxes Dilates bronchi	Smooth muscle of the bronchial tree contracts Constricts bronchi
Gastrointestinal organs	Longitudinal muscle of the alimentary tract relax and the circular muscles contract decreasing peristalsis Inhibits secretions Contracts sphincters Glycogen stored in the liver is mobilized	Longitudinal muscle of the alimentary tract contract and the circular muscle relax, increasing peristalsis Increases secretions Relaxes sphincters Contraction of smooth muscle of lower bowel
Eye	Dilator pupillae relaxes, pupil dilates Ciliary muscle relaxes, lens becomes more biconcave	Sphincter pupillae contracts, pupil constricts Ciliary muscle contract, lens becomes more biconvex
Urinary and reproductive systems	Bladder muscle relaxes, sphincter contracts Sperm ejaculation	Bladder muscle contracts, sphincter relaxes Erection
Adrenal glands	Adrenal medulla secretes adrenaline	No parasympathetic activity
Skin	Increased sweat gland secretions Hairs become erect due to contraction of the erector pilli muscles	No parasympathetic activity

Enteric nervous system

The enteric nervous system is an interconnected network of neurons organized in two cylindrical sheets embedded along the length of the gut wall. Nerves of the enteric system innervate the pancreas, liver and gall bladder (Crossman and Neary 2000; Longstaff 2005). The enteric nervous system assists in controlling peristaltic activity, glandular secretions and water and ion transfer, in essence regulating gut functioning.

1.2 Development of the nervous system

An understanding of the development of the nervous system is important because the cause of many neurological problems in infancy may be a result of a malformation that has occurred during embryological development (Padgett 2002). Following fertilization, cell division rapidly occurs and at three days a hollow ball of cells, known as a blastocyte, embeds in the uterine wall. After implantation the inner mass of the blastocyte begins to differentiate into the three primary germ layers: the ectoderm, endoderm and mesoderm. These germ layers form different structures of the body. The endoderm differentiates primarily into epithelial tissues such as the lining of the gastrointestinal tract and internal organs. The mesoderm differentiates primarily into muscles and connective tissues. The ectoderm differentiates primarily into all nervous tissue, the ear, the eye and the epidermis.

The first obvious sign of nervous system development is during the third week of embryonic life when the dorsal midline of the ectoderm thickens to form the neural plate (Padgett 2002). The lateral margins of the plate become elevated resulting in a midline depression known as the neural groove. Eventually the folds become apposed and fuse together creating the neural tube. The neural tube is completely closed by the end of the forth week of embryonic development and becomes the CNS (Longstaff 2005).

> **Points to consider**
>
> Failure of the neural tube to fuse results in abnormalities such as: anencephaly, which occurs if the rostral (or uppermost) portion of the tube fails to close and spina bifida if the caudal (or hind) portion fails to fuse.

The central fluid-filled canal persists into adulthood, the rostral portion becoming the ventricular system in the brain and the caudal portion becoming the central canal in the spinal cord. As the neural tube is forming some of the cells become isolated, grouping together to form the neural crests (Figure 1.2a). These eventually form most of the cells of the peripheral nervous system, and the sensory cells of the spinal and cranial nerves.

Development of the brain

By the fifth week of gestation the rostral portion of the neural tube undergoes extensive differentiation, with the three primary brain vesicles, the forebrain, midbrain and hindbrain, becoming identifiable. The forebrain (cerebrum) is by far the largest of these divisions and eventually gives rise to the two cerebral hemispheres and the thalamus (Figure 1.2b). The midbrain remains relatively undifferentiated. The hindbrain develops into the pons, cerebellum and medulla

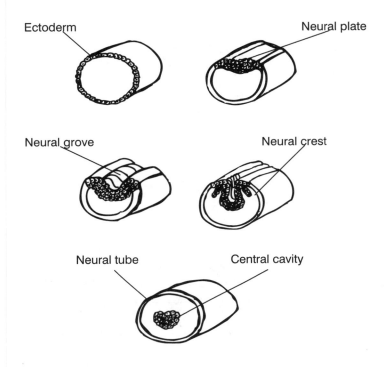

Figure 1.2a Formation of the neural tube from the embryonic ectoderm

Table 1.2a Relationship between embryonic development and final structures

Primary brain vesicles	Secondary structures	Final structures	
Forebrain:	Telencephalon	Cerebral hemispheres	
	Diencephalon	Thalamus, hypothalamus	
Midbrain:	Mesencephalon	Midbrain	Brain
Hindbrain:	Metencephalon	Pons	Stem
	Myelencephalon	Medulla oblongata	
		Cerebellum	

Source: FitzGerald and Folan-Curran 2002

oblongata. By convention the midbrain, medulla and pons are collectively known as the brain stem (Table 1.2a).

Up to about six weeks of gestation the single layer of neuroepidermal cells increase in number and are the precursors of both the supporting glial cells and the neurons. Cell differentiation and final function is determined by genetic coding and extracellular signalling, which is influenced by the position of the cells within the blastocyte (Longstaff 2005). Early neurons are known as neuroblasts, and initially proliferate at a faster rate than the glial cells (Longstaff 2005). In the final stages of differentiation the neuroblast's eventual structure, function and position are established, and during the last division neuroblasts lose the ability to divide.

The increase in cell numbers results in the formation of layers of cells, which in turn form discrete zones, the first being the inner ventricular zone (Longstaff 2005). The inner ventricular

3-4 weeks gestation

Midbrain

Hindbrain

Forebrain

Developing Heart

Spinal cord

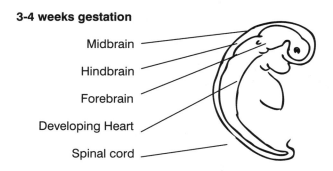

5 weeks gestation

Medulla

Developing ear

Cerebellum

Midbrain

Thalamus

Cerebral
hemisphere

Lower limb

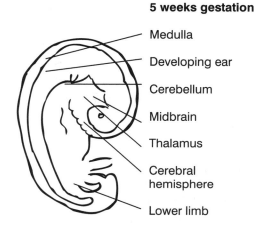

Figure 1.2b Development of the brain and spinal cord

zone is situated nearest to the neural tube. As new cells are formed at the base of the neural tube they migrate through the layers of previously formed cells, the new daughter cells adding to the rapidly expanding cerebral cortex (Figure 1.2c). Each zone of cells become specialized in their role, and the mass organization of cells eventually forms the cerebral hemispheres. This cell migration results in the development of the typical appearance of the brain: an outer cortex of grey matter (consisting primarily of cell bodies) and the white matter of the inner cortex consisting primarily of nerve tracts. Neuronal migration, which occurs as early as the second month of gestation, is controlled by a complex assortment of chemical mediators and cell signalling.

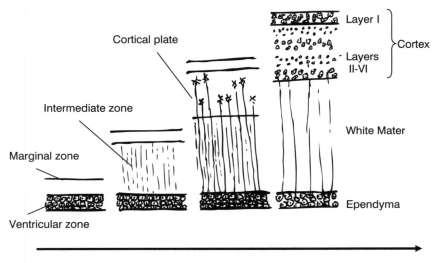

Figure 1.2c Schematic representation of cell migration and the development of the layers of the brain

Points to consider

Neuronal migration disorders, for example lissencephaly, are a group of defects caused by the abnormal migration of neurons in the developing brain. These disorders can have a profound effect upon a child's ability to develop normally.

By the 28th week of gestation the major fissures (the lateral, central and calcarine sulci) have appeared on the surface of the brain. As the brain develops, the central cavity in the rostral portion of the neural tube also undergoes considerable changes in shape and size, and forms the ventricular system (FitzGerald and Folan-Curran 2002). Although the neuronal cell numbers do not increase after birth, continued glial cell proliferation, increased neuronal connections and nerve myelination adds to the weight and size of the brain, particularly during the first years of life (Dobbing and Sands 1973). The brain has achieved most of its growth by the age of six years.

Development of the spinal cord

The spinal cord is relatively less differentiated in comparison with the brain. The brain is formed from the rostral portion of the neural tube, while the caudal portion forms the spinal cord and the central cavity becomes the central canal of the spinal cord (Crossman and Neary 2000). Unlike neuroblast migration within the brain, neuroblast cell bodies in the spinal cord remain relatively central and form the grey matter of the spinal cord. The developing cell processes grow outwards into the marginal layer that ultimately forms the white matter of the spinal cord. This gives the spinal cord its typical 'butterfly' appearance (Figure 1.8a). The first spinal reflexes are present by eight weeks of gestation, corresponding with the first embryonic movements. Nerve myelination begins to occur in the spinal cord from about 22 weeks of gestation, slightly earlier than in the brain. The process continues post-natally and is thought not to be complete until adult life (Padgett 2002).

1.3 Cells of the nervous system and their function

The two cellular components, the neuralgia (glial cells) and the neuron (nerve cells), are unique to the nervous system. Glial cells form the connective tissue of the nervous system and are essential for the normal function of neurons (Kast 2001). Glial cells outnumber neurons by a magnitude of millions. The main glial cells are: astrocytes, which provide mechanical support and help maintain the blood brain barrier; microglia, which correspond to brain phagocytes; oligodengrocytes, which form the myelin in the CNS; Schwann cells, which form the myelin in the PNS; and ependymal cells, which form the brain's epithelial cells that line the ventricles and central canal of the spinal cord (Figure 1.3a).

Neurons

The neuron is the functional unit of the nervous system (FitzGerald and Folan-Curran 2002). Neurons have highly specialized structures enabling them to receive and integrate information from sensory receptors and to transmit information to effector organs. Functionally there are three types of neurons: afferent or sensory neurons transmit nerve impulses from peripheral receptors to the CNS; efferent or motor neurons transmit nerve impulses away from the spinal cord to the effector organs; and interneurons are contained entirely within the CNS and integrate information within the CNS. Despite their diversity all neurons have a similar structure (Figure 1.3b) (Sugarman 2003).

Typically each neuron has a single cell body from which several receptive processes appear, known as dendrites. At the terminal end of the dendrites are chemical receptors capable of receiving information and transmitting impulses to the cell body. One of the processes leaving

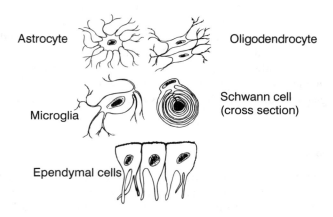

Figure 1.3a Main types of glial cells

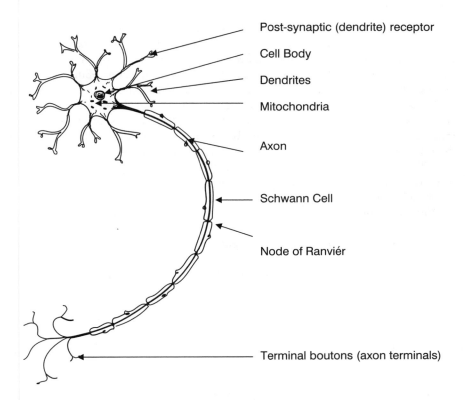

Post-synaptic (dendrite) receptor

Cell Body

Dendrites

Mitochondria

Axon

Schwann Cell

Node of Ranviér

Terminal boutons (axon terminals)

Figure 1.3b Typical neuron

the cell body is called the axon, or nerve fibre, which carries information away from the cell body. Axons end in terminal boutons, which contain vesicles that store the chemical transmitters necessary to stimulate adjacent neurons or effector organs. Transmission along dendrites and axons is unidirectional.

Nerve conduction

The most important feature of a neuron is the ability to generate and conduct electrical (nerve) impulses. Dendrites receptors can respond to a range of internal stimuli, such as the chemical mediators involved in inflammation, and external stimuli, such as touch, pressure and temperature. If the stimulus generates a nerve impulse, information about that stimulus can travel along neurons to the central nervous system for processing. This is the body's quickest means of communicating between body systems and responding to changes both internally and externally.

Continuous conduction

The ability to conduct electrical impulses is based upon the neuron's ability to maintain a difference in the ion concentration outside and inside the cell membrane (Longstaff 2005). Disruption of this ion concentration causes an ionic current flow, creating a nerve impulse. In a resting neuron the ionic balance is maintained primarily by the action of the sodium–potassium pumps, which span the cell membrane. The operation of the sodium–potassium pump is highly energy dependent. The pump transports *positive* sodium ions out of the cell in exchange for *positive* potassium ions, but at a ratio of 3:2. The difference between the ion concentrations causes an imbalance across the cell membrane. In addition to the sodium–potassium pump the cell membrane is selectively permeable, being 100 times more permeable to potassium ions. These mechanisms create a potential difference by making the outer surface of the cell membrane more positive in relation to the inner surface (Figure 1.3c). The nerve cell membrane is now polarized.

When a neuron receives an adequate stimulus a series of reactions occur:

- The part of the cell membrane adjacent to the stimulus becomes permeable to sodium ions.
- Sodium ions rapidly enter the resting cell changing the neuron's ionic balance, known as depolarization (Figure 1.3c).

a) Resting membrane

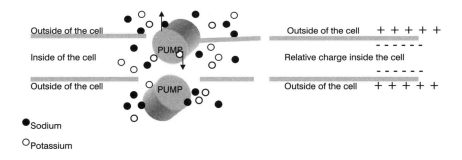

b) Reverse polarization

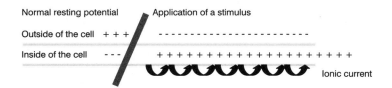

Figure 1.3c Nerve cell membrane

- As sodium ions continue to enter the cell the ionic balance reverses, known as reverse polarization.
- Reverse polarization causes a local ionic current to flow that stimulates the next part of the neuron's membrane to depolarize, resulting in the impulse passing along the length of nerve fibre (Figure 1.3c).
- Repolarization is necessary before depolarization can occur again and is achieved by restoring the cell membrane's selective permeability and reactivation of the sodium–potassium pumps.
- There is a brief period of time, known as the refractory period, when a neuron cannot respond to further stimulus because it is trying to repolarize.

This type of nerve conduction is called continuous conduction. To create a nerve impulse the stimulus must be strong enough to cause the initial cell depolarization, known as the threshold stimulus (Longstaff 2005). Once the threshold stimulus has been reached the nerve impulse is conducted along the entire neuron at a constant and maximum strength and is independent of any further stimulus, known as the all-or-nothing principle (Longstaff 2005). A stimulus weaker than the threshold stimulus cannot initiate an impulse unless several sub-threshold stimuli are applied in quick succession and their cumulative strength is greater than the threshold stimulus. Continuous conduction occurs in unmyelinated neurons.

Saltatory conduction

Both oligodendroglia and Schwann cells produce a fatty substance known as myelin which becomes wrapped around the axons of certain nerve fibres. Each myelin-producing cell forms the myelin for a short segment of the axon (Figures 1.3a and 1.3b). The myelin layer restricts the movement of ions. However, between each segment of myelin is a minuscule gap that results in an area of non-myelinated axon, known as a node of Ranvier. Membrane depolarization can occur at these nodes causing local ionic currents, which can be transmitted from node to node. The nerve impulse transmits via these nodes rather than depolarization occurring continuously along the length of the nerve fibre. This type of conduction is known as saltatory conduction

Table 1.3a Conduction velocity between different nerve fibres

Type	Diameter (nm)	Conduction velocity (m/s)	Function of neuron
A (a)	13–22	70–120	Motor and sensory impulses
A (β)	8–13	40–70	Respond to touch
A (γ)	4–8	15–40	Respond to pressure
A (δ)	1–4	5–15	Respond to pain and temperature

A fibres have the largest diameters, all are myelinated.
Have a brief refractory period and are used when a quick response is needed.

B	1–3	3–14	Relay impulses from skin and viscera

B fibres are also myelinated but conduct impulses at a much slower rate than A fibres.

C	0.2–1	0.2–2	Respond to pain from the skin and viscera.

C fibres have small diameters are unmyelinated
Have the slowest conduction times.

and greatly increases the speed of conduction. The speed of a nerve impulse is independent of stimulus strength and is normally determined by body temperature, the diameter of the fibre and the presence or absence of myelin (Figure 1.3a).

Points to consider

Destruction of myelin can have severe consequences for a child. For example in Guillain-Barré syndrome demyelination occurs because of an acute inflammation of the peripheral nerves resulting in motor paralysis. The disorder is characterized by rapid onset of weakness of the legs and arms, which progresses to the chest muscles and muscles of the face.

Synapses

Each neuron is a separate entity. Information can only be passed between neurons if their membranes are in close proximity. The junctions between neurons are known as synapses. A synapse consists of a synaptic knob (a bulge in the end of the pre-synaptic neuron), a synaptic cleft and the plasma membrane (containing dendrite neurotransmitter receptors) of the post-synaptic neuron (Figure 1.3d). Unlike neurons, impulses are transmitted across synapses chemically. This is important because it allows impulses to be graded and transmission across synapses allows the process to proceed or to be inhibited (Longstaff 2005). When a nerve impulse arrives at a synaptic end bulb, changes occur within the cellular cytoplasm causing the synaptic vesicles to release their contents (chemical neurotransmitters) into the synaptic cleft (Figure 1.3d). Calcium ions are necessary to help facilitate this process (Longstaff 2005).

Neurotransmitters

The effect a neurotransmitter has on the adjacent nerve dendrite receptor sites depends on the type of neurotransmitter and the type of post-synaptic neuron (Longstaff 2005). If the reaction causes the post-synaptic neuron to uptake sodium ions – providing the threshold stimulus has been reached – then conduction will occur and a nerve impulse will be generated. If the reaction

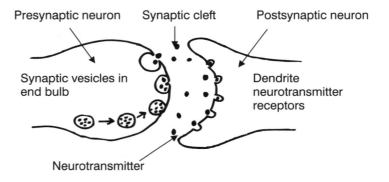

Presynaptic neuron   Synaptic cleft   Postsynaptic neuron

Synaptic vesicles in
end bulb

Dendrite
neurotransmitter
receptors

Neurotransmitter

Figure 1.3d Typical synapse

causes the post-synaptic neuron to uptake potassium ions a nerve impulse will not be generated, resulting in an inhibitory response.

Neurotransmitters can only stimulate post-synaptic dendrites, i.e. transmission is one way; this is important in maintaining homeostasis. Once the neurotransmitter activates the receptor sites they must be rapidly deactivated. Enzymes in the post-synaptic cleft deactivate the neurotransmitters. These are specific to each neurotransmitter, for example, the enzyme is acetylcholinesterase deactivates acetylcholine.

Points to consider

CNS disorders can be a result of abnormalities at synapses for example Myasthenia Gravis. This is an autoimmune disorder where antibodies block the receptor sites at the neuromuscular junctions, preventing muscle cell stimulation. The classic presentation is muscle weakness during periods of activity, which improves after rest.

There are thought to be over 30 substances in the body that can function as neurotransmitters (Longstaff 2005). Many of these have more than one function, for example in the brain noradrenalin is probably involved in the regulation of mood, dreaming and maintaining arousal but is an excitatory neurotransmitter when found at neuromuscular junctions. The most common neurotransmitter in the CNS is glutamate, which causes excitation of neurons, and gamma-aminobutyric acid (GABA), which causes inhibition of the neuronal receptors (FitzGerald and Folan-Curran 2002). The most common neurotransmitter in the PNS are acetylcholine, which is the main neurotransmitter at neuromuscular and neuroglandular junctions and causes excitation of neurons, and glutamate, which causes excitation of neurons (FitzGerald and Folan-Curran 2002). Other neurotransmitters include:

- Noradrenaline is an excitatory neurotransmitter and is concentrated in the brain stem and is released at some neuromuscular and neuroglandular junctions.
- Serotonin is an excitatory neurotransmitter and is concentrated in the brain stem. It is involved in the regulation of temperature, sensory perception, sleep and mood.
- Dopamine is an inhibitory neurotransmitter and is concentrated in the midbrain. It is involved in the regulation of emotional responses and subconscious movements of the skeletal muscles.

1.4 Anatomy of the brain

The brain accounts for about two per cent of the body's weight and lies within the cranial cavity. The forebrain, midbrain and hindbrain are the three principle anatomical divisions of the brain (Longstaff 2005). However, it is more convenient clinically to consider the brain as consisting of the cerebrum (cerebral hemispheres), diencephalon, brain stem and cerebellum (Figure 1.4a).

The cerebrum

The forebrain is situated above the brain stem and consists of the cerebrum (cerebral hemispheres) and the diencephalon (thalamus and hypothalamus). The cerebrum is by far the largest part of the brain. It consists of an outer layer, or cortex, of grey matter and an inner mass of white matter.

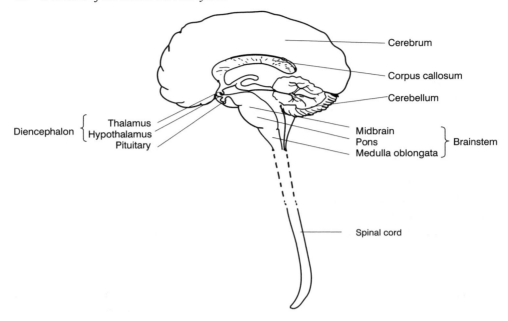

Figure 1.4a Median sagittal cross-sectional view of the brain

Grey matter consists mainly of neuronal bodies and white matter consists of axonal processes (Crossman and Neary 2000). However, deep within the white matter are large masses of grey matter (clusters of neuron cell bodies) such as the basal ganglia, thalamus and hypothalamus. These clusters usually perform specific functions, and in the case of the basal ganglia, integrate semi-automatic movements, such as walking, swimming and laughing.

The cerebrum is divided into the two cerebral hemispheres by the deep midline great longitudinal fissure. At the base of the fissure is the corpus callosum. This consists of a sheet of nerve fibres running between and allowing communication between the two cerebral hemispheres. The cerebral hemispheres are highly convoluted, maximizing the surface area. Some of the convolutions, or gyri, and fissures, or sulci, divide the cerebrum into important functional areas (Figure 1.4b).

An important principle within the central nervous system is the topographical representation of specific areas of the cortex to specific functions (FitzGerald and Folan-Curran 2002):

* The anterior part of the cerebral hemisphere or frontal lobe contains the primary motor cortex which is responsible for controlling movement. Due to the cross over (decussation) of the nerve fibres, the motor cortex in each hemisphere controls the opposite side of the body. The motor speech area is situated in the frontal lobe. In addition, the frontal lobe is also important in many higher functions including personality and behaviour.
* The posterior boundary of the frontal lobe is the central sulci which divides the frontal lobe from the parietal lobe. The parietal lobe contains the primary somatosensory cortex, and here sensations such as touch, pressure, pain and temperature are consciously perceived. Again, decussation of fibres means that each hemisphere perceives information from the opposite side of the body.

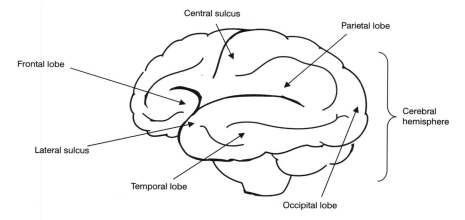

Figure 1.4b Lateral view of the brain showing the major subdivisions of the cerebral hemispheres

- The posterior part of the cerebral hemisphere or occipital lobe contains the visual cortex. Decussation of fibres at the optic chiasma means that the right visual cortex perceives sensation from the left visual field and vice versa.
- The inferior lateral areas of the cerebral hemispheres or temporal lobes, contain the auditory cortex. In addition, the temporal lobes have an important role in memory and emotions.

The diencephalon

The diencephalon consists of several specialist areas, with the two most important being the thalamus and hypothalamus (Crossman and Neary 2000). The thalamus and hypothalamus are situated deep within the brain (Figure 1.4a). The thalamus is the largest area within the diencephalon and can be thought of as the gateway to the cerebral hemispheres because many nerve impulses pass through the thalamus on the way to the cerebral cortex. The thalamus has a key role in the integration and processing of somatosensory signals and special sensory signals before ensuring they reach the appropriate areas of the cerebral cortex. Some sensations, for example pain sensations, are perceived consciously at the level of the thalamus but the location and intensity requires further processing by the sensory cortex. The thalamus also plays a part in maintaining consciousness.

The hypothalamus lies below the thalamus and is connected directly to the pituitary gland (Crossman and Neary 2000). It forms the lateral wall of the third ventricle. The hypothalamus has important autonomic, neuroendocrine and limbic functions. The hypothalamus regulates and coordinates many homeostatic functions including temperature regulation and somatic activities such as heart rate, peristalsis, papillary constrictions and dilatations. The neuroendocrine activities occur as a result of the hypothalamus directing the pituitary glands hormonal synthesis and release. The hypothalamus forms part of the limbic system which has a vital role in basic instincts such as thirst and hunger and sexual drive, and emotional behaviours such as fear.

The pineal gland is often considered with the diencephalon because of its close proximity and its association with wake and sleep cycles (circadian rhythm).

Table 1.4a Hormones of the pituitary gland and their function

Hormone	Target organ	Physiological effects
Thyroid stimulating hormone	Thyroid gland	Stimulates secretion of thyroid hormones
Growth stimulating hormone	Liver Adipose tissues	Promotes growth Controls protein, lipid, and carbohydrate metabolism
Adrenocorticotropic hormone	Adrenal gland	Stimulates secretion of glucocorticoids
Vasopressin	Kidney	Conservation of body water
Follicle stimulating hormone	Ovary and testis	Control of reproductive functions
Luteinizing hormone	Ovary and testis	Control of reproductive functions
Prolactin	Mammary glands	Stimulates milk production
Oxytocin	Mammary glands	Stimulates milk ejection and uterine contractions

Points to consider

Melatonin, which is produced naturally by the pineal gland, can be prescribed by physicians to regulate sleep cycles for neurological disorders that disrupt circadian rhythm.

The pituitary gland

The pituitary gland lies below the hypothalamus which it is attached to by the pituitary stalk. Although an endocrine organ the pituitary gland is primarily regulated by actions of the hypothalamus. The pituitary gland secretes a range of hormones which along with their functions are summarized in Table 1.4a.

The brain stem

The brain stem is a term used to describe collectively the midbrain, medulla oblongata and the pons (Figure 1.4a). The midbrain is the upper most section of the brain stem and contains part of the auditory system, cranial nerves III (oculomotor) and IV (trochlear), and the neurons which synthesize dopamine. The pons is continuous with the midbrain above and the medulla oblongata below and contains many functional structures similar to the midbrain and the medulla oblongata. In addition, a group of nerve fibres within the pons communicate information between the cerebellar cortex and the cerebral cortex. The medulla oblongata is continuous with the pons above and spinal cord below and contains numerous pathways that carry ascending information to the brain and descending information to the periphery. As the nerves transcend the medulla they cross sides.

Points to consider

Although anatomically the brain stem is a relatively small component of the brain, its importance cannot be underestimated. It contains many nuclei and tracts that are essential to key vital body functions.

The major functions of the brain stem include (Crossman and Neary 2000):

- Transmission of information between the periphery and the cerebrum, many of the fibres decussate at the level of the medulla.
- Contains the nuclei of the cranial nerves (except I and II). The cranial nerves provide somatosensory sensations to the head and neck as well as some of the special sensations such as taste and hearing. The nerves also provide motor function to the muscles of the head and neck. Some of the cranial nerves also contain autonomic fibres which help regulate blood pressure, heart rate and respirations.
- Controlling basic functions from special centres, such as heart rate and respirations, consequently if there is extensive damage to the brain rendering the cerebral hemispheres non-functioning, as long as the brain stem is intact these basic 'vegetative functions' can continue.
- Maintaining an alert state.
- Many of the nuclei located within the brain stem function collectively and form specialized systems such as the reticular activating system and the limbic system. The reticular activating system has a vital role in the maintenance of arousal and initiation of sleep, consciousness and attention. The limbic system has a vital role in basic drives such as thirst, hunger, fear and sexual drive.

Hindbrain

The hindbrain consists of the cerebellum, medulla oblongata and the pons. The cerebellum is divided into two lateral hemispheres which cover the brain stem at the base of the cranial cavity in an area known as the posterior fossa. The cerebellum is important in the integration of motor function, such as balance and gate, and coordinating motor activities. Unlike the cerebral cortex responses of the cerebellum are ipsilateral (affect the same side of the body). The cerebellum has many interconnections with other parts of the brain such as the spinal cord, brainstem and cerebral cortex; this ensures motor responses are coordinated.

1.5 The ventricular system

The inner sac of the neural tube forms the ventricular system and the central canal of the spinal cord. The ventricular system is a network of connected chambers or ventricles deep within the brain which contain cerebrospinal fluid (CSF). The ventricular system consists of four chambers: two lateral ventricles, the third ventricle and the fourth ventricle. The fourth ventricle tapers at its base and becomes the very narrow central canal of the spinal cord.

The two C-shaped lateral ventricles are situated within the cerebral hemispheres. The main body of the lateral ventricles lie below the corpus callosum and above the thalamus (Figure1.4a). The anterior horns of the lateral ventricles extend into the frontal lobes, and the posterior horns extend towards the occipital lobe. The lateral ventricles are connected to the third ventricle by a canal known as the foramen of Monro. The third ventricle is a slit-like cavity and lies at the junction of the midbrain and forebrain. The walls of the third ventricle are formed by the thalamus and hypothalamus. The aqueduct of Sylvius connects the third ventricle with the fourth ventricle. The fourth ventricle is a diamond shaped cavity located between the brain stem (pons and medulla oblongata) and the cerebellum (Figure 1.5a).

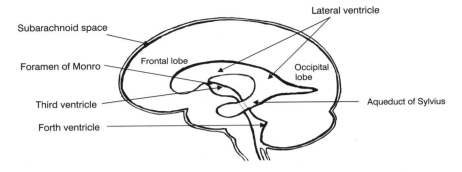

Figure 1.5a Median sagittal cross-sectional view of the ventricular system

Points to consider

The flow of CSF can be blocked at various sites within the ventricular system. Accumulation of CSF within the ventricular system causes ventricular dilatation and is known as hydrocephalus. Hydrocephalus is an important neurological condition in childhood and is explored in depth in Chapter 4.

Cerebrospinal fluid

The production of CSF occurs within specialized tissue that is composed of capillaries and ventricular lining cells (ependymal cells), known as the choroid plexus (Barker and Barasi 1999). This specialist tissue is found primarily in the lateral ventricles, with some patches of tissue in the third and forth ventricle. CSF circulation begins in lateral ventricles flowing through the foramen of Monro to the third ventricle and continuing via the aqueduct of Sylvius to the fourth ventricle (Figure 1.5a). CSF leaves the forth ventricle via the two foramina of Luschka and the foramen of Magendie, where it circulates within the subarachnoid space around the brain and spinal cord. CSF is returned to the venous circulation via indentations in the arachnoid membrane, known as the arachnoid granulations (Hendelman 2006). These project into the dural venous sinuses situated within the cerebral fissures. However, the exact mechanism for CSF absorption is unclear. It is thought the hydrostatic pressure within the subarachnoid space is higher than that in the venous sinus, which, combined with the greater colloid osmotic pressure within the venous capillaries, results in CSF being absorbed across the capillaries (Sugarman 2002).

At any given time there is approximately 150mls of CSF within the central nervous system, of which about 75mls is within the ventricular system. CSF is produced at a rate of about 20mls/ hr (Barker and Barasi 1999). Since the daily CSF production is 3–4 times the total volume (300–500mls are produced per 24 hours), a rapid increase in intracranial volume would occur if production was not balanced with absorption (Barker and Barasi 1999).

CSF is derived from the blood plasma and is a highly selective process. The composition of CSF differs from the plasma in that it has relatively higher sodium, chlorine and bicarbonate levels and lower potassium, urea, glucose and amino acid concentrations (Longstaff 2005). The protein concentration in CSF is almost negligible. CSF plays an important role in maintaining a constant intracerebral chemical environment, delivers nutrients filtered from the blood to the cells of the brain and spinal cord, and removes toxic substances produced by the brain and spinal cord (Barker and Barasi 1999). In addition, it acts as a protective shock-absorbing medium and gives the brain buoyancy.

Points to consider

Sampling CSF to detect the presence of bacteria or tumour deposits and the measurement of CSF pressure may be necessary as a diagnostic test for some neurological disorders. CSF is removed from the lumbar cistern, by inserting a trochar between the vertebrae L4–L5. The trochar must be inserted below the second lumbar vertebra because this is the level where the spinal cord terminates (Hendelman 2006).

1.6 Blood supply

The CNS is dependent on a continuous blood supply because of its vast metabolic demands and negligible store of nutrients. The brain requires a continual supply of glucose and oxygen and approximately 20 per cent of the entire cardiac blood flow reaches the brain each minute (Sugarman 2002).

Points to consider

If the blood supply to brain fails, for example following occlusion or haemorrhage of the blood vessels, neuronal death occurs. The resultant loss of function will correspond to the specific function of the area affected.

Blood vessels

Two pairs of blood vessels, the internal vertebral arteries and the carotid arteries provide the blood supply to the brain. The vertebral arteries are divisions of the subclavian arteries and enter the cranial cavity through the foramen magnum. The vertebral arteries run along the ventrolateral aspect of the medulla oblongata and eventually unite to form the basilar artery, which extends along the length of the pons. The vertebral arteries and the basilar artery, along with their distributaries, supply blood to the occipital lobe of the cerebral hemisphere, the brain stem and the cerebellum (Barker and Barasi 1999). The internal carotid arteries arise from the common carotid artery and enter the cranial cavity through the middle cranial fossa and terminate lateral to the optic chiasma. The internal carotid arteries divide to form the anterior and middle cerebral arteries (Hendelman 2006). The anterior cerebral arteries and their distributaries provide the blood supply to the medial aspect of the cerebral hemispheres. The middle cerebral arteries and their distributaries provide the blood supply to the frontal, parietal and temporal aspect of the cerebral hemispheres.

Points to consider

The vertebral arteries supply blood to the posterior of the brain, brain stem and cerebellum. The internal carotid arteries supply blood to the anterior and the middle of the cerebral hemispheres.

The two circulatory systems derived from the internal vertebral arteries and the carotid arteries are not totally independent and form part of a system of interconnecting arteries that encircle the optic chiasma and the floor of the hypothalamus and midbrain, known as the circle of Willis (Figure 1.6a) (FitzGerald and Folan-Curran 2002). The physiological principle behind the circle of Willis is that in the event of damage to one of the arteries supplying the brain there is the potential for compensation from the communicating arteries thus offering some protection from severe ischaemic damage.

Points to consider

The circle of Willis aims to protect the brain from ischaemic damage if any of the major arteries entering the brain becomes damaged. However, anatomical anomalies of the circle Willis, such as absence of connecting arteries, are common.

Venous return

Venous blood returns to the heart from the brain by a system of superficial veins, deep veins and venous sinuses. Venous return from the surface of the cerebral hemispheres occurs via the superficial veins in the subarachnoid space which drain blood into the venous sagittal sinus that eventually flows into the internal jugular vein (Crossman and Neary 2000). The deep veins of the cerebral hemispheres drain into the vein of Galen, before draining into the sagittal sinus (Barker

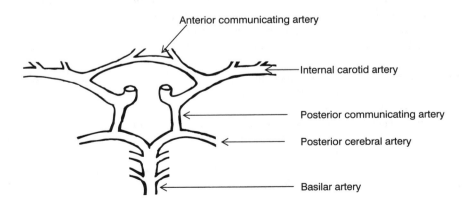

Anterior communicating artery

Internal carotid artery

Posterior communicating artery

Posterior cerebral artery

Basilar artery

Figure 1.6a The circle of Willis

and Barasi 1999). Venous sinuses are large channels inside the dural layers which convey blood from the surface of the brain into the internal jugular veins and back to the heart (Hendelman 2006). One of the major venous sinuses is the superior sagittal sinus which is situated on the upper edge of the great longitudinal fissure. Venous blood leaving the brainstem and cerebellum drains directly into the dural venous sinuses adjacent to the posterior cranial fossa (Barker and Barasi 1999).

Blood–brain barrier

The blood–brain barrier is a structural and physiological barrier between the blood vessels and the brain tissue (Hendelman 2006). The blood–brain barrier is important because it determines the exact composition of the brain's extracellular fluid. Extracellular fluid is derived from the blood but in the brain is a highly selective process because many of the blood's naturally occurring chemicals, such as catecholamines and glutamate, would be detrimental to neuronal activity (Barker and Barasi 1999). Maintaining the blood–brain barrier is a complex process that is the consequence of specific characteristics of the cerebral capillaries that prevent normal mechanisms for exchange of substances across their tight endothelial end plates (Longstaff 2005). Essential water- or lipid-soluble molecules, such as water, glucose, amino acids and oxygen, can cross the blood–barrier (Longstaff 2005). Compounds which are necessary but cannot cross the blood–brain barrier such as amino acids rely upon active transport systems within the capillary walls and compounds which are neurotoxic are excluded.

Points to consider

The selective permeability of the blood–brain barrier protects neurons from the many harmful toxins within the body and explains the selective uptake of drugs across the blood–brain barrier. For example, steroids are lipophilic molecules and can cross the barrier, while many chemotherapy agents are actively excluded from crossing the barrier.

As with all active transport systems across cell membranes the effective working of the blood–brain barrier requires a tremendous amount of energy in the form of adenosine triphosphate (ATP). ATP function is dependent on an adequate supply of oxygen. Cerebral ischemia results in an inability to maintain the blood–brain barrier, an influx of water, ions and molecules into the brain's extracellular spaces resulting in alteration in brain function (Longstaff 2005).

1.7 Protection and coverings

The brain and spinal cord are supported and protected by the bones of the skull and the vertebral column respectively, and the membranous coverings collectively known as the meninges.

The skull

The skull consists of the cranium and the bones forming the base of the skull (Figure 1.7a). The cranial fossa are hollows in the base of the cranium which accommodate particular parts of the brain. The three fossa are: the anterior cranial fossa, formed by the frontal, ethmoid and

a) Median sagittal cross- sectional view

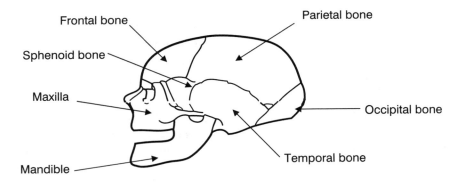

b) Dorsal view

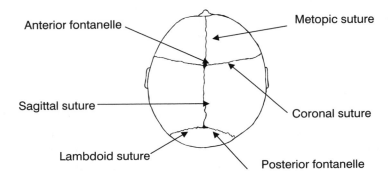

Figure 1.7a and b Bones of the skull

sphenoid bones, housing the frontal lobes of the brain; the middle cranial fossa, formed by the sphenoid and temporal bones and contains the temporal lobe; the posterior cranial fossa is formed from the occipital and petrous temporal bones and contains the cerebellum and the brain stem (Crossman and Neary 2000). The base of the skull contains holes, or foramina, that provide entry and exit points for important structures, nerves and blood vessels. The largest of these is the foramen magnum through which the medulla along with the vertebral arteries, cranial nerves XI and XII pass and becomes continuous with the spinal cord.

In children the bones of the skull remain separated at the suture sites, allowing for head malleability during birth and continuance of rapid brain growth during early life (Figure 1.7b) (Panchal and Uttchin 2003). Approximately 50 per cent of brain growth has occurred by 12 months of age, with continual growth occurring during childhood. The anterior fontanelle has completely ossified by about 18 months of age and the sutures have closed sufficiently to convert the skull into a rigid container by about 5 years of age (Padgett 2002).

Points to consider

Premature fusion of the sutures causes craniosynostosis, and is explored in depth in Chapter 6. Hydrocephalus and brain tumours in young children can cause widening of the sutures.

Meninges

The meninges consist of three layers, the pia, arachnoid and dura mater. The pia mater closely adheres to the surface of the brain. It is a microscopically thin, highly vascular membrane. The middle layer of the meninges is the arachnoid mater, which is a translucent membrane loosely surrounding the brain. It has a role in helping to maintain the blood–brain barrier. CSF flows between the pia and arachnoid mater in the subarachnoid space, which contains a network of capillaries. The exchange of water and solutes between the blood vessels and the CSF helps maintain equilibrium between the CSF and extracellular fluid.

The outer layer of the meninges is the dura mater which is a thick fibrous membrane. It lines the skull and spinal column, separating the CNS from the peripheral nervous system. The dural layer has folds which divide the cranial cavity into compartments (Hendelman 2006). The two major folds are the falx cerebri, which separates the cerebrum into the two cerebral hemispheres, and the tentorium cerebelli, which separates the cerebrum from cerebellum and brain stem. Between the arachnoid and dura maters is the subdural space through which veins draining into the venous sinuses pass. Collectively the meninges provides a physical covering that help protect the brain; CSF has a shock-absorbing effect and the blood/CSF interface contributes to maintaining the blood–brain barrier.

1.8 The spinal cord

The spinal cord is an elongated portion of the CNS and lies within the vertebral (spinal) column. Once growth and development is complete, the spinal cord is approximately 45cm in length and 1cm thick, is continuous with the medulla oblongata and terminates at the first or second lumbar vertebrae (Sugarman 2002). The central canal lies at the centre of the spinal cord and contains CSF through links with the forth ventricle. The spinal cord is the link between the brain and other organs of the body. Nerves conveying impulses from the brain to the periphery (or vice versa) descend (or ascend) through the spinal cord. The spinal cord consists of a core of grey matter (cell bodies) and an outer layer of white matter (myelinated nerve fibres). This separation of cell bodies from nerve fibres gives it the characteristic 'butterfly' shape (Sugarman 2002). Four extensions of the central grey matter protrude laterally, known as the posterior grey horns and anterior (ventral) grey horns (Figure 1.8a). Nerves enter or leave the spinal cord via the intravertebral foramina. Nerves entering the posterior horn of the spinal cord are afferent sensory nerve fibres, while the efferent pathways leaving the spinal cord via the anterior horn are primarily motor nerve fibres.

The white matter of the spinal cord contains a number of spinal cord tracts. A tract is a bundle of nerve fibres that have a common origin, function and destination. Tracts ascend and descend the spinal cord, linking the peripheral nervous system with the brain. Sensory (ascending) tracts consist of fibres that carry nerve impulse from specific regions of the spinal cord to the corresponding specific region of the brain. Motor (descending) tracts consist of nerve fibres that

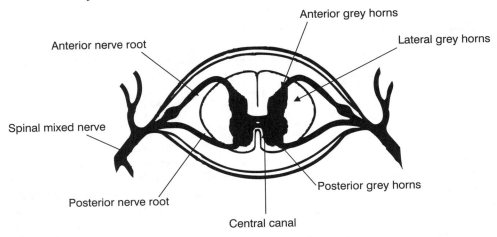

Figure 1.8a Transverse section through the spinal cord

carry information from the specific region of the brain to the corresponding specific region of the spinal cord. An example is the spinothalamic tract, a group of nerve fibres in the lateral horn of the spinal cord that ascends to the thalamus. Stimulation, for example, by pressure or heat, of peripheral nerves initiates a nerve impulse which terminates in the grey matter of the spinal cord; interconnecting neurones cross the spinal cord and connect to the spinothalamic tract which carries information to the brain.

In addition to the motor and sensory responses, the spinal cord has an important protective role through the action of the spinal reflexes. In certain situations the spinal cord can react quickly to stimuli that pose an immediate threat to the body by having the ability to respond automatically, for example moving the hand away quickly if it touches a hot object (Sugarman 2002). The simplest form of a spinal reflex is a reflex arc, where an appropriate stimulus activates a sensory neuron that directly activates an appropriate motor nerve fibre via a spinal interconnecting neuron. This results in an immediate response being initiated before the brain has opportunity to coordinate further actions.

1.9 Neuroplasticity and neuron regeneration

The traditional approach to neuroanatomy and physiology associates discrete body functions with specific brain structures (Stephenson 1996; Barker and Barasi 1999). It was thought that the brain had little capacity to grow and regain function following damage, and that neurons have limited power for regeneration. Certainly neuron cell bodies do not have centrioles and the meiotic spindles that are necessary for cell division. There are many factors that contribute to the nervous system's lack of ability to repair, including the different responses of the PNS and the CNS to injury.

The PNS has the ability to repair damage to myelinated axons and to a certain extent dendrites but this depends on:

- The severity of the damage.
- The cell body being intact.
- Schwann cells remaining active.
- The option for surgical repair.

However, the CNS is restricted in its ability to repair damage due to:

- Scar tissue rapidly developing (in an attempt to limit damage) causing a physical barrier; astrocytes are responsible for this inhibitory process.
- Oligodendrites do not response in the same way as Schwann cells and do not assist in the regeneration of myelin once damaged.

However, there is evidence to suggest that the CNS does have the capacity to return to normal function once damaged. Neurons have the ability to survive damage, regenerate new axons and form new synaptic connections (Barker and Barasi 1999). Although cell division is not possible, the process involves the ability to expand and redirect axons and dendrites creating new connections with alternative possibilities. This process is known as synaptogenesis. In response to some injuries, reactive synaptogenesis may participate in the recovery of function, but it may also hinder the process by forming aberrant connections. It is thought that early corrective rehabilitation may initiate restorative synaptogenesis in preference to simply reactive proliferation (Kaplan 1988; Stephenson 1996). More recent work with animal studies has demonstrated the ability of transplanted axons to regenerate (Davies *et al.* 1997).

An additional concept in determining the outcome of brain damage is that of neuroplasticity. Early approaches to brain functioning, which were supported by radiological imaging, suggested that the brain was a rigid map (Stephenson 1996). Each specific area was linked to a specific functional neuronal set. Evidence suggests that the brain probably functions as a 'plastic structure', this malleability results in the brain being capable of returning to a similar form and function once altered (Kaplan 1988; Rose *et al.* 1997). Therefore, although the brain appears to be organized into discrete areas associated with specific function these may not be fixed, and latent areas could take on the function of damaged areas. Plasticity makes the brain particularly vulnerable to changes in the environment but this same plasticity may provide a means to advancing recovery following damage. It has been demonstrated that reorganization of neurons can occur, for example damage to the function of the speech centre can be compensated for by the development of latent areas of the brain (Kaplan 1988, Stephenson 1996).

Points to consider

Neurological damage is a great challenge to the nervous system. Healthcare professionals working with children need to understand neuronal reorganization because it offers a physiological explanation for potential recovery and work together to prevent, where possible, maladaptation occurring.

Key messages from this chapter

- Although the nervous system functions as a whole it can be divided into the central nervous system and the peripheral nervous system
- The central nervous system consists of the brain and spinal cord
- The neural tube is completely closed by the end of the forth week of embryonic development and becomes the central nervous system
- The neuralgia (glial cells) and the neuron (nerve cells) are unique to the nervous system
- Nerve impulses are the body's quickest means of communicating between body systems and responding to internal and external changes
- The speed of a nerve impulse is independent of stimulus strength and is normally determined by body temperature, the diameter of the fibre and the presence or absence of myelin
- An important principle within the central nervous system is the topographical representation of specific areas of the cortex to specific functions
- The cerebrospinal fluid plays an important role in maintaining a constant intracerebral chemical environment
- If the blood supply to the brain fails neuronal death occurs
- The consequences of damage to the nervous system are highly variable and the body's ability to respond to damage to the nervous system is complex

Web resources

Brain Source
Aimed at sharing neuroscience knowledge
www.brainsource.com
Encyclopaedia of Life Sciences
Comprehensive coverage of a range of topics including neurosciences
www.mrw.interscience.wiley.com
PubMed
A range of biomedical and life sciences journals
www.pubmedcentral.nih.gov
National Library for Health
A range of health related resources
www.library.nhs.uk
Neurosciences for Kids
Learning resources for kids of all ages
http://faculty.washington.edu/chudler/nsdivide.html

References

Barker RA, Barasi S (1999) *Neuroscience at a Glance*. Blackwell, Oxford.

Crossman AR, Neary D (2000) *Neuroanatomy–An Illustrated Colour Text*, 2nd edn. Churchill Livingstone, Edinburgh.

Davies SJF, Fitch MT, Memberg SP *et al.* (1997) Regeneration of adult axons in white matter tracts of the central nervous system. *Nature* **390** (6661): 680–3.

Dobbing J, Sands J (1973) Quantitative growth and development of human brain. *Archives of Disease in Childhood* **48** (10): 757–67.

FitzGerald MJT, Folan-Curran J (2002) *Clinical Neuroanatomy and Related Neuroscience*, 4th edn. WB Saunders, Edinburgh.

Hendelman WJ (2006) *Atlas of Functional Neuroanatomy*, 2nd edn. Taylor & Francis, Philadelphia.

Kaplan M (1988) Plasticity after brain lesions: contemporary concepts. *Archives of Physical Medicine and Rehabilitation* **69** (11): 984–91.

Kast B (2001) The best supporting actors. *Nature* **412** (6848): 674–6.

Longstaff A (2005) *Instant Notes: Neuroscience*, 2nd edn. Taylor & Francis, Abingdon.

Padgett K (2002) Alterations of neurological function in children. In McCance KL, Huether SE (Eds) *Pathophysiology: The Biologic Basis for Disease in Adults and Children*, 4th edn. Mosby, St Louis, MO.

Panchal J, Uttchin V (2003) Management of craniosynostois. *Plastic and Reconstructive Surgery* **111** (6): 2032–48.

Rose FD, Johnson DA, Attree EA (1997) Rehabilitation of the head injured child: basic research and new technology. *Pediatric Rehabilitation* **1** (1): 3–7.

Stephenson RC (1996) Therapeutic consistency following brain lesions. *Professional Nurse* **11** (11): 738–40.

Sugarman RA (2002) Structure and function of the neurological system. In McCance KL, Huether SE, (eds) *Pathophysiology: The Biologic Basis for Disease in Adults and Children*, 4th edn. Mosby, St Louis, MO.

2 General principles of caring for the child with a neurological impairment

Understanding the principles that underpin the management of the child with a neurological dysfunction is essential to ensure the delivery of care is safe and appropriate. This chapter will outline the principles of care regarding: diagnostic procedures, managing raised intracranial pressure, intracranial pressure monitoring, the management of seizures and status epilepticus, the management of the unconscious child, rehabilitation, and meeting the emotional and psychological needs of the child and family. These general principles need to be adapted to each situation, and to the child and family's individual needs. In additional there will be a comprehensive account of undertaking a detailed neurological assessment of the child.

At the end of reading this chapter you will be able to:

Learning outcomes

- Describe in detail the purpose and key elements relating to undertaking a neurological assessment
- Outline the management of seizures and status epilepticus
- Describe the effects of raised intracranial pressure
- Appreciate the emotional and psychological needs of the child and family

2.1 Diagnostic procedures

Diagnostic procedures are vital to: assist the clinician to establish, where possible, the correct diagnosis; determine the potential prognosis for the child; and to monitor disease progression and/or the effects of treatments.

Overview of diagnostic investigations

The type of diagnostic investigations will vary depending on the child's presentation and may include:

- Blood profiling including urea and electrolytes, metabolic and immunological assays and genetic screening.
- Lumbar puncture to collect cerebrospinal fluid (CSF) samples to detect the presence of bacteria or tumour deposits and to measure CSF pressure.

- Neuroimaging techniques, which are important diagnostic procedures within neurology: the choice of technique will depend on the reason the imaging is being undertaken and the depth of detail required, balanced with the risks and availability of the procedure. Table 2.1a provides an overview of ultrasound, Computerized Axial Tomography (CT scanning) and Magnetic Resonance Imaging (MRI).
- Specialized physiological imaging techniques, such as Positron Emission Tomography (PET), which can identify areas of increased cerebral metabolic activity, and Single-Photon Emission Computerized Tomography (SPECT) can identify areas of increased cerebral blood flow, which may assist in diagnosing focal lesions such as focal epilepsy.
- Cerebrovascular studies, such as angiography, may be necessary to visualize small blood vessels and can be used to identify cerebrovascular abnormalities such as aneurysms and arteriovenous malformations. Young children may require a general anaesthetic. However, Magnetic Resonance Angiography is improving and replacing more traditional angiography techniques.
- Electroencephalogram (EEG), which records the electrical activity of the brain and is primarily used to detect changes in brain activity during seizures. EEG is often used continuously with simultaneous video recording (video telemetry), for example in children with epilepsy the pattern of seizure manifestation can be recorded and considered along with the EEG changes.

Points to consider

There are potential risks in performing a lumbar puncture in a child with high intracranial pressure as the procedure may cause brain stem compression with fatal consequences. These risks need to be balanced against the potential benefits of undertaking the procedure for diagnosis purposes.

Many procedures are only available in specialized centres. However, common imaging techniques are widely available, therefore all nurses must have appropriate knowledge of associated care related to these procedures. A summary of neuroimaging techniques, their advantages and disadvantages, the underpinning rationale and practical considerations are presented in Table 2.1a.

Preparation of the child and family for diagnostic investigations

The invasive nature, restrictions to mobility and length it takes to perform many of the diagnostic procedures can be an added source of stress for the child and family. Healthcare professionals have a duty to ensure that the child and family are suitably prepared for all procedures, no matter how routine they may seem. This begins with an explanation of the reasons the procedure is necessary. The information given should be tailored to suit the individual child and family. Information may need repeating several times because many diagnostic procedures are performed at a time of great anxiety and stress for both the child and family (Freeman *et al.* 2004). The benefits and potential risks of the procedure must be outlined and informed consent needs to be obtained. It is essential that the child and family are involved in decision-making processes about the preparation the child will require.

Table 2.1a Neuroimaging techniques: advantages, disadvantages, rationale and practical considerations

Investigation	Rationale	Advantages	Disadvantages	Practical considerations
Cranial ultrasound	Used to view central structures, ventricles and surrounding tissue in an infant	Safe Portable No sedation required Measurements can be taken	Needs open fontanelle: therefore has a limited age range Limited image, especially posterior fossa region Poor anatomical detail, grey/white matter differentiation	User dependent
X-ray	Useful in determining skull fractures and identifying mechanical ventricular shunts Used less frequently since the widespread availability of CT or MRI	Quick and relatively easy to perform Widely available	Exposes child to ionizing radiation	Children require adequate preparation due to the stressful and frightening environment Young children will require restraining to maintain position and safety Presence of a familiar adult and distraction techniques are invaluable
CT	Effective in identifying haemorrhage, ventricular size, space occupying lesions Ionizing radio opaque contrast material administered intravenously can enhance images	Widely available Produces reasonable structural detail Good identification of bones, calcification and ventricles Useful when MRI is contraindicated	Exposes child to ionizing radiation Bony interference makes certain areas such as the posterior fossa difficult to image Procedure can take 10–20 minutes, the child is required to remain motionless Effective preparation is essential, sedation or general anaesthesia may be necessary in the young child Allergic reactions to contrast mediums can occur	
MRI	Excellent at detecting brain damage and oedema The quality of the images makes it a superior technique compared with CT Contrast mediums administered intravenously can enhance images	Excellent anatomical detail such as grey/white matter differentiation No bony interference: good imaging of the brainstem and posterior fossa Images in any plane, without moving the child A range of sequences available which can assist in highlighting particular areas of the brain Angiography and venography can be performed at the same time	Procedures can take up to 40 minutes The child must remain motionless in a confined space Acute bleeding may not be detected Bony injury/malformation difficult to assess MRI can be difficult in children with metallic devices, pacemakers, implants or metal clips Specialised monitoring equipment, without metallic components, is necessary Accessibility usually limited to specialist centres	The equipment used is noisy and the child must be isolated within the scanning room Effective preparation is essential, sedation or general anaesthesia may be necessary in the young child Allergic reactions to contrast mediums can occur

Point to consider

Preparation prior to procedures decreases anxiety and promotes cooperation from both the child and the family (Wong 1995; Freeman *et al.* 2004). Without this preparation, children can develop fantasies or distorted ideas about what is going to happen. Unidentified threats amd/or unexpected stress/stresses are more upsetting to the child compared to threats that are known, understood and expected (Wong 1995).

The detailed explanation and effective preparation prior to investigative procedures is often the domain of nursing staff and play therapists. The psychological needs of the child are paramount. The majority of the preparation strategies used are informal and include the use of puppets, dolls, play, books, and videos; with no one method more effective than another. In general, young children respond better to play materials and older children benefit more from discussions, peer support and visual aids (Wong 1995). When preparing the child for a procedure the nurse should consider the child's previous experience, existing coping strategies, and age and stage of development. The child who has previous experience of the procedure needs to have their knowledge assessed, misconceptions corrected, new information supplied and new coping skills suggested if prior strategies have been ineffective (Wong 1995). The child should be approached with confidence and a belief that the procedure is expected to be successful. Parents often wish to be present during procedures and should be informed prior to the procedure where they will be allowed to stand or sit and how they can best help during the procedure, for example by providing positive distraction. During the procedure the child should be allowed to express any feelings of anger, fear or anxiety. Following the procedure the child should be praised and encouraged to express any feelings, this could be done through activities such as role play, art and writing.

For the young child or the child with limited cognition it may be necessary to perform investigations under sedation or general anaesthesia. The use of sedation is not without risks particularly for the child with raised intracranial pressure (Cote *et al.* 2000; Lawson 2000; Smith and Callahan 2001). The risk of sedating the child needs to be balanced against the need for the procedure and other alternatives should be considered, such as general anaesthetic (Lawson 2000).

2.2 Neurological assessment

The purpose of a nursing assessment includes establishing the family care that the child usually requires, the current physical and psychological condition of the child, the nursing care the child requires, and the ability of the child and family to participate in care (Casey 1988). The nursing assessment of the child and family, with specific emphasis on meeting perioperative care needs are described in Chapter 3. Caring for the child with a neurological problem including children requiring a neurosurgical procedure requires nursing staff to be skilled in performing neurological observations. These are an important component of the neurological assessment and essential if changes in neurological function are to be detected. In many instances these changes are subtle, however if acted upon promptly, can mean the difference between a good or poor recovery or even between survival and death.

Points to consider

The purpose of a neurological assessment includes:

- Identifying the child's normal abilities and developmental stage.
- Providing a baseline record of the child's neurological status at the time of admission.
- Identifying the presence and effects of neurological dysfunction.
- Detecting life-threatening situations.
- Identifying changes promptly through serial observations.
- Influencing management decisions by monitoring overall improvements or deteriorations in the child.
- Assisting in the prediction of the eventual outcome of the neurological insult.

(Hickey 2003a)

Neurological observations

Neurological observations include the assessment of conscious levels, pupil reactions, motor function and other parameters including cardiovascular observations.

The assessment of conscious levels

Consciousness is a state of awareness and in general can be thought of as two components: arousal and wakefulness, and cognitive functioning. Cognition is the combination of several interconnected processes, such as perception, thinking, remembering and organizing information, and requires the integration of a range of sensory stimuli. Consciousness depends on effective brain function, particularly the interactions between the brain stem and cerebral cortex (McLeod 2006). Consciousness is a sensitive indicator of neurological functioning (Hickey 2003a). The assessment of consciousness is an essential skill required by healthcare professionals working with the neurologically compromised child because acute changes can be life threatening.

The first and the most frequently used numerical scale for assessing conscious levels is the Glasgow Coma Scale (GCS) (Teasdale and Jennett 1974). It was developed to reduce the subjectivity and ambiguity when assessing a patient's conscious level. Prior to the introduction of the GCS, the language used to grade a patient's responsiveness, such as confusion, drowsiness, lethargy, delirium and stupor, were open to different interpretations. The GCS assesses three components: eye opening, verbal response and motor response, with a numerical score given for the most appropriate response within each component (Table 2.2a). These components assess a patient's awareness of the environment.

The reliability of the GCS has been questioned particularly when used by inexperienced staff (Fielding and Rowley 1991; Ellis and Cavanagh 1992). It is, therefore, important to ensure healthcare staff are adequately educated and develop the skills necessary to undertake a neurological assessment effectively (Smith 1999). The GCS has also been criticised for not being sensitive enough to detect changes in children (Westbrook 1997). The GCS has undergone several adaptations for use in children, including the Adelaide scale (Reilly *et al.* 1988) and the James' adaptation (James and Trauner 1985) which will be described below.

Table 2.2a Components of the Glasgow Coma Scale

Component	Score	Parameters
Eye opening	4	Eyes open spontaneously in response to normal environmental activities
	3	Eyes open in response to direct commands
	2	Eyes open in response to a painful stimulus
	1	Absence of eye opening despite application of a painful stimulus
Verbal response	5	Answers appropriately to questions
	4	Converses but confused
	3	Makes little sense
	2	Incompressible sounds
	1	No verbal response despite the application of a painful stimulus
Motor response	6	Obeys commands
	5	Localisation of a painful stimulus and purposefully moves in an attempt to locate the stimulus and remove it
	4	Withdrawal from the painful stimuli in an attempt to move away from the stimulus but it is not a purposeful movement
	3	Flexion response to a painful stimulus
	2	Extension to a painful stimulus
	1	Flaccidity, there is no detectable movement or change in tone of the limbs despite repeated and varied stimulation

Source: Teasdale and Jennett 1974

Points to consider

Important considerations when assessing conscious levels include:

- Prior to approaching the child observe the child from a distance to determine; if their eyes are open, they are vocalising as appropriate for their age and if there is any motor activity. If parents or familiar person are present establish if they consider the child's activities to be normal for the child
- Always record the best response, for example if the motor response is better in one limb record this response recorded
- Consciousness cannot be assessed in children who are receiving anaesthetic agents. Consciousness can be assessed in children receiving sedation; however, the score may not reflect the patient's best abilities
- Consciousness can be viewed as a continuum from a fully alert state to an unresponsive state (McLeod 2006). The stimulation required to elicit a reaction in the child can also be viewed as a continuum; from spontaneous, auditory stimuli through to the application of a painful stimulus
- Failure to response spontaneously or to an auditory stimulus/ light tactile pressure requires application of a painful stimulus. The site for the application of the painful stimulus must reflect that the GCS is assessing brain function and not spinal reflexes. To test for localisation of pain a central pressure must be applied for example supraorbital pressure (Teasdale and Jennett 1974). The application of nail bed pressure and trapezium squeeze may elicit a flexion reflex response (Price 2002)

Points to consider

The National Paediatric Neuroscience Benchmarking group within the UK (Tatman *et al.* 1997; Warren 2000) and the National Institute for Health and Clinical Excellence (NICE 2007) advocate using the James' adaptation because it is easy to use, the scoring system has a maximum of 15 and minimum of 3, is internationally recognized and it takes into account the developmental level of the child.

Eye opening

Across all ages eye opening is a spontaneous response to normal environmental activities. It is a positive sign and indicates that the arousal mechanisms in the brain stem are functioning. Spontaneous eye opening in response to normal environmental activities scores 4. Eye opening in response to direct commands scores 3, and indicates that the cerebral cortex is processing information. Eye opening in response to a painful stimulus scores 2 and suggests lower than normal brain function. Absence of eye opening despite the application of a painful stimulus scores 1 (Table 2.2a). Absence of eye opening despite application of a painful stimulation implies a marked degree of depression of the arousal systems within the brain (Teasdale and Jennett 1974). However, in a persistent vegetative state, spontaneous eye opening is usually present and is probably due to a primitive ocular reflex rather than an expression of environmental awareness. The eye opening response is an important component of the neurological examination because it can often assist in differentiating between coma due to metabolic causes and coma due to structural causes. In a metabolic coma it is not uncommon for patients to have spontaneous eye opening but diminished verbal and motor responses on the GCS.

Verbal response

The verbal response of a child will depend on their stage of language and cognitive development. Where possible, the child's stage of verbalization should be ascertained from the child's normal carer prior to undertaking the first assessment, which will enable the child's optimal score to be documented. It is the deviation from the child's norm that will assist in determining the child's conscious level. It is possible to assess the verbal component of the GCS for all children and if the scale being used has been adapted for use with infants, all children can potentially achieve the maximum score of 5. The score given should reflect age-appropriate responses and consider the child's normal developmental stage. Table 2.2b outlines the verbal component of the GCS adapted for use in infants and children. Children should be asked questions in a language familiar to them or, where possible, by a familiar adult. If the child does not respond to a verbal stimulus then a painful stimulus should be applied. Response only to deep pain or no response is an indication of significant depression of the nervous system (Teasdale and Jennett 1974). The addition of the grimace score to the verbal response has made the assessment of verbal response suitable in intensive care settings (Warren 2000) (Table 2.2b). It is important to record if the child is unable to speak on the assessment chart, for example the presence of a tracheostomy or damage to speech centre.

Table 2.2b Verbal component of the neurological assessment adapted for use in children

Score	Verbal response		
	Infant/young child	Older child/adult	Grimace – all ages
5	Alert, babbles, coos/ uses words or sentences/ usually ability	Orientated	Spontaneous normal facial/ oro-motor activity
4	Less than usual ability or spontaneous irritable cry	Confused	Less than usual facial/oro-motor spontaneous activity or only response to touch stimuli
3	Cries inappropriately	Inappropriate words	Vigorous grimace to pain
2	Occasional whimpers/moans	Inappropriate sounds	Mild grimace to pain
1	No response	No response	No response

Source: Warren 2000

Best motor response

The final component of the GCS assesses the ability of the child to respond to an instruction that requires the child to undertake a motor action. If the child can obey a simple command a maximum score of 6 will be achieved (Table 2.2a). This requires the child to have an appropriate level of understanding to interpret and act on the instructions given. In a babies or young infants who do not have the cognitive ability to respond to instructions, a maximum score of 6 would be recorded if there are normal spontaneous movements. If there is no evidence of a normal spontaneous movement or the ability to respond to a simple instruction a stimulus must be applied.

A purposeful movement is an attempt by the child to locate and remove the painful stimulus and scores 5. Applying nail bed pressure is inappropriate because a flexion reflex response to pain may be initiated rather than purposeful movement and may overestimate the child's neurological functioning. Localizing to pain indicates the brain is able to receive and process information. If the child's level of consciousness becomes depressed the child may simply withdraw from the painful stimulus and indicates the presence of neurological damage. In this instance when a painful stimulus is applied the child makes some attempt to avoid it but does not try to remove the stimulus and the score is recorded as 4. Flexion and extension to painful stimuli, score 3 and 2 respectively, and imply further impairment of neurological responsiveness (Figure 2.2a). Flaccidity is the most severe impairment of the motor component and is recorded as a score of 1. This is only recorded when repeated and varied stimulation elicits no detectable movement or change in tone of the limbs (Teasdale and Jennett 1974). A score of 1 indicates severe depression of the brain stem and ability to process information. Motor response *cannot* be assessed in patients who are receiving paralysing agents.

Points to consider

In infants of less than 6 months of age the normal motor response to stimulation is flexion; young infants cannot localize to pain (Brett and Kaiser 1997).

Bilateral withdrawal of limbs (flexed): arms flexed, legs flexed, knees come up

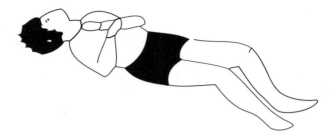

Bilateral extension of the limbs (decerebrate): arms extended, external rotation of the wrists, legs extended, internal rotation of the feet

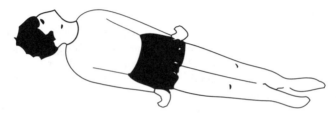

Figure 2.2a Flexed and extended limb positions

Summation of the components of the Glasgow Coma Scale

Summation of the three components of the GCS provides a summary of the child's conscious state and can act as a quick reference guide when reviewing the child's condition (Watson *et al.* 1992). The summation of the score for each component, known as the Glasgow Coma Score, ranges in value from 3 to 15, with 15 indicating full consciousness. The score becomes lower as the degree of neurological impairment increases. Coma is usually defined as a score of 8 or less (Kraus *et al.* 1987). This definition of coma will only be appropriate for children if a modified paediatric scale is used. If an adult tool is applied to young children the best score they will be able to achieve is 9 because of their stage of development.

Summation of the GCS has been criticised for not accurately depicting the patient's condition and concealing the whole picture (McNett 2007). For example, a number of different combinations of the three components can result in the same score. Summation of the scores makes the assumption that each component has equal significance, which may not be accurate in terms of predicting long-term outcome of the neurological injury particularly following traumatic brain injury (McNett 2007). However, in an acute intracranial catastrophe all three components of the GCS are usually depressed.

Additional components of a neurological assessment

The original neurological observation chart produced by Teasdale and Jennett (1974) incorporates the assessment of pupil size and reaction to light, motor function and vital signs.

Pupil responses

The assessment of pupil functioning provides a valuable insight into the physiology of the brain stem and in particular the optic (cranial nerve II) and oculomotor (cranial nerve III) nerves. The optic nerve transmits impulses from sensory light receptors that are situated in the retina of the eye to the oculomotor centre in the midbrain which is responsible for coordinating the pupillary reflex light and the occipital cortex where the stimulus is perceived as vision. The oculomotor nerve extends from the oculomotor centre to the pupillary muscles of the eyes. It is a mixed nerve with sympathetic and parasympathetic activity: the sympathetic activity results in contraction of the pupilodilator muscles resulting in enlargement of the pupils; and the parasympathetic activity results in contraction of the pupiloconstrictor muscles resulting in constriction of the pupils. The normal pupil response to a direct light stimulus is an immediate brisk constriction of the pupil, and a brisk dilation of the pupil once the light source is removed (Hickey 2003a). Normal pupils are usually round, between 2–6mm in diameter and fairly equal in size but there may be slight discrepancies between the two pupils.

The assessment of pupils should include size, equality and reactivity to light (Hickey 2003a). Although each eye is examined independently, the response should be observed in both eyes. Light directed into one eye will constrict the pupil in the opposite eye due to the consensual light reflex. When assessing the pupils they should be observed for size and equality prior to shining a bright light into the eye and observing the reaction in both eyes. Wherever possible external light sources should be eliminated. The assessor should allow a few seconds to pass before testing the opposite eye to allow recovery from the consensual light reflex response. The pupillary response is graded as to the degree of response and is usually termed brisk, sluggish or fixed (unreactive). The size of the pupil is recorded as pinpoint, small, moderate or dilated.

Points to consider

The assessment of the pupil responses is important because:

- Pupil responses can be undertaken on patients who are receiving anaesthetic or paralysing agents
- Extremely small pupils can indicate narcotic overdose or direct lower brain stem compression
- A large pupil or unequal pupils usually indicate compression of the midbrain and consequently the oculomotor nerve. A dilated, fixed pupil is an ominous finding and suggestive of a terminal state (Hickey 2003a). These findings should arouse immediate concern and be reported immediately to medical staff
- An irregular or oval pupil may indicate raised intracranial pressure and could be the first sign of oculomotor nerve compression due to transtentorial herniation
- Drugs that either constrict or dilate the pupils should be accurately recorded.

Motor function

Evaluating limb responses can assist in determining the site of brain damage as specific deficits will correlate to the specific area of brain damage. Damage to the motor cortex and cerebellum will result in abnormalities in motor function. Assessing motor function is not the same as assessing the best motor response, which is one of the key components of the GCS. The assessment of motor function aims to provide an overview of the function (muscle strength, muscle tone, posture and the coordination of movements) of each of the four limbs independently (Peters 2007). A developing weakness, or hemiparesis, can indicate damage to one side of the motor cortex due to raised intracranial pressured in one hemisphere.

Muscle strength, muscle tone, posture and the coordination of movements can be assessed by observing the child and recording the position of the limbs and the range of movements the child is able to perform spontaneously. The child can be given age-appropriate activities in order to observe the ability to coordinate movements. Muscle strength and tone are assessed by asking the child to raise each limb against the pressure of the assessor's hand and usually recorded as normal, mild weakness or severe weakness.

Vital signs

Alterations in the body's vital signs can indicate pathophysiological changes within the brain, particularly the brain stem, and may warn of impending neurological deterioration. Cardiovascular observations are particularly important because of the relationship between cerebral haemodynamics and cerebral functioning (Hickey 2003a). Compromises to the cerebral blood flow will result in a vasomotor response, with blood being diverted from other body systems to maintain an adequate cerebral perfusion. The resultant rise in arterial blood pressure, in association with an increased intracranial pressure, is known as Cushing's reflex or response (Hickey 2003a). Tachycardia will initially occur as a result of mild hypoxia. Significant compromises to cerebral blood flow will cause further increases in blood pressure resulting in a compensatory bradycardia, suggestive of a dangerously high intracranial pressure and usually denotes an impending intracranial catastrophe.

Changes in respiratory rate and rhythm can occur with neurological dysfunction. Breathing is a complex process with the neurochemical control of ventilation depending on the interaction between the respiratory centre (situated in the brain stem), central and peripheral chemoreceptors, and the autonomic innervation of the bronchial smooth muscles (Brashers 2002). Changes in respiratory rate and rhythm can be due to many pathological processes. However, alterations to normal respirations, such as hyperventilation, shallow breathing or irregular breathing, should raise concerns in a child with a neurological problem. Rapidly expanding lesions, such as intracranial haemorrhage, direct medulla damage or brain stem herniation, are likely to cause respiratory arrest (Hickey 2003a). Lesions that expand slowly such as cerebral tumours are likely to affect the respiratory rate less dramatically.

Body temperature is regulated by the hypothalamus and neurological impairments can result in both hypothermia and hyperthermia. Hyperthermia is probably more common (Hickey 2003a) and can be due to infective and non-infective conditions. Central fever as a result of neurogenic aetiologies is typically associated with brain tumours, trauma and following neurosurgery.

Additional components of the neurological assessment should include observation of the adequacy of the cough and gag reflexes and the detection of seizures. The signs and symptoms of raised intracranial pressure are outlined below. Depression of the cough and gag reflexes can follow widespread brain damage. A child with a diminished cough or gag reflexes will be at risk of an ability to maintain their own airway, which has potentially serious consequences. Any type of insult on the brain has the potential to cause seizures, which require appropriate monitoring and management because the resultant hypoxia will compound existing problems.

2.3 Normal and raised intracranial pressure

Intracranial pressure (ICP) is a normal phenomenon that is the result of the pressure exerted by the cranial contents on the skull, which in the older child and adult is a fixed non-expandable box. The intracranial contents consist of the brain (80%), CSF (10%) and blood (10%) (Kanter and Narayan 1991).

Points to consider

Typically intracranial pressure is between 5–15mmHg, although these values are probably slightly lower for infants and young children (3–7mmHg) (Chitnavis and Polkey 1998; Bullock *et al.* 2000).

Transient changes to the normal values occur in response to vascular dynamics, coughing, straining during defecation and body position. Maintaining the ICP within normal limits depends on the correct functioning of the physiological mechanisms that ensure a stable intracranial volume, in particular cerebral haemodynamics.

Cerebral haemodynamics

Cerebral blood volume accounts for approximately 10 per cent of the intracranial contents. An adequate blood flow and oxygen supply to the cerebral tissues is essential to maintain normal neuronal function. Cerebral haemodynamics is the relationship between the cerebral blood volume, the cerebral blood flow and cerebral perfusion pressure and is necessary to ensure adequate cerebral oxygenation (Boss 2002). Cerebral blood flow (CBF) is dependent on an adequate blood pressure and cardiac function, with blood viscosity being a contributing factor. However, excessive increases in blood volume will cause a rise in ICP. The body's ability to sustain a stable cranial blood volume by regulating the CBF through a range of arterial blood pressures is an important aspect of maintaining the ICP within narrow parameters. Usually cerebral blood flow can remain fairly constant if the mean arterial pressure is between 50–160mmHg. This is an intrinsic regulatory process known as autoregulation. Autoregulation is a major homeostatic and protective mechanism that is the result of the ability of the smooth muscles of the arterioles to constrict or dilate as a result of changes in the intraluminal pressure. Adjusting the diameter of the cranial blood vessels maintains a fairly constant CBF. However, as with most homeostatic systems, there becomes a critical point when normal mechanisms are overcome, for example following local or diffuse injury, ischaemia, inflammation and chronic hypotension or hypertension.

Chemical and metabolic activities have a strong influence on CBF, particularly carbon dioxide and oxygen levels, and the pH of both the blood and local tissue. Carbon dioxide, as the end product of metabolism has a profound effect on CBF, and if levels are high, CBF increases. Other products of cell metabolism such as hydrogen ions, lactic acid and pyruvic acid, if high, will increase the CBF. Increased metabolism results in a low pH (acidosis) causing arteriole vasodilation, further increasing CBF.

The cerebral perfusion pressure (CPP) is the pressure gradient between the blood capillaries and cerebral tissues, and is of vital importance in ensuring that the brain cells are properly perfused with blood. It is generally accepted that a CPP above 60mmHg ensures adequate cerebral perfusion (Rosner and Daughton 1990; Giulioni and Ursino 1996).

Points to consider

To maintain the cerebral perfusion pressure (CPP) above 60mmHg the mean arterial pressure (MAP) needs to be considerably greater than the intracranial pressure (ICP):

$$CPP = MAP - ICP$$

This is an important equation in the management of the neurologically compromised child because inadequate cerebral perfusion eventually results in cell death and the ability to measure both MAP and ICP allows the CPP to be calculated. This will be discussed later in this chapter and in Chapter 5.

Cerebrospinal fluid

Cerebrospinal fluid, although not having the same degree of regulation as cerebral blood flow is an important component of the intracranial volume. There is approximately 150mls of CSF within the central nervous system, of which about 75mls is within the ventricular system and is produced at a rate of about 20mls/hr (Barker and Barasi 1999). Adjustments to the CSF volume are limited but can compensate for slight changes in cerebral blood flow. For example, if cerebral blood flow increases CSF can be 'squeezed' from the ventricles into the subarachnoid space where the dura mater has some degree of elasticity to accommodate changes. Longer term increases in intracranial volume can be offset to a limited extent by an increase in CSF absorption in the arachnoid villa (Boss 2002).

Monro-Kellie doctrine

As early as the 1780s the Monro-Kellie doctrine has acknowledged that the rigidity of the skull restricts any increase in intracranial contents (Chitnavis and Polkey 1998). The principle is based on the fact that the sum of the contents of the intracranial cavity is fixed, with the total volume of all the components of the cranial cavity remaining fairly constant. In other words, any change in the volume of either the blood, brain or CSF must be compensated for by a reciprocal reduction in another component.

Points to consider

Under normal circumstances the intracranial cavity is in a state of dynamic equilibrium, which can be represented by the following equation:

$$_{intracranial}Volume = Vol_{brain} + Vol_{CSF} + Vol_{blood}$$

Once the limited compensatory mechanisms, primarily a reduction in CSF volume and some reduction in the blood volume, have failed a volume–pressure response occurs (Kanter and Narayan 1991). In other words, there is little tolerance to further changes in the volume of the intracranial contents without a dramatic rise in ICP which can be represented by the pressure–volume curve (Figure 2.3a), and an uncompensated state evolves.

Points to consider

The point at which a critical volume expansion is reached is influenced by:

- The speed of the increase, for example with very slowly expanding lesions there can be a great deal of accommodation before the intracranial pressure rises (Chitnavis and Polkey 1998)
- The total increase in volume change (Kanter and Narayan 1991)
- Any underlying brain pathology, for example additional space within the cranial vault will be available in the atrophied brain (Kanter and Narayan 1991)

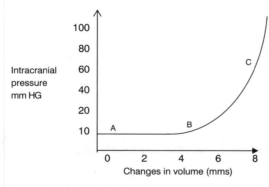

A =   increases in brain volume can be compensated for without a rise in ICP
B =   this is a critical point where there is no change in the ICP but further increases in volume cannot be compensated and will result in changes in increase in ICP
C =   This is an uncompensated state where small changes in volume have a disproportional effect

Figure 2.3a Volume–pressure curve

A vital aspect of caring for the neurologically compromised child is detecting an increase in intracranial pressure. For those children without invasive ICP monitoring healthcare practitioners must rely on the clinical assessment of the child. However, a neurological assessment cannot detect the position of the child's clinical state in relation to the pressure–volume curve. If volume changes within the brain were plotted on the pressure–volume curve (Figure 2.3a), the child could present with the same clinical picture at positions A and B. However, at position B if the intracranial volume continues to increase there would be a dramatic increase in ICP with potentially life threatening consequences for the child. The importance of accurate and timely neurological assessment is a vital component of the child's care and has been described in detail in Section 2.2.

Raised intracranial pressure (RICP)

RICP is usually described as an ICP above 20mmHg sustained for five minutes or more (Miller and Dearden 1992). Pressures above 20mmHg may result in tissue ischaemia. Changes to the normal pressure waveforms, in particular the development of 'A' or 'plateau' waves (Figure 2.3b), can also indicate a reduction in brain compliance and a progressive rise in ICP (Chitnavis and Polkey 1998).

i   The normal ICP waveform has a recognisable pattern of rhythmical peaks that gradually taper. These correspond predominantly to arterial blood pulsations and to a lesser degree the respiratory cycle

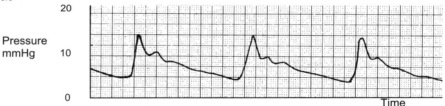

ii 'A' or plateau waves are clinically the most important of Lundberg's classification of ICP waves (Chitnavis and Polkey 1998). These occur when there is reduced brain compliance, and begin with a slow rise in ICP values typically 10-20 mmHg but can increase significantly higher, and have a characteristic plateau that increases in length as the brain's compliance reduces

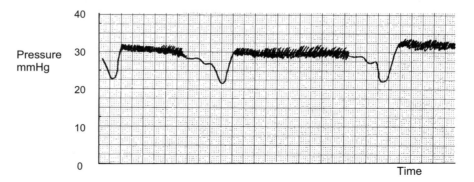

Figure 2.3b Normal ICP waveform and plateau waves

A range of neurological insults can result in an inability of normal mechanisms to maintain the intracranial pressure within acceptable limits. The causes of raised intracranial pressure include:

- Conditions which increase the brain volume
  - space occupying lesions such as tumour, abscess or haematoma
  - cerebral oedema for example following traumatic brain injury or cerebral infection
- Conditions which increase the blood volume or blood flow
  - obstruction to venous outflow
- Conditions which compromise normal CSF levels
  - blockages within the ventricular system causing hydrocephalus
  - conditions which increase CSF levels are rare but could include tumours of the choroid plexus.

Points to consider

The signs and symptoms of RICP include:

- Alterations in conscious levels; irritability, lethargy, confusion, decreased responsiveness
- Dilated pupils, decreased response to light
- Abnormal motor activity or reflexes
- Headaches, nausea and vomiting
- Cushing's response (increased blood pressure with a compensatory bradycardia) or bradycardia on its own and apnoea are late and ominous signs

(Hazinski *et al.* 1999)

The signs and symptoms of RICP in an infant, prior to fusion of the skull sutures, usually occur late because an increase in volume forces the membranes between the skull bones to splay, accommodating pressure changes. The infant will present with more insidious signs and symptoms such as irritability, poor feeding, general developmental delay, large and tense anterior fontanelle even when the infant is in the sitting position, and increased head circumference (Brett and Harding 1997).

Once the ICP starts to rise, additional volume changes – no matter how small – have a great impact on the pressure (Figure 2.3a). Eventually a cycle of events occurs: as the ICP increases, cerebral blood flow decreases, leading to tissue hypoxia, increasing pCO_2 levels and decreasing pH levels resulting in cerebral vasodilation and oedema, which in turn leads to further increases in ICP (Figure 2.3c). The cascade of events perpetuates and a malignant cycle develops (Rosner and Daughton 1990).

It is essential that the child at risk of entering this cycle is transferred to a paediatric intensive care unit, where healthcare professionals are experienced in the care of the child with acute neurological problems, to ensure RICP is appropriately managed.

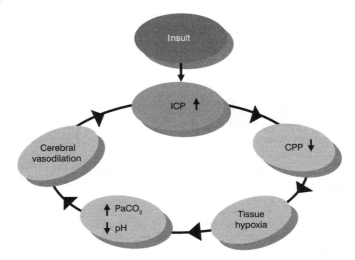

Figure 2.3c Malignant progressive brain swelling: cascade of events (Source: adapted from Hudak *et al.* 1998)

Factors that can contribute to an already increasing intracranial pressure include:

- Hypoventilation
- Hypercapnia ($PaCO_2$ greater than 6kpa)
- Hypoxaemia (PaO_2 less than 6.5kpa)
- Head down position and compression of the neck
- Seizures
- Fever
- A fall in mean arterial pressure, for example if there is hypovolaemia, cardiogenic or septic shock, hypothermia, vasodilatory drugs, e.g. anaesthetic agents
- Stimulation, e.g. invasive procedures, physiotherapy, suctioning
- Inadequate sedation in the ventilated child.

The management of RICP in a child following traumatic brain injury will be discussed in Chapter 5.

Consequences of untreated RICP

Folds in the relatively rigid dura naturally divide the brain into compartments. Two important dural folds are the tentorium cerebelli, which is a tent-like structure that separates the occipital lobes from the cerebellum and the brain stem, and the falx cerebri that forms the deep great longitudinal fissure dividing the cerebral hemispheres into two halves above the corpus callosum (Figures 1.4a and 1.4b) (Hickey 2003b). Once the pressure in one compartment reaches a critical level, brain tissue will shift from the area under pressure into an area of less pressure. For example, the effects of an expanding lesion in one cerebral hemisphere would result in the brain tissue being displaced to the opposite side of the brain. This shifting of brain tissue results in structures being damaged as a result of compression, traction forces and shearing of tissues. Damaged tissues will malfunction or cease to function.

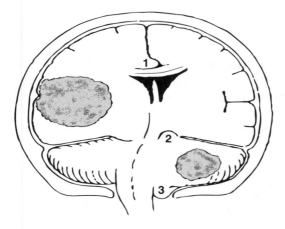

1 Subfalcine shit (midline shift)

2 Transtentorial herniation

3 Infratentorial herniation

Figure 2.3d Common sites for brain herniation

If a primary lesion above the tentorium continues to expand, increasing the intracranial volume, eventually the brain contents herniate through the tentorial notch, an oval opening in the tentorium through which nerves and blood vessels descend into the infratentorial compartment. A progressive increase in pressure in the infratentorium results in a downward displacement of the brain stem into the foramen magnum, the opening at the base of the skull through which the spinal cord passes. Continued pressure increases eventually culminate in the medulla oblongata being projected into the foramen magnum. Herniation of the medulla oblongata is catastrophic because the medulla contains vital centres that regulate breathing, blood pressure and cardiac function. Figure 2.3d highlights the common cites of brain herniation.

Transtentorial herniation

The specific signs and symptoms of transtentorial herniation will depend on whether the cerebrum as a whole is shifting downwards or predominantly one hemisphere is being displaced. Signs of lateral (uncal) transtentorial herniation include (Hickey 2003b):

- The ipsilateral pupil will become dilated and sluggish and eventually becomes fixed and dilated as the ICP continues to rise.
- Ipsilateral ptosis, progressing to paralysis of extraocular muscles.
- Initially there may be restlessness but there can be quick progression to a coma.
- Contralateral limb weakness which may develop into a hemiparesis.

Signs of central transtentorial herniation include (Hickey 2003b):

- Initially both pupils may be small and reactive and eventually become fixed and dilated as ICP continues to rise.
- An increasing difficulty with upward gaze.
- Initially the child may be restless but there can be quick progression to a coma.
- May have bilateral limb weakness which eventually develops into decorticate (flexion of the upper limbs and extension of lower limbs) and decerebrate (extension of all of the limbs) posturing.

Points to consider

Progression of both lateral and central herniation will result in changes in the child's vital signs, such as bradycardia, elevated systolic blood pressure, elevated temperature, Cheyne-Stokes respiration and eventually cessation of respiration.

Infratentorial herniation

The signs and symptoms of infratentorial herniation include rapid onset of a coma, pupillary changes, motor dysfunction, impaired brain stem reflexes (corneal, gag, swallow), changes in vital signs and compression of the medulla oblongata which will cause respiratory arrest (Hickey 2003b).

Points to consider

In the ward environment the management of a child at risk of developing acute raised intracranial pressure (RICP) must be aimed at detecting and promptly acting on changes in the child's neurological state. This includes understanding and interpreting neurological assessments (Section 2.1) and applying the knowledge of the reasons RICP may develop to each individual child. The management of RICP in a child who has sustained a traumatic brain injury is outlined in Chapter 5, Section 3.

2.4 Principles of intracranial pressure monitoring

Continuous ICP monitoring has become a valuable aid in the assessment of a child with a neurological problem. In an acute situation ICP monitoring is used in children who have sustained major neurological trauma, where neurological changes cannot be readily observed due to the child requiring ventilatory support, and drugs that paralyse and sedate. These children should be cared for in a paediatric intensive care unit. However, ICP monitoring is not necessarily exclusive to intensive care. ICP monitoring is used as a diagnostic tool for example in determining hydrocephalus in children with craniosynostosis and for children with hydrocephalus where the decision to insert a shunt is not straightforward or there are complex problems with the functioning of the shunt system (Chitnavis and Polkey 1998). Several factors need to be considered when considering ICP monitoring, these include: the benefit to the child undergoing the procedure; if the results will influence treatment options; the type of monitoring system available locally; the skills of the health professional team; and to ensure the safety of the child (Germon 1994).

There are a variety of monitoring techniques available to record continuous ICP and which can be classified by the location of the probe or the system used to transmit data (Germon 1994). Germon (1994), Chitnavis and Polkey (1998) and Hickey (2003b) provide a detailed review of the different types of ICP monitoring and their relative merits. There are two main types of ICP monitoring equipment: a fluid-filled catheter attached to an external transducer (such as a ventricular or subdural catheter); or a catheter which has an intracranial transducer in the tip (such as a fibre-optic probe) (Hickey 2003b). Both types of catheters are inserted via a burr hole made through the skull and are usually sutured in place; fibre-optic probes are usually secured to an outer casing (often referred to as 'the bolt'), which is screwed to the burr hole. In both situations the catheters are then attached to a display monitor.

Common catheter or probe positions include:

- *Intraventricular:* A catheter or fibre-optic probe is inserted into the ventricles within the brain. It is considered the gold standard for ICP monitoring due to the pressure recording being taken from deep within the brain and it is thought to be a better reflection of the whole brain pressure. Excellent waveforms can be obtained and CSF can be sampled. However, insertion may be difficult and CSF leakage and infection are potential complications.
- *Intraparenchyma:* A catheter, either fibre-optic transducer or electronic strain-gauge, is placed directly into the brain tissue via a bolt device. Catheters are quick to place, provide good waveforms and are easy to maintain. CSF sampling is not possible.
- *Epidural/subdural/subarachnoid:* Catheters connected to transducers can be inserted into the epidural, subdural or subarachnoid space. The waveforms are not as good as intraparenchymal monitoring and catheters easily occlude. In general, intraparenchymal monitoring has replaced these systems.

Children's units should have clear policies relating to the management of ICP monitoring and strict criteria for the suitability of nursing these children in a ward environment. For the non-ventilated child consideration needs to be given to the age and developmental stage of the child. If the child is at risk of developing an acute RICP, intensive care may be a more appropriate environment. Strategies must be in place to minimize the risk of the child pulling out the catheter. These may include having a nurse present at all times, arm restraints or sedation. Care must be taken when sedating a neurologically compromised child because the effects of the sedative can potentially accelerate a rising ICP (Cote *et al.* 2000; Selbst 2000). If the ICP is to have meaningful value, particularly as part of investigative procedures prior to further cranial surgery, then it is paramount that all of the child's activities are recorded and correspond to the time frame on the ICP tracing.

The frequency of neurological assessment will to some extent depend on the reasons for undertaking ICP monitoring. However, when used, ICP recordings should form part of the neurological assessment. The child must be monitored for potential complications of ICP monitoring, which include infection, haemorrhage, increased cerebral oedema, occlusion of the catheters or sensors, mechanical failure of the monitor and accidental removal. Infections are the most common complication and have been reported to be as high as 40 per cent (Hickey 2003b). Infection is more likely to occur with intraventricular catheters, ICP devices *in situ* for more than 5 days, repeated flushing of the system, CSF leakage, concurrent system infection and repeated replacement of catheters (Hickey 2003b).

2.5 Managing acute seizures and status epilepticus

Status epilepticus is described as a disorder in which epileptic activity – a seizure or series of seizures – persists for 30 minutes or more (Scott *et al.* 1998; Tasker 1998). However, from a clinical perspective most seizures that do not spontaneously cease within 5 minutes progress for 30 minutes or more, therefore treatment is usually commenced at 5 minutes (Scott *et al.* 1998; Tasker 1998; Appleton *et al.* 2000). Seizure activity dramatically increases the brain's metabolic

Points to consider

Rapid management of acute seizures and convulsive status epilepticus treatment has the potential to minimize the associated morbidity and mortality (Scott *et al.* 1998; Scott and Neville 1999).

needs, which are initially met by a physiological response that increases the cerebral blood flow thus meeting the brain's demands for oxygen and glucose. This initial compensatory phase can only be maintained for about 30 minutes, after which compensatory mechanisms fail, resulting in cerebral oedema, metabolic acidosis and circulatory collapse and an increasing risk of cerebral damage (Verity 1998; Shorvon 2001). The potential outcomes of prolonged seizures include death and severe neurological sequelae, and are more likely to occur in children with underlying acute or progressive neurological problems (Verity 1998).

Causes of acute seizures in children include (Shorvon 2001):

- Acute cerebral disturbances
  - Trauma
  - Infection
  - Tumours
  - Cerebrovascular disease
  - Metabolic disturbances
  - Febrile seizures
- Pre-existing epilepsy
  - Drug withdrawal
  - Progression of the underlying disease
  - Acute illness
- Pre-existing neurological abnormalities for example cerebral palsy.

Children who have repeated episodes of convulsive epilepticus may need an adapted acute protocol which reflects their individual response to treatments and consideration can be given to potential drug interactions with the child's regular anti-convulsants (Tasker 1998; Scott and Neville 1999). Individual protocols will require the inclusion of parental home treatment regimens, where appropriate.

Points to consider

The aim of management of acute seizure and status epilepticus is to control the seizure activity before cerebral damage and life-threatening sequelae occur (Scott *et al.* 1998; Tasker 1998). The prompt and consistent management of seizures and status epilepticus depends on healthcare staff responding and implementing structured interventions promptly (Tasker 1998; Scott and Neville 1999; Appleton *et al.* 2000; Shorvon 2001). Clear evidence-based protocols must be available to support and guide clinical decisions (Table 2.5a).

Table 2.5a Principles of managing acute seizures and status epilepticus

Stage	Action	Rationale
Immediate assessment and stabilization	Rapid cardiopulmonary assessment- AIRWAY, BREATHING, CIRCULATION If necessary maintain and secure the airway and give oxygen Monitor vital signs, including temperature and pulse oximetry Check capillary glucose Neurological assessment and confirm presence of seizure Obtain information about the child's past medical history/history of seizures	Recognize respiratory failure and shock Airway obstruction will compound hypoxia Ensure management is appropriate for the individual child
Immediate seizure control (5–10 minutes)	Administer fist line anti-convulsant: If intravenous (IV) access available administer IV lorazepam If there is no IV access administer either rectal diazepam or intramuscular midazolam or intramuscular paraldehyde. Secure IV or intraosseous access if not available and obtain bloods for electrolytes and glucose, and blood levels for anti-epileptic drugs. Commence intravenous fluids. Repeat further IV dose of lorazepam if no response after 10 minutes Repeat cardiopulmonary assessment Prepare for intensive support	Lorazepam has a longer duration of action compared to diazepam and lower risk of drug accumulation. It may be less effective in children taking regular benzodiazepine anti-convulsants Paraldehyde may result in abscess formation at injection site
Second stage treatment (15 minutes onwards)	If no response after 15 minutes start phenytoin infusion Intubate and ventilate, transfer to intensive care	Phenytoin is effective within 10–30 minutes and has a long duration of action and may prevent recurrent seizures
Intensive care management	Ventilate, monitor pulse/BP/temperature/urine output, EEG Penobarbitone infusion If no response consider IV bolus of midazolam or thiopentone	Phenobarbitone is effective but may take time to reach therapeutic levels and may cause lowering of the blood pressure. Midazolam is water soluble and easy to administer, less irritant to veins and appears to be effective in stopping seizures that have been unresponsive to other drugs

Source: Tasker 1998; Scott and Neville 1999; Appleton *et al.* 2000; Shorvon 2001

2.6 Care of the unconscious child

Unconsciousness is a lack of awareness of one's self and the environment, lack of cognitive functioning and an inability to respond to sensory stimuli (Hickey 2003c). There are a myriad of neurological conditions that result in unconsciousness, with the depth and duration lasting for seconds (e.g. during a seizure) to months (e.g. following traumatic brain injury).

Children with impaired levels of consciousness and who are unable to maintain their own airway are at risk of hypoxia and hypercarbia, with potential respiratory failure and, therefore, will require intensive care facilities (Hazinski *et al.* 1999). However, many children who have impaired levels of consciousness do not require intensive care facilities but are dependent on the healthcare team to meet their needs. The major goals in caring for these children include:

- Ensuring essential functions, such as airway, breathing and circulation are maintained to sustain life.
- Preventing complications relating to immobility.
- Maximizing the restoration of functions.
- Providing support to the family.

Table 2.6a outlines the care required for the child with impaired levels of consciousness to maintain essential activities of daily living and prevent complications as a result of being unconscious. The emotional and psychological needs of the child and family, and principles of rehabilitation are discussed in Sections 2.7 and 2.8.

Table 2.6a Care of the child with impaired levels of consciousness

Actual/potential problems	*Nursing interventions*
Altered neurological functioning due to cerebral dysfunction	Monitor neurological functioning through regular assessment Manage alterations in sleep patterns and periods of irritability through structuring activities appropriately, having planned rest periods, using relaxation techniques such as aromatherapy and massage Drugs such as melatonin may be prescribed for sleep disturbances – review their use regularly Ensure stimulation activities are planned and appropriate for the child's age and condition Assess and manage pain appropriately
Risk of altered respiratory function due to underlying cerebral dysfunction, inability to maintain airway and immobility Potential problem of atelectasis and chest infection	Assess respiratory function and identify risk of airway obstruction, ensure position does not compromise the airway, use airway aids and suctioning as appropriate Appropriate monitoring such as respiratory rate and effort, colour, peripheral perfusion and pulse oximetry Assess gag and swallow reflexes, in conjunction with a speech and language therapist, keep the child nil by mouth until these reflexes have returned Ensure regular chest physiotherapy, ensure position changes and passive movements are incorporated into care activities Monitoring for signs of chest infection by recording temperature and changes in the amount and colour of secretions
Unable to maintain nutrition and hydration Potential problems of malnutrition, anaemia, electrolyte disturbances, and gastric ulcers	Assess nutritional status, including monitoring of the child's weight Provide a good nutritional intake by appropriate methods that meet the needs of the child, enteral feeding via a naso-gastric/jejunal tube may be necessary. A gastrostomy tube may be more appropriate if long-term enteral feeding is required Ensure nutritional intake reflects increased calorific intake, liaise with the dietician to ensure the correct composition and volume of feed
Unable to maintain nutrition and hydration Potential problems of malnutrition, anaemia, electrolyte disturbances, and gastric ulcers (continued)	Monitoring intake and output, observing for signs of under/over nourishment and dehydration If gag and swallow reflex have been assessed to be adequate and there are no other contra-indications oral food and fluids should be encouraged. The re-introduction of oral feeding may need to be supplemented by enteral feeding because neurological problems may result in oral–motor difficulties, reduced alertness and increased fatigability contributing to inadequate nutritional intake Consider the child's needs in relation to positioning and supportive seating, taste and textures, likes and dislikes, choice of utensils, and effective age appropriate communication

continued…

Table 2.6a continued

Actual/potential problems	Nursing interventions
Unable to maintain self-care needs	Ensure care is appropriate in meeting individual needs and considers usual family practices in relation to maintain hygiene needs There needs to be particular emphasis on the assessment of the mucous membranes of the eyes and oral cavity for dryness, take appropriate action to keep clean and moist: • corneal dryness will require instillation of artificial tear drops or gels such as hypomellose drops • protecting the eyes by the use of patching if the child is unable to completely close the eyes • assessing oral hygiene needs and involvement of dental hygienist/ dentist as appropriate, ensure frequent teeth brushing, consider the need to use suction techniques to prevent aspiration
Potential complications of immobility including: Skin breakdown	Assess pressure areas using a recognised child appropriate assessment tool. Implement preventative measure based on the assessment to ensure the integrity of the skin is maintained
Muscular skeletal deformities; muscle wasting, muscle contractures, peripheral nerve impairment and poor muscle tone	Liase with the therapy team to establish individual positioning regimes. Principles include maintaining the child's head in neutral position, with the spine and hips positioning in alignment with the head, maintaining flexion of the limbs and preventing extension of the ankles Ensure staff and child safety by using appropriate moving and handling equipment and techniques Ensure correct positioning is used at all times and use splints where appropriate
Poor circulation and inadequate lung functioning	Undertake passive exercises and regular position changes in order to improve circulation, relieve pressure, facilitate lung expansion, prevent urinary stasis, improve gut mobility and minimise muscle atrophy Anti-coagulant therapy and anti-embolism stockings will be necessary in older children
Infections particularly chest and urine infections	Ensure regular chest physiotherapy, ensure position changes and passive movements are incorporated into care activities Monitoring for signs of chest infection by recording temperature and changes in the amount and colour of secretions Minimising the risk of urine infection; where appropriate nurse the infant child in nappies and older child in pads; ensure meticulous skin care. An indwelling catheter is a potential sources of infection, if required maintain local policies in relation to the care of indwelling catheters and apply the principles of universal infection precautions Assess for the risk of infection by observing colour, smell and concentration of urine and measurement of body temperature
Constipation	Monitor bowel motions and manage constipation appropriately including high fibre diet or supplements, adequate hydration and use of suppositories as necessary

2.7 Emotional and psychological needs of the child and family

The diagnosis of a neurological disorder is devastating for the child and family and has far-reaching effects that can potentially affect the physical, cognitive and affective (behaviour, personality) functions of the child (Hickey 2003d). Changes in cognitive and affective functions can be particularly difficult for the child and family to accept and have the potential to alter all dimensions of family life and change the anticipated expectations parents may have for their child. It is vital that the emotional and psychological needs of the child and family are considered and incorporated into care because normal coping abilities may become ineffective. Although the child and family will require support from the multidisciplinary team, the presence of nurses over the 24-hour care period often results in emotional and psychological care becoming a nursing responsibility. Depending on the diagnosis, the child and family will need to adjust to a range of situations and issues, including (Hickey 2003d):

- Threat to the survival of the child.
- Threat to quality of life of the child as a result of:
  - Motor paralysis
  - Bowel and bladder dysfunction
  - Communication difficulties
  - Sensory deficits
- Potential behavioural problems.
- Future ability of the child to live independently.
- Future ability of the child to form relationships.
- Future education and career prospects.
- A dependent child may require parents to review current care arrangements, which may result in a reduction of income and alteration in lifestyle.
- Reaction and needs of siblings.

The family will have many questions about the child's condition; why and how the neurological problem occurred. In addition, there may be overwhelming feelings of guilt or inadequacy. These feelings may be compounded in situations where there is no definitive diagnosis, the injuries are a result of an accident or the child's condition is life threatening. Parents may feel frustrated and isolated. Extensive investigations and unpleasant treatments will add to the general despair. The family may be angry that vague signs and symptoms have gone unnoticed. There will be fears regarding the prognosis and long-term outcomes. The family may be experiencing difficulty in accepting the changes in their child and grieve for the child they know, love and who has been an integral part of their lives. The family may also find that strain is placed on family relationships and, consequently, may find it difficult to support each other, especially if family members are at different stages of grieving and accepting their child's condition. These emotions will affect the family's ability to comprehend information given to them.

Points to consider

Nurses have an important role in meeting the emotional and psychological needs of the child and family. It is essential to establish the usual coping strategies and support systems used by the child and family. Long-term support should be aimed at supporting and developing existing mechanisms.

Nursing interventions should be an integral part of everyday practice and can aid in supporting the emotional and psychological needs of the child and family. Nursing interventions include:

- Ensuring the family is given enough opportunity to ask questions and giving responses that are clear, accurate and honest.

- Providing and reinforcing information regularly, keeping the family updated.
- Including the child in discussions at a level appropriate to their age and stage of development.
- Providing support by listening to the family's anxieties and concerns.
- Providing the family with information about support groups and parent to parent self-help groups.
- Ensuring a non-judgemental approach to care respecting the cultural, religious and spiritual beliefs of the family.
- Assisting the family to make realistic goals about their child's care.
- Ensuring care is family-centred, all aspects of care are discussed and care planning is negotiated with the family and child where appropriate.
- Involving parents practically in all aspects of caring for their child while in hospital, for example washing, dressing, bathing, feeding, medication, communicating with their child.
- Ensuring appropriate community care is arranged and that necessary equipment and adaptations to the home have been made prior to the child going home.
- Offering support for siblings and encouraging parents to be open and honest with them.
- Referring to social services for anxieties regarding money, parents taking time off work, housing issues.
- Recognizing there will be extreme anxiety if a child requires care in a different setting; ensuring systems allow for smooth transfers.
- Recognizing when there is a need to refer to other members of the multidisciplinary team.

Points to consider

The input and support the child and family requires will vary depending upon the unique needs of the child, the diagnosis, and stage and response to treatment (Freeman *et al.* 2000). The information shared with the child and family must be communicated effectively between multidisciplinary team members to prevent confusion and ensure a consistent approach to care. This can be achieved through shared goals and regular team meetings.

Providing support to a child and family at a stressful time can be a daunting and stressful task for the nurse, who may feel inadequate and lacking in information especially while waiting for a diagnosis on the child. It is important for the nurse to spend time establishing a relationship with the child and family. Research relating to living with a sick child in hospital, found that parents valued nurses who were warm, friendly, patient and unhurried in their interactions with the child and family; they also appreciated nurses who gave them the time to talk about issues that were important to them and to express their feelings openly (Darbyshire 1994). Creating a comfortable environment for families and children is important (Freeman *et al.* 2004).

2.8 Principles of rehabilitation

Traditional models of care focusing on disease and its treatment are not always appropriate for a child with a neurological problem, particularly for those children where the neurological damage has resulted in significant loss of function. The philosophy underpinning rehabilitation is to enable an individual to circumvent impairments to minimize disability (Neumann 1995). Programmes of care must be individually designed and strongly influenced at encouraging the child to reach their full potential, working within a developmental context, to integrate the children back into their family, school and community (Roffe 1989). This can only be achieved through a structured, caring and safe environment with all members of the multidisciplinary team adopting a child- and family-orientated approach to care. The care given will be provided for by a variety of disciplines, the team must have common goals with care integrated into the child's daily routines.

Best practice recommendations

Clearly defined care pathways or protocols should be available for children who have sustained a brain injury to ensure effective multidisciplinary working, and appropriate services should be mobilized at each stage of the child's and family's journey. Care pathways will need clear guidance relating to:

- Role and function of members of the rehabilitation team, including an outline of the role of key worker, the format and function of multidisciplinary meetings
- Child and family assessment strategies
- Goal planning with the child and family
- Liaison with local services and professionals from healthcare, education and social services
- Discharge planning processes
- Transition to adult services.

Nurses are a vital component of the multidisciplinary team and their roles include: assessment of the child, particularly regarding actual or potential problems relating to activities of living; coordination of care and maintaining effective links with all team members; providing technical and physical care; integrating therapies initiated by other professionals into every ay care; providing emotional support to the child and family; and involving the family in care (Long *et al.* 2002). In the early rehabilitation phase preventing limb deformities through correct limb positioning and maintaining muscle tone is a key component of care. It is vital that nurses liaise with the physiotherapist and occupational therapist regarding appropriate positioning, type and frequency of passive stretching exercises and the use of splinting if necessary.

The importance of effective family-centred care and parental involvement in care is particularly important for the child rehabilitating from a neurological disorder because of the potential life-changing consequences of the condition for the child and family and the long-term nature of care requirements. If the child is to be successfully integrated back into the family, the family must understand the process of rehabilitation and be involved in goal setting and monitoring their child's progress. The progress and psychological adjustment of the child may be improved if family-centred care is effective (Siebes *et al.* 2007).

Parents have highlighted that to be effectively involved in their child's rehabilitation they need to participate in goal setting, treatment decisions and multidisciplinary team meetings (Siebes *et al.* 2007). In addition, the timing of meetings and ability to be involved in care delivery requires healthcare professionals to recognize and consider the usual family practices and other family commitments (Siebes *et al.* 2007). One way of achieving effective goal setting between the multidisciplinary team and the child and family is through the use of a rehabilitation progress chart (Figure 2.8a). Charts should be constructed in a user-friendly format using appropriate language.

Core activities \ Score	1	2	3	4	5	6	7
Understanding	Non apparent	Appears to listens to familiar sounds	Responses to familiar sounds	Identifies people and objects	Needs prompting to understand and respond to simple requests	Understands and responds to simple requests	Understands general conversations
Talking	Non apparent	Makes noises when upset/ uncomfortable	Uses sounds to communicate	Uses sounds, gestures, picture board to communicate	Uses words	Uses simple sentences	Understands general conversations
Mobility	Immobile	Sits with support	Stands with support	Takes steps with support	Stands unaided	Walks unaided	Walks up and down stairs unaided
Socialization	No apparent awareness	Appears aware of people and surroundings	Responds to familiar people	Initiates interactions with familiar people	Responds to strangers	Initiates interactions with strangers	Joins in small group activities
Play/Education	No apparent interactions	Observes play/ activities	Engages in solitary play/activities	Engages in play/ activities along side others	Interactive play/ activities with others	Contributes to group activities	Initiates own activities
Fine movement	No apparent fine motor control	Palmer grasp and transfer	Pincer grasp points with index finger	Manipulates objects	Holds pencil	Picks up small objects	More controlled movements such as threading beads
Dressing	Dose not assist	Helps by holding out limbs prior to dressing	Takes off garments but unable to replace them	Puts on some items of clothing	More active in helping with all aspects of dressings	Can dress and undress but may need help with complex tasks such as fastening	Can dress and undress unaided
Feeding and drinking	Enteral feeding only	Some semi-solid foods taken from a spoon	Thickened drinks from a cup	Finely chopped food taken from a fork or spoon	All fluids from a cup	Finger foods managed	Eats and drinks appropriate for age and stage of development
Toileting	Unaware of toileting needs- wears protective nappies/ pads	Aware when wet	Indicates need for the toilet	Asks to use the toilet	Gains bladder control	In general had both bladder and bowel control	Toileting is appropriate for age and stage of development

Figure 2.8a Rehabilitation core activities (Source: Tyler 1980; Nash *et al.* 1998)

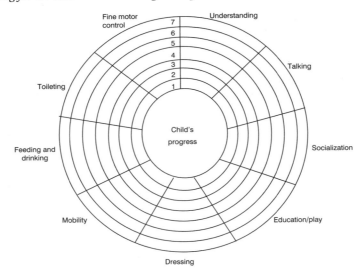

Figure 2.8b Progress evaluation chart (Source: adapted from Tyler 1980; Nash *et al.* 1998)

In the example outlined each core rehabilitation activity is broken down into seven components: 1 identifying the minimal skills and 7 the maximum achievable. Shading the appropriate segment on the progress document (Figure 2.8b), when achievements are made assists in monitoring the child's progress. Progress charts should be reviewed regularly by the multidisciplinary team and in conjunction with parents to form the basis of ongoing goal setting.

For many children with a neurological problem, rehabilitation is a long and ongoing process and will continue once the child has been discharged from hospital. Effective discharge planning is central in preparing the child and family for ongoing care, and ensuring community care provision is established prior to discharge (DfES/DH 2004). Transferring the child's care from the hospital to community setting can be a stressful time for the family, particularly for children with complex needs (Lewis and Noyes 2007). Expectations that parents will take on the role of parent and care giver are usually assumed rather than negotiated and may reflect the reality that there is lack of alternative care (Kirk 2001). The aim of effective transfer of the child's care to the community is to ensure parents are prepared for their child's discharge, including being competent in any ongoing aspects of care that need to be maintained post-discharge and ensuring community support systems are in place. A home assessment may be necessary if the child's physical functioning is limited and should include access into the home, access to toilet/ bathroom and bedroom and the ability of the home to accommodate any equipment that the child may require. Where possible, home visits with the child are desirable and the length of time the child is away from the hospital setting should be gradually increased in the period prior to full discharge. Any potential home adaptations will need to be identified early and have the potential to delay the child's discharge from hospital to home.

Service providers need to ensure funding decisions and service level agreements are in place to support the child with complex needs being discharged from hospital and the transfer of care to the community setting (Lewis and Noyes 2007). Where there is a significant number of children who are discharged from hospital an integrated discharge planning team can support the patient and healthcare team in coordinating the child's care (DH 2003). If an integrated discharge planning service is not available a key worker should be named to coordinate the transfer process

(Lewis and Noyes 2007). For many children issues relating to future education and schooling may be major considerations which require detailed assessment and advanced planning.

Points to consider

The goals for effective discharge planning include:

- Actively engaging family members in the process of transferring care from hospital to home
- Ensuring parents are involved in decisions about the potential change in their roles, which may require a significant extension of usual parenting responsibilities
- Ensuring parents receive appropriate training to become competent in the skills needed to care for their child at home
- Having knowledge of local support services and facilities
- Developing effective communication between primary, secondary, social care and education providers
- Beginning the process of transition to community care early, with trial periods out of the hospital to highlight any unidentified needs.

(Lewis and Noyes 2007)

The child may require ongoing input and support from welfare systems into adulthood. The transition from child to adult services can be a period of instability for the child and family. Transition planning needs to be flexible in its timing, have a designated named key worker, involve the young person, utilize care plans with clear aims linked to each stage of the transition process, and there needs to be robust auditing of the transition process (RCN 2004).

Key messages from this chapter

- Diagnostic procedures are vital in helping to make the correct diagnosis and in monitoring the progression of the disease
- A vital aspect of caring for the neurologically compromised child is detecting an increase in intracranial pressure. For those children without invasive ICP monitoring healthcare practitioners must rely on the clinical assessment of the child
- Neurological observations, including the assessment of conscious levels, pupil reactions, motor function and other parameters, including cardiovascular observations, are essential for nurses caring for children with neurological problems
- The child with impaired levels of consciousness will require healthcare professionals to maintain essential activities of daily living and prevent complications as a result of being unconscious
- The diagnosis of a neurological disorder is devastating for the child and family with far-reaching effects that can potentially affect the physical, cognitive and affective (behaviour, personality) functions of the child
- For many children with a neurological problem rehabilitation is a long and ongoing process and will continue once the child has been discharged from hospital.

Web resources

National Institute for Health and Clinical Excellence
provides national guidance on the promotion of good health and the prevention and treatment of ill health, and produces guidance relating to: public health (promoting good health and the prevention of ill health for those working in the all healthcare sectors), health technologies (guidance on the use of new and existing medicines, treatments and procedures), and clinical practice guidance (appropriate treatment and care of people with specific diseases and conditions)
www.nice.org.uk
Scottish Intercollegiate Guidelines Network
develops and disseminates national clinical guidelines, derived from systematic reviews of the scientific evidence, to ensure practice is based on current evidence.
www.sign.ac.uk
National Library for Health
provides a range of health related resources
www.library.nhs.uk

References

Appleton R, Choonara I, Martland T *et al.* (2000) The treatment of convulsive status epilepticus in children. *Archives of Disease in Childhood* **83** (5): 415–19.

Barker RA, Barasi S (1999) *Neuroscience at a Glance.* Blackwell Science, Oxford.

Boss B (2002) Concepts of neurological dysfunction. In McCance KL, Huether SE (eds) *Pathophysiology: The Biologic Basis for Disease in Adults and Children*, 4th edn. Mosby, St Louis, MO.

Brashers VL (2002) The pulmonary system. In McCance KL, Huether SE eds) *Pathophysiology: The Biologic Basis for Disease in Adults and Children*, 4th edn. Mosby, St Louis, MO.

Brett EM, Harding BN (1997) Hydrocephalus and congenital anomalies of the nervous system other than myelomeningocele. In Brett EM (ed.) *Paediatric Neurology*, 3rd edn. Churchill Livingstone, London.

Brett EM, Kaiser AM (1997) Neurology of the newborn. In Brett EM (ed.) *Paediatric Neurology*, 3rd edn. Churchill Livingstone, London.

Bullock R, Chestnut RM, Clifton G *et al.* (2000) Guidelines for the management of severe traumatic brain injury. *Journal of Neurotrauma* **17** (6/7): 451–3.

Casey A (1988) A partnership with child and family. *Senior Nurse* **8** (4): 8–9.

Chitnavis BC, Polkey CE (1998) Intracranial pressure monitoring. *Care of the Critically Ill Child* **14** (3): 80–4.

Coté CJ, Notterman DA, Karl HW, Weinberg JA, McCloskey C (2000) Adverse sedation events in pediatrics: a critical incident analysis of contributing factors. *Pediatrics* **105** (4 pt 1): 805–14.

Darbyshire P (1994) *Living with a Sick Child in Hospital. The Experiences of Parents and Nurses.* Chapman and Hall, London.

Department for Education and Skills/Department of Health (2004) *National Service Framework for Children, Young People and Maternity Services.* The Stationery Office, London.

Department of Health (2003) *Discharge from Hospital: Pathway, Processes and Practice.* The Stationery Office, London.

Ellis A, Cavanagh SJ (1992) Aspects of neurological assessment using the Glasgow Coma Scale. *Intensive and Critical Care Nursing* **8**: 94–9.

Ferguson-Clark L, Williams C (1998) Neurological assessment in children. *Paediatric Nursing* **10**: 29–33.

Fielding K, Rowley G (1991) Reliability and accuracy of the Glasgow Coma Scale with experienced and inexperienced nurses. *Lancet* **337**: 535–8.

Freeman K, O'Dell C, Meola C (2000) Issues in families of children with brain tumors. *Oncology Nursing Forum* **27** (5): 843–4.

Freeman K, O'Dell C, Meola C (2004) Childhood brain tumors: parental concerns and stressors by phase of illness. *Journal of Pediatric Oncology Nursing* **21** (2): 87–97.

Germon K (1994) Intracranial pressure monitoring in the 1990s. *Critical Care Nursing Quarterly* **17** (1): 21–32.

Giulioni M, Ursino M (1996) Impact of cerebral perfusion pressures and autoregulation on intracranial dynamics: a modeling study. *Neurosurgery* **39** (5): 1005–15.

Hazinski MF, Headrick C, Bruce D (1999) Neurological disorders. In Hazinski MF (ed.) *Manual of Pediatric Critical Care*. Mosby, St Louis, MO.

Hickey JV (2003a) Neurological assessment. In Hickey JV (ed.) *The Clinical Practice of Neurological and Neurosurgical Nursing*, 5th edn. Lippincott, Philadelphia, PA.

Hickey JV (2003b) Intracranial hypertension: theory and management of increased intracranial pressure. In Hickey JV (ed.) *The Clinical Practice of Neurological and Neurosurgical Nursing*, 5th edn. Lippincott, Philadelphia, PA.

Hickey JV (2003c) Management of the unconscious neurological patient. In Hickey JV (ed.) *The Clinical Practice of Neurological and Neurosurgical Nursing*, 5th edn. Lippincott, Philadelphia, PA.

Hickey JV (2003d) Behavioural and psychological responses in neurological illness. In Hickey JV (ed.) *The Clinical Practice of Neurological and Neurosurgical Nursing*, 5th edn. Lippincott, Philadelphia, PA.

Hudak C, Gallo BM, Morton PG (1998) *Critical Care Nursing: A Holistic Approach*, 7th edn. Lippincott, Philadelphia, PA.

James HE, Trauner DA (1985) The Glasgow Coma Scale. In James HE, Anas NG, Perkin RM (eds) *Brain Insults in Infants and Children*. Grune & Stratton, Orlando, FL.

Kanter MJ, Narayan RK (1991) Management of head injury. Intracranial pressure monitoring. *Neurosurgery Clinics of North America* **2** (2): 257–65.

Kirk S (2001) Negotiating lay and professional roles in the care of children with complex health care needs. *Journal of Advanced Nursing* **34** (5): 593–602.

Kraus JF, Fife D, Conroy C (1987) Pediatric brain injuries: the nature, clinical course and early outcomes in a defined United States' population. *Pediatrics* **79** (4): 501–50.

Lawson GR (2000) Sedation of children for magnetic resonance imaging. *Archives of Disease in Childhood.* **82**: 150–4.

Lewis M, Noyes J (2007) Discharge planning for children with complex needs. *Paediatric Nursing* **19** (4): 26–9.

Long AF, Kneafsey R, Ryan J, Berry J (2002) The role of the nurse within the multi-professional rehabilitation team. *Journal of Advanced Nursing* **37** (1): 70–8.

McLeod A (2006) Intra and extracranial causes of alterations in level of consciousness. In Woodward D (ed.) *Neuroscience Nursing: Assessment and Patient Management*. Quay Books, London.

McNett M (2007) A review of the predictive ability of Glasgow Coma Scale Scores in head-injury patients. *Journal of Neuroscience Nursing* **39** (2): 68–75.

Miller JD, Dearden NM (1992) Measurement, analysis and the management of raised intracranial pressure. In Teasdale GM, Miller JD (ed.) *Current Neurosurgery*. Churchill Livingstone, London.

Nash J, Appleton R, Rowland B *et al.* (1998) Immediate medical and nursing needs. In Appleton R, Baldwin T (eds) *Management of Brain-injured Children*. Oxford University Press, Oxford.

National Institute for Health and Clinical Excellence (2007) Head Injury. *Triage, Assessment, Investigation and Early Management of Head Injury in Infants, Children and Adults.* NICE, London.

Neumann VC (1995) Principles and practices of treatment. In Chamberlain MA, Neumann VC, Tennant A (eds) *Traumatic Brain Injury Rehabilitation Services, Treatment and Outcomes*. Chapman and Hall Medical, London.

Peters A (2007) Neurological observations. In Glasper EA, McEwing G, Richardson J (eds) *Oxford Handbook of Children's and Young People's Nursing*. Oxford University Press, Oxford.

Price T (2002) Painful stimuli and the Glasgow Coma Scale. *Critical Care Nurse* **7** (1): 19–23.

Reilly PL, Simpson DA, Sprod R, Thomas L (1988) Assessing the conscious levels of infants and young children: a paediatric version of the Glasgow coma scale. *Children's Nervous System* **4**: 30–3.

Roffe J (1989) The role of the nurse in paediatric rehabilitation. *Paediatric Nursing* **1**: 11–13.

Rosner MJ, Daughton S (1990) Cerebral perfusion pressures, management in head injury. *Journal of Trauma* **30**: 933–40.

Royal College of Nursing (2004) *Adolescent transition care. Guidance for Nursing Staff*. RCN, London.

Scottish Intercollegiate Guidelines Network (2004) *Safe Sedation of Children Undergoing Diagnostic and Therapeutic Procedures: A National Clinical Guideline*. SIGN, Edinburgh.

Scott RC, Neville BG (1999) Pharmacological management of convulsive status epilepticus in children. *Developmental Medicine and Child Neurology* **41**: 207–10.

Scott RC, Surtees RA, Neville BG (1998) Status epilepticus: pathophysiology, epidemiology, and outcomes. *Archives of Diseases in Childhood* **79** (1): 73–7.

Selbst SM (2000) Adverse sedation events in paediatrics: a critical incident analysis of contributing factors. *Pediatrics* **105** (4): 845–65.

Shorvon S (2001) The management of status epilepticus. *Journal of Neurology Neurosurgery and Psychiatry* **70** (suppl 2): 22–7.

Siebes RC, Wijnroks L, Ketelaar M et al. (2007) Parent participation in paediatric rehabilitation treatment centres in the Netherlands: a parents' viewpoint. *Child: Care, Health and Development* **33** (2): 196–205.

Smith J, Callaghan L (2001) Development of clinical guidelines for the sedation of children. *British Journal of Nursing* **10** (6): 113–17.

Smith J (1999) Specialist courses: education for the future. *Paediatric Nursing* **11** (4): 19–21

Tasker RC (1998) Emergency treatment of acute seizures and status epilepticus. *Archives of Diseases in Childhood* **79** (1): 78–83.

Tatman A, Warren A, Williams A, Powell JE, Whitehouse W (1997) Development of a modified paediatric coma scale in intensive care clinical practice. *Archives of Diseases in Childhood* **77** (6): 519–21.

Teasdale G, Jennett B (1974) Assessment of coma and impaired consciousness. A practical scale. *Lancet* **2**: 81–3.

Tyler S (1980) *Keele Pre-School Assessment Guide*. NFER-Nelson, Windsor.

Verity CM (1998) Do seizures damage the brain? The epidemiological evidence. *Archives of Diseases in Childhood* **78** (1): 78–84.

Warren A (2000) Paediatric coma scoring researched and benchmarked. *Paediatric Nursing* **12** (3): 14–18.

Watson M, Horn S, Curl J (1992) Searching for signs of revival: uses and abuses of the Glasgow Coma Scale. *Professional Nurse* **7** (10): 670–3.

Westbrook A (1997) The use of a paediatric coma scale for monitoring infants and children with head injuries. *Nursing in Critical Care* **2** (2): 72–5.

Wong DL (1995) The child with cognitive, sensory, or communication impairment. In Wong DL (ed.) *Whaley and Wong's Nursing Care of Infants and Young Children*, 5th edn. Mosby, New York.

3 General principles of caring for the child requiring neurosurgery

The principles of care that apply to every child requiring surgery are also important for the child undergoing neurosurgery. This chapter will provide an overview and underpinning rationale of the care required for the child and family where the child is undergoing neurosurgery. The child's needs specific to the underlying neurosurgical condition are outlined in subsequent chapters. Terminology relating to neurosurgical procedures is provided in Appendix I.

At the end of reading this chapter you will be able to:

Learning outcomes

- Describe the principles of perioperative care for the child and family
- Explain the management of shock and haemorrhage
- Discuss the principles of acute pain management in children
- Outline the principles of surgical incision wound management
- Prepare the child and family for discharge home following neurosurgery.

3.1 Perioperative care

There are few specific perioperative requirements relating to cranial surgery. The main goals of care are to minimize potential complications of the surgical procedure and effects of the anaesthetic by ensuring the child and family are prepared appropriately and safely for surgery and recovery needs are met. Surgery and anaesthesia disrupt normal functioning, homeostatic mechanisms and are potentially life-threatening.

Points to consider

- The purpose of general anaesthesia is to ensure surgery can proceed under optimal conditions and to keep the child comfortable
- Principles of anaesthesia are to induce unconsciousness, achieving effective muscle relaxation and the provision of suitable analgesia
- The drugs and techniques used affect all body systems. The ability to detect sensations, such as pain, touch, temperature and body position are lost
- The challenges of anaesthetizing children relate to the physiological, anatomical and psychological differences from adults, such as a lower residual respiratory capacity, a higher minute ventilation and cardiac output, a higher metabolic rate and a large body surface area in relation to weight
- Pathophysiological changes, such as hypoxia, hypercarbia, hypovolaemia and hypothermia can occur quickly in children
- Complications of anaesthesia in children are largely confined to high-risk groups, where children have complex and multiple problems or adverse drug reactions.

(NCEPOD 1999)

Although interlinked, perioperative care is usually divided into three general phases: pre-, intra- and postoperative care (Leinonen and Leino-Kilpi 1999). Nurses are a vital link in ensuring continuity in care across the perioperative period and promote care that is child and family focused (Cowan 1998).

Best practice recommendations

The key role of the nurse relating to the perioperative care of the child includes ensuring:

- Accurate, comprehensive and concise information relating to the child and family is obtained and shared with all healthcare professionals caring for the child
- There is a record of care required, any problems encountered, interventions and the effectiveness of care
- Baseline observations (including physical measures) relating to the child's preoperative condition are recorded and available for comparison during and post-anaesthesia
- Care is of a high quality which can be achieved by setting, maintaining and promoting perioperative care standards.

Neurosurgical procedures that have a high potential for acute oedema or extensive blood loss postoperatively, or the duration of the procedure is lengthy, may require the child to be nursed in intensive care postoperatively. In addition to the general principles of intra-operative care described subsequently the specific needs of the child in intensive care relating to ventilatory support will apply. It is not within the scope of this text to provide details of care of the child or family nursed in intensive care.

Preoperative care

Preoperative care can be divided into three general areas: the psychological preparation of the child and family, optimizing the health of the child prior to surgery and ensuring the physical safety of the child (Heath 1998).

Optimizing the health of the child prior to surgery

The aim of preoperative assessment is to ensure the child is in optimal health prior to anaesthesia and surgery (Heath 1998). The preoperative assessment requires a multidisciplinary approach and although primarily involves the surgeon, the anaesthetist and nursing staff, can involve all members of the multidisciplinary team, depending upon the child's individual needs.

Essential care

The preoperative assessment should:

- Establish the child's current health and the need for surgery. This may include specific investigations depending on cause of neurological problem for example assessment of pituitary function will be necessary in children with pituitary tumours
- Screen for the presence of unknown underlying abnormalities, which have the potential to influence the outcome of anaesthesia
- Plan to manage existing diseases such as diabetes mellitus
- Identify the child and parent's understanding of the surgery and any health education needs
- Identify any psychological and social circumstances that may have an impact upon the care needs of the child and family.

Preoperative assessment involves history taking and physical assessment (Rushforth *et al.* 2000). Taking the child's health history includes: establishing the child's current condition and its effects; current treatments (including complementary therapies) and medications; past medical history and ongoing health problems; previous anaesthetic history and complications; and identification of any known allergies (ASA 2002). The physical examination should include an assessment of the airway, heart and lungs, and measurement and documentation of vital signs (ASA 2002). One of the major dilemmas for anaesthesiology in children is the decision relating to anaesthetizing children who present with an upper respiratory tract infection (URTI) (Tait *et al.* 2001; Brown *et al.* 2000). The presence of URTI is associated with increased intra-operative complications such as bronchospasm, laryngospasm and oxygen desaturation (Brown *et al.* 2000). For the majority of children with a URTI anaesthesia can proceed because associated complications do not have any long-term effects (Tait *et al.* 2001). However, consideration needs to be given to the whole clinical picture including the presence of a productive cough, fever, history of respiratory disease such as asthma, presence of a wheeze and general malaise (Tait *et al.* 2001; Brown *et al.* 2000).

Requesting preoperative investigations, such as chest X-ray, electrocardiogram, blood samples and urinalysis for all patients undergoing surgery is now deemed unnecessary (Munro *et al.* 1997). Investigations should only be requested in the presence of a specific clinical condition or defined risks due to the nature of the surgical procedure (Munro *et al.* 1997; ASA 2002). However, children undergoing neurosurgery will as a minimum require preoperative blood sampling, urea and electrolytes and full blood count and cross-match because of the potential for blood loss during surgery.

Best practice recommendations

A comprehensive review of the preoperative evidence and criteria for selecting an investigation in relation to patient characteristics have been published by the American Society of Anesthesiologists Task Force on Preanesthesia Evaluation (ASA 2002) and the UK Health Technology Assessment Programme (Munro *et al.* 1997).

Point to consider

It is vital that the rationale for preoperative investigations is clear to avoid unnecessary procedures for the child.

A nursing assessment will assist in identifying the specific needs of the child and family, allowing information about the surgery and its implications to be tailored to meet the needs of the child and family. The child and family should be given the opportunity to ask questions and express concerns with the nurse's aim being to reduce fears and anxieties.

Points to consider

The purpose of a nursing assessment is to establish:

- Family care that the child usually requires
- Current condition of the child both physically and psychologically
- Nursing care the child requires in relation to both current diagnosis and general health needs
- Ability of the child and family to participate in care required.

(Casey 1988)

Taking a history from the child and family and conducting a thorough assessment is the start of the process of systematically planning care, which leads to ensuring interventions are appropriate to the individual needs of the child and family. In addition, care must be evaluated to assess the effectiveness of interventions and provide opportunity to review the needs of the child and family. Effective documentation is a vital component of care.

Best practice recommendations

Good record keeping is a professional requirement and ensures:

- Safety and well-being of the patient
- Accurate, comprehensive and concise information relating to the child and family is available
- A record of care required, any problems encountered, interventions and the effectiveness of care
- A baseline upon which the child's condition can be compared
- A means to set and maintain standards and promote quality care
- Better dissemination of information between members of the healthcare team.

(NMC 2007)

The child and family must be prepared for the immediate postoperative period including the probability of being nursed in intensive care. Where possible the child and family should be offered the opportunity to visit intensive care facilities. The child's postoperative appearance should be explained to the child and family and should include descriptions of the wound/ bandages, drains, facial swelling, hair removal and the range and function of monitoring equipment.

Consent, written or verbal is required for a patient, of any age, before medical treatment can be given (DH 2001). For invasive procedures like surgery it is usual practice for healthcare professionals to obtain written consent. The type of consent form will reflect local practices. Consent forms are becoming much more detailed, which aids in ensuring the child and family are fully informed about the potential risks and benefits of the surgery. In addition safety can be promoted if specific consent forms are used, for example correct site surgery and blood transfusion consent forms. Where appropriate sensitive issues, such the possibility of retaining samples for research purposes, requires discussion with the child and family and formal consent obtained. Obtaining formal consent is usually the role of the surgeon performing the operation. However, nurses caring for a child will require knowledge and understanding of the law relating to children obtaining consent for nursing procedures which can be expressed or implied and is usually obtained verbally.

Essential care

Legalities relating to consent in children:

- In England, Wales and Northern Ireland there is no statute that gives children under 16 years of age the right to consent to treatment (British Medical Association 2001). The person with parental responsibility must provide consent for any medical treatment on behalf of a child under 16 years of a age (Family Law and Reform Act, 1969).
- In Scotland children under the age of 16 years can consent to treatment where, in the opinion of a qualified medical practitioner, the child is capable of understanding

the nature and possible consequences of the procedure or treatment (Age of Legal Capacity (Scotland) Act 1991).

- Children can legally consent to surgical, medical or dental treatment at or over 16 years of age in the United Kingdom (Family Law and Reform Act, 1969; Age of Legal Capacity (Scotland) Act, 1991. This is a statutory right and has the same standing as consent given by an adult. It is not necessary to obtain consent from a parent or guardian. There are exceptions to this statutory right, e.g. individuals who are deemed incapable of consenting for treatment due to 'disability'.
- Consent for treatment is not necessary in life-threatening situations.
- Children can consent to treatment at any age provided that they are deemed to have sufficient understanding and intelligence to fully understand treatments being proposed (Gillick v. West Norfolk and Wisbech Area Health Authority 1985). Those with parental responsibility cannot override this decision, although the decision can be overridden by a court of law.
- If a child refuses medical treatment the decision can be overridden by the person with parental responsibility for that child and by the court, even if the child has sufficient understanding of their actions and the subsequent consequences of their actions (Re W 1992; Re E 1993).

Healthcare professionals must understand who may have parental responsibility for consent. Individuals deemed to have parental responsibility are (DH 1989):

- Legal parents; the child's biological parents.
- The child's legally appointed guardian.
- A Local Authority authorized person who has been designated parental responsibility in a care order in respect of the child.
- A Local Authority authorized person who holds an emergency protection order in respect of the child.

Points to consider

Both parents do not necessarily have parental responsibility; parental responsibility applies to both the mother and father if they were married at birth or some time after birth. If the parents have never married, the mother alone has parental responsibility, although a father can apply for parental responsibility. For children born before December 2003, unmarried fathers can obtain parental responsibility by: marrying the mother; obtaining a parental responsibility order form from the court; or registering parental responsibility with the court. Since 2003, law has changed in line with European Union family polices, and unmarried fathers can obtain parental responsibility by: registering the child's birth with the mother at the time of birth; re-registering the birth; marrying the mother; obtaining a parental responsibility order form from the court; or registering parental responsibility with the court.

Preparation of the child for theatre

A key role of the nurse caring for the child and family, where the child requires surgery, is preparing the child for theatre and ensuring safety protocols are maintained. Many procedures relating to physical preparation of children for theatre appear to be lacking in evidence or clear rationale.

> **Points to consider**
>
> When preparing the child for theatre a balance must be achieved between procedures that have safety implications and those that have no apparent value. It is inappropriate to prepare a child for something that is unnecessary, both in terms of the potential distress for the child and family and wasting valuable resources. All aspects of care must be fully explained with appropriate rationale offered, negotiated with the child and family and where possible choices given.

Surgeons are responsible for ensuring the correct surgical site is clearly marked with a skin marker. If a decision is made with parents not to mark the skin this must be clearly documented. It is usual practice to wash the hair in a povidone-iodine hair wash prior to theatre. The guidelines for hair removal from the US Centers for Disease Control and Prevention advocate that hair removal should only be performed if hair is present at the incision site (Mangram *et al.* 1999). Hair removal for cranial surgery is usually restricted to a minimum, for example the immediate area around the incision site. This prevents the hair becoming entangled with sutures or embedded within the wound which has the potential to cause tissue reaction and the formation of a granuloma. Prior to craniotomy, hair removal needs to be discussed sensitively with the child and family. The timing and method of hair removal must be considered. Clipping or shaving the hair should be carried out immediately prior to the procedure (Briggs 1997; Mangram *et al.* 1999). Children may find hair removal procedures unpleasant and it may be more sensitive to undertake these procedures once the child is anaesthetized.

There is limited evidence regarding the most appropriate choice of clothing for theatre procedures. Traditional theatre gowns have been used because it is presumed they are clean, easy to remove if necessary, flame resistant and prevent the patient's own clothing from the risk of damage due to any spillages that may occur in theatre. Children should be permitted to wear their own clothing to theatre and part of the preoperative preparation must include providing information relating to the suitability of clothing to bring to hospital (loose, cotton nightwear) (Hogg 1994; Hogg and Cooper 2004). If hospital policy dictates, or the child (and family) wishes to wear a special gown, these should be designed specifically for children, be available in a range of sizes and protect the privacy and dignity of the child. Children who are distressed should not be coerced into wearing a theatre gown. Despite these recommendations, a survey carried out by the Royal College of Nursing Children's Surgical Nurses Forum, indicated that many children are not given a choice of what to wear to theatre (Smith and Dearmun 2006).

Jewellery is a hazard because of its potential to become caught on theatre equipment and may cause unnecessary injury to the child and theatre personnel. Furthermore, it may act as a conductor and cause skin damage when electrical equipment, such as diathermy, is used. The need to remove jewellery should be explained to the child and family. If items of jewellery have religious significance, removal must be negotiated with the child and parents, alternatively it may be possible to cover the items with surgical tape to minimize the risk of injury. Ideally all makeup and nail varnish should be removed because of the potential to mask a child's natural colour and react with any substances used in theatre. It is important that any dental bridges or braces are removed, and any loose teeth or capped teeth are recorded and highlighted to the anaesthetist because of the risk of accidental dislodgement, and potential airway aspiration during intubation.

The anaesthetist will have discussed and assisted the child and family in making choices relating to the delivery of the anaesthesia, which is usually inhalation induction for infants and young children and intravenous induction for older children and adolescents. Gaining the trust and cooperation of the child and family will greatly assist in ensuring a smooth induction.

Essential care

Preparation for cannulation and venepuncture should include:

- Providing information about the procedure, which should describe the visual, auditory, tactile and olfactory sensations that the child may experience. Honesty is important, and any potential discomfort should be explained
- Ensuring a child friendly environment such as involving parents, and a positive, unhurried and supportive attitude of the healthcare professional
- Teaching the child coping strategies such as using distraction techniques (appropriate to the child's age) and positive reinforcement
- Using topical anaesthetic creams.

(Smalley 1999)

To maximize the potential of local skin analgesia it is vital that healthcare professionals choose and apply creams appropriately and are aware of limitations and complications of topical anaesthetic agents. EMLA® (a eutectic mixture of two anaesthetic agents: Lidocaine and Prilocaine), developed in 1980, is probably the most well known of the topical anaesthetic creams and produces a dermal nerve block if applied to the skin for a minimum of 60 minutes (Fetzer 2002). EMLA has two main limitations, namely: the recommended application time of 60–90 minutes (Fetzer 2002; Wolf *et al.* 2002) and not being licensed for use in children under 1 year of age (Meakin and Murat 2000). The potential complications of EMLA include mild local reactions such as skin irritation and pallor or erythema, and in the young child ingestion/aspiration of the occlusive dressing and cream (Norman and Jones 1990). This can be minimized by applying a secure outer bandage. The more severe complication of methaemoglobinaemia, which although rare, has a higher potential for developing in children under 1 year with the incidence increasing as age decreases (Frayling *et al.* 1990). The drawbacks of EMLA have resulted in the use of AMETOP® gel (topical cream containing tetracaine formally known as amethocaine) becoming the more favoured topical anaesthetic cream of choice. AMETOP has a shorter action time (30–45 minutes) (Lawson *et al.* 1995) and can be used on children over 1 month of age. Minimal side effects, such as local erythema have been reported with AMETOP use (Meakin and Murat 2000). A secure outer bandage applied over the occlusive dressing is vital for the child at risk of inadvertently displacing the dressing and therefore ingesting the cream (Norman and Jones 1990).

Traditionally, premedications were administered to improve the safety of anaesthesia (Meakin and Murat 2000). The frequency in which premedications are used within the UK has seen a general decline (Mirakhur 1991). However, the original rationale for premedications has become less relevant with improved airway management, sophisticated anaesthetic techniques, the development of new anaesthetic agents and the use of muscle relaxants. The main aims of using a premedication are reducing anxiety and increasing the cooperation of the child (Meakin and Murat 2000). The use of sedatives have the potential to exacerbate intracranial pressure in a child with acute raised intracranial pressure.

Points to consider

Other drugs that may be prescribed preoperatively include:

- Anticholinergic drugs, for example atropine, which prevents reflex bradycardia and reduces airway secretion, may be appropriate for children with excessive secretions or anticipated difficulties in airway management, e.g. children with cerebral palsy
- H_2 antagonists, for example ranitidine, which reduce gastric volume and acidity, and may be appropriate in those children at risk of vomiting and regurgitation during anaesthetic induction such as children with gastro-oesophageal reflux. It is usual practice to give ranitidine on induction of anaesthesia to children with posterior fossa tumours because of the increased risk of gastric aspiration
- Pre-emptive analgesics are becoming increasingly popular (McQuay 1992), in particular non-steroidal anti-inflammatory drugs, which are effective if given preoperatively (Rømsing and Walther-Larsen 1997)
- It is usual practice to give hydrocortisone on induction of anaesthesia to children with pituitary tumours because of alterations to endocrine response.

Preoperative fasting is universally accepted as essential to reduce the risk of regurgitation of the stomach contents into the oesophagus during anaesthesia (Ferrari *et al.* 1999; Sethi *et al.* 1999; Splinter and Schreiner 1999). Unfortunately the effects of preoperative fasting include hunger, thirst, headache, irritation and discomfort (Sethi *et al.* 1999), which can be distressing for the child and family. Minimizing the length of time children fast has physiological and psychological benefits (Splinter and Schreiner 1999). Physiological benefits include: less acidic gastric contents; decreased risk of hypoglycaemia; improved fluid homeostasis and, therefore, decreased risk of dehydration; decreased lipolysis (Splinter and Schreiner 1999); and possible reduced postoperative nausea and vomiting (Smith *et al.* 1997). Psychologically, the child will be less irritable due to an intake of calories, less thirsty and there will be increased child and parent satisfaction (Splinter and Schreiner 1999). It is therefore understandable that there has been increased liberalization of preoperative fasting times for children in recent years. However, the risk of endangering the safety of the child (primarily the potential for aspiration) must be offset against the need to ensure the child's comfort and to prevent complications, such as dehydration and hypoglycaemia (Emerson *et al.* 1998).

Best practice recommendations

Guidelines produced by the Royal College of Nursing (2005) and the Association of Anaesthetists (2001) within the UK recommend the following fasting guidelines for children undergoing elective surgery:

- Neonates and infants: 2 hours clear fluids, 4 hours breast milk, 6 hours formula milk and solids before induction of anaesthesia
- Children: 2 hours clear fluids, 6 hours formula milk and solids before induction of anaesthesia
- Children should be encouraged to take unlimited clear fluids as close as possible to two hours preoperative fasting times. (Volume of fluids does not have an impact on patients residual gastric volume and gastric emptying.)
- Regular medications taken orally should continue preoperatively. Up to 0.5ml/kg (30mls total) of water may be given orally to help children take medications
- Pre-medications, such as benzodiazepine can be given (H_2-receptor antagonists are not recommended for healthy children)
- Delayed operation by more than 2 hours necessitate giving clear fluids orally
- If excessive fasting has occurred consider offering the child a drink and scheduling operation later on the operation list
- Chewing gum should not be permitted on the day of surgery
- Sweets including lollipops are considered to be solid food.

Fasting guidelines ensure children are not excessively fasted. However, it is imperative each child is assessed as an individual.

Points to consider

The incidence of perioperative pulmonary aspiration is rare and more likely to be associated with:

- Emergency surgery
- Surgery performed out of normal working hours
- Presence of factors which delay stomach emptying, such as obesity, raised intracranial pressure, gastrointestinal disease, stress, pain, trauma
- Conditions where there is increased risk of regurgitation such as with gastro-oesophageal reflux, renal failure and diabetes
- Impaired bronchial clearing, such as with altered consciousness, bulbar palsy
- Inexperienced anaesthetist.

(Phillips *et al.* 1994)

Certain medications may have an effect upon gastric emptying, and is relevant to both premedications and the child's regular medication (Splinter and Schreiner 1999). For example, opioids and anticholinergic drugs are thought to delay stomach empty. Certain premedications such as trimeprazine appear to reduce gastric contents, while midazolam (another premedication) does not appear to have any effect on gastric contents. For children at risk of regurgitation, the anaesthetist should consider procedures that minimize potential complications (Phillips *et al.* 1994; ASA 1999) such as increasing the length of the fasting period, gastric aspiration via a nasogastric tube, using an H_2 antagonist (e.g. ranitidine), using antacids (e.g. sodium citrate), rapid sequence induction and tracheal intubation, as appropriate to the clinical situation.

Points to consider

The majority of children should continue to take their regular medication as normal prior to surgery. Any doubts should be discussed with the appropriate anaesthetist.

Comprehensive, concise and easily accessible documentation is essential if there is to be effective communication between the ward and operating theatre to ensure the safety of the child while anaesthetised (Nash and O'Malley 1997). This is often achieved using a theatre checklist, which may appear to be a task orientated approach to care but is essential for the safety of the child.

Best practice recommendations

A theatre checklist should include:

- Demographic details of child and identification number
- Identification bracelets securely attached to the child
- Proposed operation
- Summary of the preoperative information
  - Fasting details
  - Medications including premedication
  - Known allergies
  - Results of investigations
  - Child's physical parameters: height and weight recordings are essential for drug and fluid calculations, baseline temperature, pulse, respirations, blood pressure and neurological observations allow for comparisons both intra- and postoperatively
  - Presence of loose teeth/prosthesis/glasses/jewellery
- Summary of intra-operative information
  - Type of anaesthetic agent and muscle relaxants
  - Position of child during the procedure and potential sites where undue pressure has occurred
  - Skin closure/instillation of creams or ointments in the wound/type of dressing used

- Summary of recovery
  - Pain relief given and prescribed
  - Intravenous fluid requirements
  - Observations (temperature/pulse/respirations/oxygen saturations/sedation score/ pain score/neurological observations)
  - Specific postoperative care requirements.

To ensure seamless care, maintain safety and encourage parental involvement, it is essential that cohesive protocols exist for transporting children to theatre, and that there is effective interdepartmental communication. It is essential that the journey to theatre does not contribute to the child's anxiety (Hogg 1994). Therefore it is vital that the child is offered appropriate choices, which should be appropriate to their age and condition. Children who have had a sedative premedication are required to be escorted on a theatre trolley or on their own bed. Theatre trolleys can be made interesting for the young child, for example depicting children's characters such as Thomas the Tank Engine. It has become increasingly common for children who have not had a sedative premedication to walk to theatre or if an infant carried by their parent. The use of motorized toy cars can be an exciting prospect for the pre-school child. Parents should be given the choice of accompanying their child to theatre, and the child should be encouraged to take their favourite toy, book or comforter with them.

Intra-operative care

Prior to the child leaving the ward it is essential to ensure the correct child is being escorted to theatre for the correct operation, that all preoperative requirements have been met and the identification of the child is confirmed. This information should be confirmed again prior to induction of the anaesthesia (Walker and Lockie 2000). During handover of the child to theatre staff, ward staff must highlight information relating to each individual child, such as any known allergies, pain relief already administered, and specific details relating to the child and family which may be of value to the theatre staff in the intra-operative phase. The actual intra-operative phase begins when the child arrives in the anaesthetic room and ends when the child leaves the recovery room.

The core role of the nurse in the theatre environment is to ensure the surgical, anaesthetic and recovery needs of the patient are met (Wise 1999; Cowan 1998). This is achieved by coordinating the activities of the multidisciplinary team, supervising the total experience of the child, and assessing, planning, implementing and evaluating care (Wise 1999; Cowan 1998). This requires nurses having the knowledge and skills relating to: anaesthetic and surgical techniques; post-anaesthetic care including caring for a child following neurosurgery; infection control management; maintaining a safe environment; risk assessment; and pain management. In the child health setting the role will include being an advocate for the child and family, ensuring guidelines are appropriate to meet the needs of the child and are audited, being competent with equipment specifically designed for children and keeping up to date with current child care issues and practices. This is more likely to be achieved by nurses qualified in caring for children (Smith and Dearmun 2006).

Best practice recommendations

The core principles within *Surgery for Children: Delivering a First Class Service* (Children's Forum of the Royal College of Surgeons 2007) and *Guidance on the Provision of Paediatric Anaesthetic Services* (Royal College of Anaesthetists 2001) include:

- Care must be delivered by appropriately trained medical and nursing staff
- Special facilities should be available for certain groups of children, such as neonates (less than 44 weeks gestation), children with significant co-morbidity and children with complex surgical needs including major trauma
- A consultant who regularly anaesthetises children should lead the anaesthetic service
- There must be a child-centred approach to care, which includes facilities separate from adult patients, parental involvement in all aspects of care, appropriate consent and consideration to the rights of the child
- Appropriate paediatric equipment must be available
- There should be a properly funded and staffed acute pain service specifically for children
- Occasional paediatric practice is unacceptable.

The child's physiological systems are placed under stress during surgery because of the impact of anaesthetic agents and the surgical procedure, and the potential for drug reactions and latex allergies (Burns 1997). The safety of the child, minimizing risks and the early detection of complications, effective monitoring and prompt interventions are vital components of care within the theatre environment.

Essential care

Safety issues within the theatre environments include:

- Staff having appropriate skills relating to airway management, and responding to and managing emergency situations
- Implementing infection control measures
- Minimizing heat loss and maintaining body temperature
- Skilled in detecting changes in the child's condition, ensuring effective observation and monitoring of the child
- A range of equipment will be used for monitoring the child's physical condition. It is essential that equipment maintenance adheres to safety legislation and that all staff are competent in the use of the equipment within their area
- Ensuring the correct positioning of the child and implementing interventions to prevent injury and relieve pressure during procedures.

The need to maintain a patent airway is a vital part of the care of the child both intra- and postoperatively. Maintaining the airway during surgery is the primary concern of the anaesthetist. However, the potential for airway problems in children means that all staff, including nurses caring for the anaesthetized child and the child recovering from anaesthesia require the knowledge and skills to manage potential airway problems across age ranges. Furthermore, to support the anaesthetist, familiarity with airway management techniques is vital in ensuring the smooth management of the child in the theatre environment. The choice of airway management in the anaesthetized child will depend upon the age of the child, the surgical procedure, ventilation requirements and the presence of any pre-existing airway/respiratory problems. The main types of airway management include facemask (with or without an airway), laryngeal mask and endotracheal intubation (Walker and Lockie 2000).

Observations of the child's physiological status will include monitoring the heart rate and rhythms, blood pressure, respiratory rate and effort, skin colour, oxygen saturation levels, conscious levels and temperature. Infants and children do not have the same ability as adults to maintain body temperature (Noble *et al.* 1997) due to the higher ratio of surface area to body weight, less subcutaneous fat, thinner dermis and epidermis. Intra-operatively, the ability to maintain a normal body temperature is compromised because (Imrie and Hall 1990):

1   General anaesthetic agents impair normal thermoregulatory responses, probably due to alterations of hypothalamic functions. The underlying neurological condition may already have affected the child's ability to control body temperature; this will be further compounded during anaesthesia.
2   There is a reduction in the metabolic rate.
3   There are increased thermal losses due to skin exposure, which can be significant in the young child.
4   Low ambient temperatures in the operating suite.
5   The administration of cold intravenous fluids, drugs and skin preparation fluids.
6   There is risk of developing malignant hyperthermia, which can be triggered by some anaesthetic agents.

Children who become hypothermic during surgery are at a greater risk of hypoxaemia and hypercapnoea and have a more prolonged recovery period (Olsson 2000). Measures should be instigated to reduce heat loss such as ensuring the child is adequately insulated with blankets, use of warming mattresses, use of radiant heaters, minimal exposure of skin surfaces, anaesthetic gases and fluids are warmed, the ambient temperature is appropriate and the child's temperature is regularly monitored (Imrie and Hall 1990). In an ideal situation and to estimate total body temperature, both core and peripheral temperatures would need to be recorded. In practice this rarely occurs (Imrie and Hall 1990). Oesophageal, rectal, tympanic membrane and axilla skin probes are commonly used to estimate body temperature (Noble *et al.* 1997).

Essential care

Practices that help to minimize wound contamination include:

- Ensuring the environment is cleaned thoroughly, including all surfaces, walls and floors
- Dealing with spillages promptly and appropriately
- Maintaining ventilation systems in guidance with manufactures recommendations
- Adhering to policies and procedures relating to clothing, wearing of masks, gowns and use of gloves, and guidelines on managing infections
- Maintaining strict asepsis and equipment sterility during operations
- Minimizing the movement and number of personnel within theatres
- Ensuring adequate skin preparation.

(Gould 2001)

An important role for theatre staff will include ensuring procedures relating to infection control are instigated and maintained because the major source of postoperative wound contamination appears to occur during the actual surgical procedure (Horwitz *et al.* 1998).

Immediate recovery from anaesthesia

The aim of care in the initial postoperative period is to prevent potential life-threatening complications following anaesthesia and surgery (Heath 1998). It is essential that staffing levels reflect the dependency level of the child, therefore the child's initial care will usually be in a designated recovery area within the theatre suite. Staff caring for children in this early recovery period must have excellent skills in the assessment and management of airway obstruction, hypoxaemia, haemorrhage (internal and external), agitation/delirium, hypothermia, and nausea and vomiting (Watcha 2000). Following surgery the child will require assessment of the following: sedation levels, respiratory rate and effort, oxygen saturation levels, cardiovascular monitoring (skin colour, skin temperature, pulse and blood pressure), body temperature and the wound (dressings and drains). In addition, children who have undergone neurosurgery will required a detailed neurological assessment to detect any rise in the intracranial pressure (see Chapter 2, Sections 2 and 3). The frequency of observations will depend on the initial assessment of the child, duration and type of neurosurgery and intra-operative drugs given but are usually recorded every 15 minutes in the early postoperative period with continual monitoring of the pulse and oxygen saturation levels via a pulse oximeter.

Although most children will be breathing spontaneously on arrival in the recovery area, the residual effects of drugs administered during anaesthesia may still be present and the child may not have complete control of the airway and may be at risk of airway obstruction. Until the gag and cough reflexes return to normal the child will be unable to clear the airway, and pooling of secretions may further compromise the airway. A child who is unconscious but maintaining their own airway should be placed in the recovery position, unless contradicted by the surgical procedure (Figure 3.1a), to prevent the tongue from falling back and obstructing the airway. It may be necessary to modify techniques in the infant and small child, such as providing a support placed in the hollow of the back to maintain the position. However, the principles of

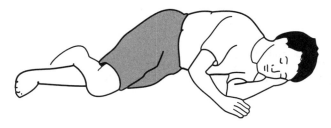

Figure 3.1a Recovery position

the recovery position, placing in a true lateral position, allowing the airway to remain open to facilitate drainage of secretions and easy access of airway should be maintained (Resuscitation Council UK 2005). For a child who has a compromised airway or is unconscious/unresponsive but breathing, maintaining a patent airway is vital. In the absence of airway adjuncts this can be achieved using the chin lift, jaw thrust or placing the child in the recovery position. Recovery nurses must be familiar and competent with the use of airways adjuncts such as the oropharyngeal (or Guedel) airway and the nasopharyngeal airway.

An additional component to airway management is the removal of secretions, blood or vomit which may pool in the upper airways. Removal of oropharyngeal, nasopharyngeal or tracheal secretions by using a suction catheter may be necessary. Removal of secretions using suctioning is not without risks which include hypoxaemia, cardiac dysrhythmia, trauma, bleeding and infection (Hackeling *et al.* 1998; Kapadia *et al.* 2000). These risk factors are compounded by the poor knowledge of many nurses relating to suctioning procedures (Day *et al.* 2001, 2002).

Essential care

The principles of suctioning in an acutely ill child include:

- Assess the child for the need for suctioning including the presence of secretions and chest auscultation
- Pre-oxygenation via bag and mask prior to the procedure may be necessary
- Maintaining a sterile procedure
- For tracheostomy or tracheal suctioning the external diameter of the catheter should not exceed one-half the diameter of the tube
- Catheters should be flexible and cause minimal trauma
- A minimal negative pressure, between 80–150mmHg, should be applied only on withdrawal of the catheter for a maximum of 10–15 seconds.

(Wood 1998; Day *et al.* 2001)

Inability to maintain the airway because of the residual effects of anaesthesia and blood loss during the operation will compromise the amount of oxygen available to perfuse the cells of the body. Following neurosurgery it is particularly important to prevent cerebral anoxia which has the potential to add to brain swelling postoperatively, Chapter 2, Section 3. Therefore, oxygen therapy is a high priority in the overall management of the child in the recovery room. The techniques used to administer oxygen must meet the clinical needs of the child in the immediate recovery area and include simple face masks, partial rebreather masks and non-rebreather bags.

In the immediate postoperative period all children should be monitored using pulse oximetry because it is invaluable in providing a continuous method of estimating arterial oxygen saturation (Chameides and Hazinski 1997; Chandler 2001) and is an effective and frequently used method of monitoring oxygen saturation levels in children (Chandler 2000; Urschitz *et al.* 2003). A pulse oximeter measures arterial blood oxygen saturation (SpO_2), by estimating the oxygen saturation of haemoglobin when two light emitting diodes and a photosensitive detector are placed across a tissue bed, typically across a finger or toe (Chameides and Hazinski 1997, Chandler 2000). The normal range for oxygen saturation levels is between 94–100 per cent (Urschitz *et al.* 2003). Accurate recordings are dependent upon a pulsatile blood flow and thus will not provide reliable information in a child in shock or with poor peripheral perfusion (Chameides and Hazinski 1997). Although oxygenation can be monitored using pulse oximetry it is vital to observe the effectiveness of respirations (rate and depth), essential to eliminate carbon dioxide. Hypoventilation leads to hypercapnoea ($PaCO_2$ greater than 6kpa) an important factor that can contribute to an increase in intracranial pressure, discussed in Chapter 2, Section 3.

Haemorrhage is a potential complication of surgery and some blood loss during surgery is inevitable (Watcha 2000). Failure to adequately cauterize blood vessels during surgery will result in continued blood loss in the immediate postoperative phase (Dealey 1999). Large amounts of blood loss should be obvious because of leakage through dressing. Slow insidious leakage of blood or internal loss may be less obvious, therefore routine checking of wounds should be continued with postoperative observations.

Essential care

The early detection of haemorrhage is an essential component of postoperative care, and includes:

- Careful observations of wound site, dressing and drains, if present, for excessive oozing and fluid loss
- Cardiovascular monitoring (pulse, blood pressure, colour), observation of respiratory rate and effort
- Neurological observations to detect a rise in the intracranial pressure which may be a result of bleeding within the cranial cavity.

Effective pain management is an essential component of the care of the child undergoing neurosurgery. Although effective pain management is dependent upon a multidisciplinary approach, in practice the overall responsibility of postoperative pain management is often devolved to the paediatric anaesthetist, certainly in terms of immediate postoperative planning and prescribing analgesia regimens (Howard and Lloyd-Thomas 2000). Postoperative pain assessment should begin as soon as the child arrives in recovery to ensure that the child receives prompt and appropriate care, as the presence of pain will complicate recovery. Leaving pain management until the child reaches the ward is not acting in the best interests of the child (DH 1989) and as pain intensity increases the management becomes much more difficult. Recovery staff must ensure assessment and interventions are documented and that pain management plans are clearly documented and articulated to the nurse taking over the care of the child following discharge from recovery. The management of pain in children who have undergone a neurosurgical procedure is discussed in detail in Section 3.2.

As soon as practically possible the child should be returned to the familiar ward environment. However, the child should only be discharged from recovery when able to maintain their own airway, has regained a satisfactory level of consciousness, and all physiological parameters are stable. The handover to the ward staff must be of sufficient depth to ensure that communication (both written and verbal) relating to the specific condition and postoperative needs of the child, including pain management plans, are clearly articulated to the member of staff accepting responsibility of the child. There should be a policy for the transfer of the child from the recovery to the ward, including type of equipment available on the transporting trolley (at least oxygen and suction), and the level and experience of escorting staff, who must be capable of dealing with any emergency situation that may arise during transfer.

Meeting the child's and family's psychological needs within the theatre environment

Nurses have raised concerns about the poor implementation of policies relating to the overall well-being of the child and family where the child is admitted for a surgical procedure; particularly parents not being given the choice of escorting their child to the anaesthetic room or having the opportunity to be with their child in the recovery area (Smith and Dearmun 2006). Nurses should have knowledge of current policy directives relating to the care of the child such as the *National Service Framework for Children, Young People and Maternity Services: Change for Children, Every Child Matters* (DH 2004) and policies specifically relating to anaesthesia and surgery such as *Surgery for Children: Delivering a First-Class Service* (Children's Forum of the Royal College of Surgeons 2007) and *Guidance on the Provision of Paediatric Anaesthetic Services* (Royal College of Anaesthetists 2001). Nurses can play a key role in ensuring guidance, standards and principles relating to children are implemented to ensure a quality perioperative service for the child and family.

In general, children are usually escorted directly to the anaesthetic room from the ward. However, some theatre suites use a holding bay to reduce delays between cases. It is essential these areas consider the psychological well-being of the child; the environment must be child friendly with a range of play facilities/activities to meet all ages. The area should be separate from adult waiting areas and parents should be made to feel welcome. The waiting time for children following arrival in the theatre suite and induction of the anaesthetic should be kept to a minimum (Hogg and Cooper 2004). The anaesthetic room should not be a threatening environment and the manner in which procedures are carrier out should minimize the anxiety of the child and parents (Hogg 1994). Therefore sights, smells and sounds that may be distressing to the child should be minimized. The decor should be child friendly, unnecessary medical equipment should not be visible and there should be a range of appropriate and suitable play/distraction activities. Parents should be encouraged and supported but not pressured to remain with the child during induction of the anaesthetic (Hogg and Cooper 2004). This requires the area having enough space to accommodate the parent and a ward nurse, while maintaining a safe environment in which theatre staff can work effectively.

The practice of offering parents, if they wish, to be present in the recovery area as soon as practicably possible is a relatively new concept. The benefits include: providing comfort and reassurance to the child, reduced anxiety in the child and facilitates an altogether less traumatic experience for the child and family (Brown 1997, 1995; Fina *et al.* 1997). However, there appear to be concerns relating to the provision of information to the parent if the procedure has not gone according to plan (Brown 1995). One of the first questions a parent will undoubtedly ask is if the procedure went without complications. This will occur regardless of whether the parent is united with their child on the ward or recovery area. It is usual practice for the surgeon who has carried out the procedure to explain to parents the nature and potential outcome of any complications. It is essential this communication takes place as soon as possible and, in practical terms, is often much easier to do in the recovery area where the surgeon can be on hand prior to the next case starting, with only minimal disruption to the theatre list (Brown 1995). To ensure their presence is maximized parents should have clear expectations of their role within recovery and an understanding of what to expect. Other considerations within the recovery area include ensuring there is adequate space to accommodate parents to ensure that safety of the child is not compromised, equipment and décor should be appropriate for the child and children should have a recovery area separated from adult patients (Hogg *et al.* 2004).

Postoperative care

The postoperative needs of the child following cranial surgery should focus on the prompt detection of complications from the anaesthesia and the surgical procedure. Receiving a child back from theatre to the ward begins prior to the child's arrival, with preparation of the bed space and necessary monitoring equipment. As a minimum this should include ease of access from the theatre trolley to the bed, and should include ensuring oxygen and suction are readily available and in working order. Specific equipment, such as infusion stands, monitoring equipment, drain and catheter holders, and relevant documentation, should be anticipated for the planned procedure and prepared. Consideration needs to be given to the visibility of the child on the ward, which must be appropriate for the child's needs and for the predicted level of observation required.

Essential care

The immediate assessment of the child on return to the ward must include:

- Ability to maintain airway
- Presence of swallow and gag reflexes
- Sedation level
- Neurological observations including vital signs (blood pressure, pulse, respirations and temperature) recorded at least hourly, or more frequently depending on the specific procedure, until risks of raised intracranial pressure have diminished
- Colour and oxygen saturations, the rate of administration of oxygen, if still required
- Immediate blood loss from the wound/amount of blood in wound drains, if present
- Child's pain level and administration of analgesia
- Presence of nausea and vomiting
- Type of intravenous fluids being given and the rate of administration of intravenous infusions.

(Zeitz and McCutcheon 2002)

Although the potential for adverse events relating to anaesthesia and surgery will decrease with time, it cannot be assumed that discharge from recovery occurs when the child is completely free from potential risk of airway obstruction, shock and haemorrhage. Following the initial assessment of the child on return to the ward setting, the aim of postoperative observations is to detect complications early and ensure that physiological functions altered during anaesthesia are returning to normal values (Zeitz and McCutcheon 2002). There is a lack of published guidance relating to the frequency of observations in children post-surgery, however half- to one-hourly seems normal practice. When making decisions about the frequency to undertake observations the nurses should consider: specific procedure type and length of time in theatre, responsiveness of the child upon returning to the ward, presence of advanced analgesia systems (such as opioid infusions) and the age and stage of development of the child. For example, neonates are at increased risk of apnoea and bradycardia due to their immature physiological responses (Steward

Table 3.1a Overview of immediate care of a child following neurosurgery

Actual/potential problems	Nursing interventions
Potential airway obstruction and inadequate oxygenation due to depressed conscious levels and the effects of prolonged anaesthesia	Maintain the child's airway by positioning in the recovery position/use airway aids Assess and monitor respiratory effort and oxygen saturation levels Maintain oxygen therapy, ventilatory support may be necessary Assess the child's neurological status
Potential cardiac and respiratory instability due to neurological depression and effect of prolonged anaesthetic, particularly following surgery to the posterior fossa area, which contains vital control centres	Assess and monitor the child's respiratory effort, oxygen saturation levels and vital signs Ventilatory support and invasive blood pressure monitoring may be necessary Assess and report changes in the child's neurological status
Altered neurological functioning due to potential risk of intracranial pressure increases as a result of generalised cerebral oedema and haemorrhage	Regular neurological assessment in order to detect neurological changes, which may indicate a rise in ICP Management of RICP (outlined in Chapter 5, Section 3) Monitor for signs of haemorrhage including observing wound bandages and drains, if present, for excessive blood loss, changes in conscious levels, raised pulse, falling blood pressure, changes in peripheral perfusion The child may require blood transfusion therapy and/or surgical control of bleeding/removal of haematoma if bleeding is excessive The position the child's head is nursed in is important and usually dependent on the procedure and surgeon's preference, in general nursing a child with the head elevated at 30°C and head in the midline is the norm which facilitates good venous return. However, with some surgical procedures for example certain types of shunts nursing the child upright may result in the development of a subdural haematoma due to rapid drainage of the cerebrospinal fluid
Potential fluid and electrolyte disturbances due to an inability to take oral fluids	The child's fluid intake and output must be monitored In the early post-operative period the child will have an intravenous infusion Unless there is potential damage to the ninth and tenth cranial nerves, which may affect swallowing, the child may begin oral fluids as soon as consciousness is regained. It may be necessary for the child to undergo assessment by a speech and language therapist prior to commencing oral fluids

continued…

Table 3.1a continued

Actual/potential problems	Nursing interventions
Maintaining fluid and electrolytes in children who have undergone cranial surgery is a balance between ensuring adequate circulatory blood volume in order to maintain good cerebral perfusion and preventing over-hydration, which will add to cerebral oedema	The management of fluids will be influenced by the type of surgery and tolerance of oral fluids, with the type and amount of fluids administered specific to each child's needs and urea and electrolyte profile Where prolonged intravenous fluid are required the child will need regular blood sampling (including serum osmolality), circulatory assessment (pulse, blood pressure, capillary refill, temperature gradient difference between core and periphery)
Potential problem of inappropriate antidiuretic secretion or diabetes insipidus following surgery to the posterior fossa area	Measure and monitor urine output, test and record specific gravity Samples will be required in order to measure urine and blood osmolarity
Potential inability to maintain normal thermoregulation	Monitor the child's temperature regularly
Hyperpyrexia can be a result of hypothalamus dysfunction and/or irritation of cerebral tissues for example the direct contact of blood with cerebral tissues	Manage pyrexia appropriately because any increase in core temperature increases cerebral metabolic rate, increases cerebral perfusion and potentially adds to any rises in intracranial pressure
Vomiting, as a direct result of RICP and potential side effects of anaesthetic agents	Administer anti-emetics. If vomiting persists the child will require continuation of intravenous fluids and a detailed nutritional assessment. Ranitidine may be prescribed to prevent gastric irritation
Pain as a result of wound incision, positioning in theatre, stretching of the meninges and RICP	Assess pain and administer regular analgesia, Chapter 3, Section 2 Intravenous opioids may further compromise respiratory effort, oral or rectal codeine may be a suitable alternative Unresolved pain may hinder the ability to undertake an affective neurological assessment
Potential for the development of seizures due to cerebral inflammation/irritation	Observe the child for signs of seizure activity In the unconscious child this may require continuous EEG monitoring Follow seizure management guidelines (outlined in Chapter 2, Section 5)
Promote wound healing following surgical incision Potential wound infection	Maintain universal infection control measures Wound bandages are usually present for the first 24–48 hours and assist in reducing swelling at the wound site and help secure any drains that may be present Prophylactic antibiotics are rarely recommended Observe wound for redness, hardness and presence of exudate, which may indicate presence of infection and leakage of CSF Monitor the child's temperature Clips are often used to secure the wound and usually removed 7–10 days post-operatively

1982; Welborn *et al.* 1986). These infants will require more frequent observations and continuous monitoring to detect apnoeic episodes and episodes of bradycardia compared to older children.

Early postoperative complications and care

The most likely early postoperative complications are haemorrhage, nausea and vomiting, pain, dizziness and excessive drowsiness (Watcha 2000). The immediate care needs of the child post-neurosurgery are outlined in Table 3.1a.

It is important to observe the child for the signs and symptoms of haemorrhage, and if detected early the child can be appropriately managed and rapidly stabilized. Nurses should maintain observations of wound dressings and drains, if present, for excessive oozing and fluid

Essential care

The care of the child who has significant blood loss and is hypovalaemic includes:

- Rapid cardiopulmonary assessment: airway, breathing and circulation
- Administration of face mask oxygen
- If venous access is lost re-establishing, if it is not possible to insert a wide-bore peripheral vascular catheter then an intraosseous needle must be inserted (the preferred site being the tibial tuberosity)
- Restore circulatory volume; fluid resuscitation necessitates rapid infusion of volume expanders at a rate of 20ml/kg over 20 minutes, followed by reassessment and further fluid boluses as necessary
- The initial management is either an isotonic crystalloid solution such as 0.9 per cent saline or a colloid solution such as 4.5 per cent albumin. Saline has the advantage of being readily available but results in a transient expansion of circulating fluid, therefore large quantities are necessary. Colloids remain in the intravascular compartment longer but are more likely to cause sensitivity reactions
- Large volumes of dextrose containing fluids should not be given because resultant hyperglycemia causes osmotic diuresis, which effectively causes fluid to be withdrawn from the circulatory system, exacerbating the hypovolaemia and causing hypokalaemia
- Blood should be ordered and given as soon as possible; blood transfusion is paramount because although resuscitation fluids will help in restoration of the intravascular volume, loss of haemoglobin will severely reduce the ability to maintain tissue oxygenation and blood clotting factors will become depleted
- In all but minor haemorrhages surgical intervention will be necessary to control the bleeding
- Where possible, external pressure to wound site should be applied
- A child who is hypoglycaemic (determined by blood glucose levels) should receive a bolus of high concentration glucose (for example 10–20mls/kg of 5 per cent dextrose)
- Insertion of a urinary catheter and measurement of urine output.

(Ratcliffe 1998)

loss, and should monitor cardiovascular output until the risk of haemorrhage has reduced. Blood losses of over 15 per cent of the total circulatory volume will result in detectable signs of circulatory failure, namely: tachycardia, decreased peripheral pulses, delayed capillary refill and cool extremities (Chameides and Hazinski 1997). Hypotension will be a late sign and probably not occur until blood loses are within the region of 20–30 per cent of total circulatory volume. If there is significant postoperative bleeding the child will become hypovolaemic. Hypovolaemia is a characteristic of all forms of shock because, independent of the cause, as shock progresses there is always a resultant vasodilatation, increased capillary permeability and plasma loss into the interstitial fluid spaces.

It is estimated that postoperative nausea and vomiting (PONV) occurs in 40–50 per cent of people undergoing anaesthesia (Cohen *et al.* 1990; Lerman 1992). PONV is more likely (Burns 1997):

- To occur in children than in adults.
- Where there has been high levels of preoperative anxiety, in association with certain surgical procedures.
- With the use of opioids.
- When there has been insufflation of the stomach during anaesthesia.

Minimizing PONV is a vital component of care for the child undergoing anaesthesia (Watcha 2000). In absence of evidence to support guidance regarding the timing and type of fluid/foods to be offered to a child postoperatively then common sense needs to prevail; PONV can be reduced by:

- Avoidance of premedications and anaesthetic agents that are known to increase the risk of PONV.
- Considering alternative pain management to opioids, which are known to increase PONV, particularly for day surgery and minor procedures, such as local anaesthetic and nerve blocks, and non-steroidal anti-inflammatory drugs.
- Administration of antiemetic drugs prophylactically intra-operatively for procedures where there is a high risk of PONV.
- Providing sufficient fluid intra-operatively.
- Not rushing a child to drink postoperatively, while not withholding fluids in a distressed child (unless surgery indicates the child must remain nil by mouth).
- Preventing large volumes of fluids being ingested over a short span of time and, where possible, avoiding fluids with increased acidity such as fruit juices or fizzy drinks.

PONV is a major source of distress for the child and family and if severe PONV can put additional strain on the wound, contribute to bleeding and lead to dehydration. The child and family will require support and reassurance. Treatment with intravenous fluids and antiemetic drugs may be necessary.

Complications following neurosurgery

In addition to the general complications following surgery, the child's care must consider the potential complications that may be a result of neurosurgery. Complications include:

- Cerebral haemorrhage (subdural, epidural, intracerebral and intraventricular).
- Raised intracranial pressure due to general tissue swelling or haemorrhage.
- Seizures.
- Cerebrospinal fluid leakage.
- Pneumocephalus.
- Hydrocephalus.
- Meningitis.
- Metabolic imbalances.
- Neurological deficits, such as diminished level of consciousness, communication difficulties, motor and sensory deficits, diminished swallow and gag reflexes and visual disturbances (Hickey 2003).

The care related to minimizing and managing these complications are outlined in subsequent chapters relating to specific conditions requiring neurosurgery. Oral phenytoin may be prescribed in the immediate postoperative period if there is an increased likely hood of seizures developing. This will be influenced by location of the surgery – for example surgery in the frontal lobe is more likely to result in postoperative seizures compared to other craniotomy sites.

Ongoing care and discharge from acute services

There is lack of consensus relating to many aspects of general care following surgery such as when the child can mobilize, eat and drink, bath and return to school. In general, and unless contraindicated because of the specific surgical procedure, small volumes of non-acidic fluid can be given when the child had regained consciousness and is thirsty. Food can be introduced once oral fluids have been tolerated. The child should be allowed to rest and not rushed into early mobilization. Generally, there are no restrictions on mobilization following neurosurgery, unless deficits in limb function have been detected as a consequence of the surgery. Care should be taken when mobilizing children immediately postoperatively because momentary dizziness may occur.

Preparation for discharge is an ongoing process, which starts on admission – or in some cases prior to admission – where information gathered relating to the child and family will influence and help predict subsequent care needs (Heath 1998; Hogg and Cooper 2004). Preparation for discharge includes providing the child and family with information about the specific care the child will require relating to the specific neurosurgical procedure the child has undergone, and, where appropriate, a clear indication of subsequent healthcare interventions. Parents may be extremely anxious about taking their child home and will require detailed information relating to general caring skills, such as eating and drinking, bathing, resuming normal activities, and specific care details, such as giving medications and wound care (Bailey and Caldwell 1997). Wound care is discussed in Section 3.

The child may require ongoing care in the home environment following discharge. The child and family may be required to learn and become competent with technical aspects of care because of the child's condition or as a result of the surgical procedure. For these children discharge to home can be complex. The number and range of healthcare professionals involved at discharge, can often be overwhelming; therefore it is essential that there is effective communication within the team. Where available, a specialist children's nurse who has an understanding of the needs of the child and family can coordinate the discharge process and provide ongoing support once the child is at home. The nurse specialist can bridge the gap between services where the child requires referral to other healthcare teams such as endocrine or cancer services. The information provided to the child and family must be accurate, consistent, delivered in an appropriate manner and documented (Bradford and Singer 1991). Verbal advice should, wherever possible, be supported with written advice. However, written advice is only of added value if it is clear, unambiguous, written in terms appropriate for the child and family and in a language the family understands.

Neurological deficits may require the child to have a programme of care that shifts from managing acute surgical needs to one of rehabilitation. In this case, a named worker should coordinate the process and there should be early referral and liaison with the community nursing team. In cases where the child has a pre-existing neurological condition, a home care package may already be in place. It is vital that the named worker informs all members of the multidisciplinary team of the child's impending discharge and of the child's current care needs. When a child is discharged from a specialist paediatric neurology centre, the local community services where the child lives will need to be involved in the ongoing care of the child and will need to be involved in planning the child's discharge home (Hogg and Cooper 2004). It is paramount that the family feels confident to take the child home into their care and are competent with any specialized care prior to discharge. It is also essential that the child's main carers are fully informed of discharge and follow-up arrangements and provided with contact details of appropriate healthcare professionals should they have cause for concern or issues they wish to discuss.

3.2 Postoperative pain management

Any surgical procedure will cause pain due to the inflammatory response, damaged nerve cells and enhanced pain sensations in the damaged tissue and area surrounding the incision (Fitzgerald and Howard 2003). It is therefore vital that all children who have undergone a neurosurgical procedure have their pain assessed and managed appropriately.

Points to consider

It is important to recognize that some children with neurological conditions may have chronic pain associated with the underlying diagnosis, e.g. headaches and gut motility and musculo-skeletal problems (Hunt *et al.* 2003).

Pain can be defined as 'an unpleasant sensory and emotional experience associated with actual or potential tissue damage' (International Association for the Study of Pain 1992: 2). Acute pain is of recent onset, has limited duration and highlights to the individual that they have sustained an injury or points to the presence of disease (IASP 1992: 2). While less precise, McCaffery's (1968: 11) definition of pain as 'whatever the person experiencing it says it is, and existing whenever the person says it does' is popular because it reflects the individuality of the experience. Neither definition is entirely appropriate for children because the child's level of cognition will inevitably affect how they verbalize, localize and display pain. In addition, there are many myths and misconceptions about the pain experience and management of pain in children.

Points to consider

Myths and misconceptions about the pain experience by children include:

- Infants cannot feel pain because of an immature nervous system
- Children do not feel as much pain as adults
- Narcotic use is dangerous in children
- Active children cannot be in pain
- Sleeping children cannot be in pain
- Children engaged in play cannot be in pain
- Pain results in children crying
- Children always tell the truth about their pain
- Injections are not painful
- Giving a child an injection results in hostility towards the carer.

(Eland 1990; Burr 1993; Byrne *et al.* 2001)

Acute pain has the potential to delay and complicate the recovery of the child who has undergone a surgical procedure. Therefore, pain management is a vital component of the care of a child following surgery. Unfortunately, many children in hospital continue to suffer unnecessary pain because of inadequate recognition and consequently management of their pain (Cummings *et al.* 1996; Stevens and Koren 1998; Twycross 1998a).

Points to consider

The potential consequences of unrelieved acute pain include:

- Psychological problems such as recurrent nightmares and increased anxiety
- Bronchiectasis and atelectasis due to inadequate lung expansion
- Alkalosis due to increased respiratory rate and shallow breathing
- Chest infection due to increased secretions accumulating from inadequate cough and lack of spontaneous movement
- Rapid respirations, increased heart rate, increased perspiration and increased metabolic rate will increase fluid losses.

(Eland 1990)

Nurses have a vital role in ensuring children's pain is managed effectively. However, concerns have been raised about nurses' attitudes towards the recognition of pain in children including: if a child had not voiced any concerns they must not be in pain; parents not being believed when expressing concerns about their child's pain; and denying the reality of pain experienced by children in an attempt to protect themselves from emotional stress, which compromises the provision of effective pain management (Byrne *et al.* 2001; Simons *et al.* 2001). Nurses are more likely to provide effective pain management if they have experience of their own child experiencing pain, work in acute and critical care units, and have undertaken higher levels of nurse education (Twycross 1998a, 2002).

The inability of young children to verbalize their needs and the lack of valid and reliable assessment tools across the age spectrum compound the difficulties for staff trying to relieve children's pain (Jackson 1995). Furthermore, young children adopt many coping strategies such as avoiding interactions, resisting behaviours and self-protection behaviours, which to the uninformed could lead to misinterpreting the child's needs (Woodgate and Kristjanson 1995). To understand a child's perception of pain it is essential that healthcare professionals consider the child's developmental stage and relate these to visual, physiological and behavioural cues the child might be displaying (Buckingham 1993). For the child with a neurological problem, additional communication problems may exist and some children may not be able to express pain because of nerve or muscle damage (Hunt *et al.* 2003).

Points to consider

Many factors influence the child's ability to express pain including:

- Age and previous experience: younger children will have much less experiences to draw upon and will be less likely to have the ability to anticipate the outcome of the pain and therefore decide how to plan effective coping strategies. This heightened anxiety may intensify the perception of pain
- The child's cognitive ability will influence how they interpret and express pain
- Linguistic abilities the words 'pain' and 'hurt' may be entirely absent from a young child's vocabulary and expressive language
- Personality
- Family and cultural beliefs.

(Thompson and Varni 1986; Carter *et al.* 2002a)

Assessment of pain in children

Good pain management is fundamentally linked to effective assessment and serves two main purposes: to ensure interventions are appropriate; and to evaluate the effectiveness of interventions (Carter 1994). The QUEST framework was developed for assessing pain in children and involves: questioning the child; using a pain rating scale; evaluating behaviours and physiological changes; securing family involvement; taking the cause of the pain into account; taking action and evaluating response (Baker and Wong 1987).

Question the child and secure family involvement

Effective pain assessment is a crucial component of preoperative care for all children undergoing surgery. The child and family should be questioned about the child's previous experiences of pain, any specific behaviours the child may display which could indicate the presence of pain, the child's understanding of pain and the child's developmental stage. There needs to be an understanding of the family's attitudes towards pain, which should include the potential influence of cultural, religious and spiritual beliefs. This information, in conjunction with knowledge of the type of surgery and the predicted intensity of post operative pain, will enable healthcare professionals to discuss and plan with the child and family the type and mode of delivery of postoperative analgesia. Where possible the child should be involved in deciding the pain assessment tool, and the child and family should have a detailed explanation about its use.

Pain assessment tools

Without the ability to directly measure pain, assessment tools are a vital component of the assessment process. Despite difficulties in producing a pain assessment tool that is practical, versatile and free from individual bias, their use is recommended because they are associated with increased administration of analgesia and, therefore, a reduction in pain (RCN 1999). Pain assessment tools should be based upon the following criteria: ratio scaling properties, relatively free from individual practitioner bias, provide immediate and accurate information, reliable and generalizable, sensitive to changes in pain intensity, simple and easy to use (Schofield 1995). Clinical practice guidelines relating to the recognition and assessment of acute pain in children are available (RCN 1999).

Best practice recommendations

Principles of recognizing and assessing acute pain in children include:

- Choosing an assessment tool appropriate to the child's developmental stage, personality and condition. No one tool will 'fit' all
- Using a self-report tool for those children who can communicate. These are the gold standard because a child's own subjective account is the single most reliable indicator of the intensity of pain
- Using an assessment tool that is fairly accurate, easy to understand and quick to use such as a one-dimensional pain intensity tool. Examples include visual analogue scales, verbal rating scales, numerical rating scales, verbal descriptor scales, behaviour rating scales, body diagrams and picture scales
- Remembering that verbal descriptors of pain may be inappropriate below 8 years of age
- Observing for alterations in behaviours which may suggest the presence of pain, such as the child becoming restless, having sleep disturbances, not easily distractible or shortened attention span, and refusal to eat
- Observing for physiological changes that may suggest the presence of pain such as elevation of heart rate, decreased oxygen saturation levels, increased respiratory rate, slight increase in blood pressure and increased palmer sweating.

(RCN 1999)

Pain assessment tools need to be appropriate to the age of the child:

1   Infants and toddlers (preverbal)
     Children unable to verbalize will be unable to use a self-report assessment tool. Tools for assessing pain in the preverbal child include: CHEOPS (Children's Hospital of Eastern Ontario Pain Scale); LIDS (Liverpool Infant Distress Score); the NFCS (Neonatal Facial Coding System); PIPP (Premature Infant Pain Profile) tools (RCN 1999). These tools

Score	Appearance/behaviours
0	Laughing, smiling, contented Gurgling, cooing, chatting Actively playing, contented/restful sleep
1	Distracts easily Articulating pain, moaning, complaining in general Grimaces on movement
2	Able to distract for short periods only Withdrawn miserable Touching area of body repeatedly, uncomfortable, restless
3	Difficult to distract Miserable, moaning crying Irritable, sensitive to handling, guarding
4	Unable to distract Screaming, aggressive, persistently grimacing Abnormally still, body rigid/tense position, sleep exhausted

Figure 3.2a Example of a behaviour pain tool

rely upon the assessor's interpretation of the child's behaviour, and make an assumption about the presence and nature of 'pain'. This can place considerable demands on healthcare professionals in distinguishing between normal behaviours and pain behaviours (Carter 1994). Behaviour pain assessment tools incorporate variables related to facial expression, crying and body posture aspects, see Figure 3.2a.

2 Young children

A variety of pictorial scales have been designed for use with young children, 3–7 years of age, such as that of Wong and Baker (1988) and faces pain scales of Bieri *et al.* (1990) which express various emotions which correlate to pain intensity. Faces scales are easy to use and user friendly, however younger children tend to choose faces at the extremities of the scale (RCN 1999). Figure 3.2b is an example of a faces pain tool.

3 Older children

A range of pain assessment tools are suitable for older children. Visual analogue scales consist of a vertical line, usually 10cm, with the words 'no pain at all' and 'worst possible pain' written at opposite ends of the line (Figure 3.2c) (Taylor 1998). The child is asked to mark on the line the level of their pain. Although the scale can be used with children where language is limited (the child's own words can be substituted), the child must have the ability to think abstractly to translate the pain experience to a visual line. It is therefore

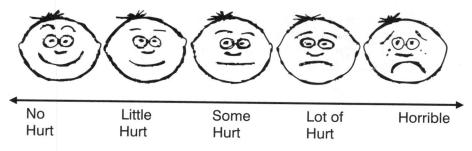

No	Little	Some	Lot of	Horrible
Hurt	Hurt	Hurt	Hurt	

Figure 3.2b Example of a faces pain tool

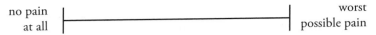

Figure 3.2c Example of a visual analogue assessment tool

inappropriate for preoperational children. Verbal rating scales are a similar design to the visual analogue scale, however there is a list of descriptors, such as 'no pain', 'mild pain', 'moderate pain', 'severe pain', 'very severe pain' along the line; these may be associated with a numerical value. Numerical rating scales are again similar tools but the line is divided into a scale, usually 1 to 10.

Children with a neurological disorder may have associated cognitive, behavioural and emotional difficulties. It is vital to consider individual requirements for these children because the less able and inarticulate child may receive sub-standard care and less analgesia than their able counterpart (Twycross *et al.* 1999). Although for many of these children, pain may have become an intrinsic part of the child's life, when additional factors contribute or change this, for example following surgery, normal tolerance to pain may become exacerbated. Parents may have devised their own frameworks for assessing the child's pain, which should be incorporated into nursing care plans. They will also require guidance from healthcare professionals regarding the acute nature of postoperative pain.

Family involvement

It is essential that healthcare professionals involve parents in the process of managing their child's pain. Assessing pain in children with special needs is particularly challenging because the child often has communication difficulties and may have different pain perception (Carter *et al.* 2002b). For children with neurological problems parents often have very detailed knowledge of their child's normal expressions and behaviours which an understanding of is vital in determining if the child is experiencing pain (Hunt *et al.* 2003).

Points to consider

Ensuring family involvement in managing their child's pain is important because:

- Parents are an invaluable source of information about a child's normal behaviours and can therefore assist in the assessment of pain, particularly non-verbal cues
- Parents have intimate knowledge of a child's usual coping mechanisms
- The presence of parents greatly reduces the anxiety provoked by hospitalization
- Parents will know the child's normal comforters
- Involving parents in managing pain is essential in light of early discharge from hospital which necessitates that pain management continues at home

  (Twycross 1998a; Hogg and Cooper 2004).

Parents must be supported and helped to become involved in the care of the child when the child is in pain. Unfortunately, parental involvement in pain management appears to occur at very superficial levels, with parents having passive roles in the overall management of their child's pain (Byrne *et al.* 2001; Simons *et al.* 2001; Pölkki *et al.* 2002).

Essential care

Including parents in their child's pain management can be achieved by:

- Introducing issues relating to pain management and potential parent roles during the admission procedure
- Providing written information relating to pain management
- Providing parents with guidance on non-pharmacological methods of pain management
- Ensuring emotional support is provided to prevent parents from feeling isolated and helpless.

(Byrne *et al.* 2001; Simons *et al.* 2001; Pölkki *et al.* 2002)

Parents inevitably take on the responsibility for ongoing care of the child following discharge (Ireland and Rushforth 1998). This can be a daunting prospect for many families and for many children will include the need to manage the child's pain. Prior to discharge the child and family will require detailed advice on pain management including explanations of at-home analgesia and education relating to non-pharmacological strategies which may alleviate the child's pain (Kankkunen *et al.* 2003).

Methods of pain control in children

It is essential that postoperative pain is managed promptly and efficiently to reduce the distress of the child and improve the outcome of surgery. Providing effective pain management is not only an integral component of nursing care (Nursing Midwifery Council 2002a), but also one of the basic rights for all children as recognized by the United Nations Convention on the Rights of the Child (Newell 1991). Acute pain can be an anticipated result following surgery. Pain management can be planned in advance, taking into consideration the type of surgical intervention. Pain following neurosurgical procedures occurs as a consequence of muscles and soft tissue damage at the site of the surgical incision. The severity of the pain experienced is linked to the site of the craniotomy; frontal lobe surgery is associated with lower pain intensity compared to occipital and posterior fossa approaches (Thibault *et al.* 2007). An integral part of the strategies for managing pain in children will involve choosing the best pain control interventions. Multi-modal interventions are important but in the management of acute postoperative pain non-pharmacological interventions should be used only as an adjunct to pharmacological agents.

Pharmacological interventions

The type of drug given will depend upon several factors: the pain assessment, cause of the pain, the therapeutic action of the drug, intensity and location of the pain, and the individual child's needs (Broadbent 2000). An analgesic ladder is a useful concept in that drugs of similar potency can be grouped together (Figure 3.2d). An analgesic ladder should simplify and guide in the prescription of analgesia but be flexible and sensitive enough to meet a child's individual needs

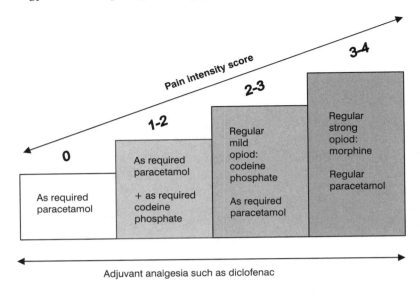

Figure 3.2d An example of an analgesic ladder

(Moriarty 1998). This can be achieved by having four drug choices that have a range of actions and potencies, such as paracetamol, diclofenac, codeine phosphate and morphine (Moriarty 1998). Adjunctive therapies are particularly useful, for example non-steroidal anti-inflammatory drugs such as diclofenac, and muscle relaxants such as baclofen. The ladder should be used in a step-wise approach; if a drug is ineffective, move to the group of drugs on the next step of the ladder, which may have the desired effect. It is important to start on the correct step of the ladder, for major surgery this may be stage 4 (Figure 3.2d).

Paracetamol is the most commonly prescribed analgesic in children (Carter 1994). Despite this it is often used inappropriately; it is only suitable for relieving mild pain or as an adjunct to more potent analgesics (Moriarty 1998). A non-steroidal anti-inflammatory drug such as diclofenac given as an adjuvant with regular paracetamol can often provide effective analgesia (National Prescribing Centre 2000). Oral paracetamol is dependent on effective gastrointestinal functioning. However, choices about the mode of delivery of paracetamol are improving and paracetamol is now a viable option for children who are nil by mouth or suffering from postoperative nausea and vomiting. Paracetamol is available as fastmelts which dissolve on the tongue, suppository and intravenous formulas (British Medical Association 2006). Paracetamol is effective if given by suppository but this mode of delivery may be unacceptable to some children and their wishes should be respected. Care must be taken not to exceed the recommended maximum daily dose, calculated on body weight, due to potential liver damage. This is an important consideration if paracetamol is given on discharge as many over the counter preparations (for colds and influenza) contain paracetamol and the number of trade names could be misleading for parents (Broadbent 2000).

Diclofenac is a non-steroidal anti-inflammatory drug with analgesic, anti-inflammatory and antipyretic properties. Non-steroidal anti-inflammatory are contraindicated if there is renal impairment, hypovolaemia, low platelets or tendency to bleed, liver disease, gastric ulceration, or for children under 6 months of age, immunocompromised children, and should be used with caution in children with asthma (Moriarty 1998). Diclofenac is available in a range of oral forms including a suspension, making it suitable for small doses, and in suppository form dosage will need to be calculated on body weight. Diclofenac is useful for mild to moderate pain and as an adjunct to other analgesics.

Opioid analgesics are used for moderate to severe pain. Codeine phosphate is a weak opioid, effective at relieving mild to moderate pain, and is best used in conjunction with diclofenac and paracetamol (Moriarty 1998). Codeine phosphate is available in a wide range of oral, suppository and injectable forms. Intramuscular injection only is recommended because intravenous injection results in apnoea and severe hypotension (Yaster and Deshpande 1988). A major limiting factor with codeine phosphate is its constipating effect. Codeine phosphate had traditionally been the drug of choice following neurosurgery (Thiabault *et al.* 2007; Roberts 2005). The rational for using codeine following major neurosurgery is related to codeine being less likely to cause respiratory depression than stronger opioids and therefore safer in patients at risk of acute rises in intracranial pressure (Roberts 2005).

Morphine is available in a wide range of preparations and can be given orally, rectally, intramuscularly, subcutaneously and intravenously. Excessive sedation and respiratory depression is an undesirable side effect of morphine and remains a concern because of the potential for eventual respiratory arrest. Other side effects of morphine include nausea and vomiting, constipation, itching and urine retention. Children's fear of injections (Eland 1981, Mather and Mackie 1983) and the peaks and troughs associated with intermittent intramuscular injections has made continuous intravenous morphine infusions a standard approach in the management of postoperative pain following major surgery (Bray *et al.* 1986; Maikler 1998). The risk associated with the use of continuous morphine infusions can be reduced if weight-related doses are used and children are appropriately monitored (Walco *et al.* 1994). Morphine sulphate is the gold standard opioid against which all other analgesic drugs are compared and is the drug of choice when managing severe pain (Moriarty 1998). Despite morphine being used widely in the majority of surgical specialities, its use following major neurosurgery is variable (Roberts 2005). Side effects, such as respiratory depression, can be detected early if the child is regularly assessed and oxygen saturation levels are monitored continuously because respiratory slowing occurs well before there is severe respiratory depression. If respirations slow, appropriate interventions such as reducing or stopping the infusion can be implemented. In addition, antidotes such as naloxone can be administered as these quickly reverse the effects of opioids. Naloxone should always be prescribed alongside the morphine prescription.

Points to consider

The choice of route and method of administration of analgesia will depend on many factors including:

- The pain score
- Cause of the pain (e.g. trauma, surgery) and predicted duration of acute pain
- The child's cognitive level and abilities, this is particularly important when considering patient-controlled analgesia systems
- Physical status, e.g. oral medication is not suitable if a child is vomiting or has impaired gut motility; subcutaneous may not be suitable if there is poor tissue perfusion; and intravenous administration may not be appropriate if venous access is problematic
- Ability to monitor the child

- Time available to prepare the child and family, this is particularly important in patient-controlled analgesia systems
- Support available from anaesthetic services/pain services
- Local practice, policies and guidelines.

Non-pharmacological interventions

There is no evidence to support the sole use of non-pharmacological interventions in acute situations. Children manage and cope with pain by using a range of strategies such as resting, applying pressure, patting, rubbing, sleeping and distraction (watching television, colouring, reading) (Unruh *et al.* 1983; Woodgate and Kristjanson 1995). Therefore non-pharmacological interventions for relieving pain are particularity suitable for using with children to support pharmacological interventions.

Points to consider

Non-pharmacological interventions suitable for use in children include:

- Provision of appropriate information
- Play and activity therapy
- Distraction
- Application of heat and cold packs
- Non-nutritive sucking in neonates and infants
- Relaxation techniques
- Imagery
- Massage
- Therapeutic touch
- Aromatherapy
- Transcutaneous electrical nerve stimulation (TENS)
- Acupuncture
- Hypnosis.

(Eland 1990, Carter 1994, Twycross 1998b)

Many of these techniques do not have a strong evidence base to support their effectiveness, and responses will be variable between children and across the age span. Some of these techniques may be more suitable in the management of chronic pain and may require specialist training.

Pain services

Acute postoperative pain should be managed by an acute pain team (Hogg 1994; Lloyd-Thomas and Howard 1994; Royal College of Paediatrics and Child Health 1997; RCN 1999; Royal College of Anaesthetists 2001, 2000; Sanders and Michel 2002). Pain services should consist of an interdisciplinary team responsible for the development and implementation of guidelines and protocols relating to the management of pain in children (Royal College of Paediatrics and Child Health 1997).

Points to consider

The function of an acute pain team includes:

- Developing protocols for the assessment of pain
- Developing systems for including the child and family in the assessment process and subsequent management strategies
- Developing and providing child and parent information in a variety of formats
- Ensuring pain assessment tools link to guidelines on analgesia choices (e.g. a pain ladder)
- Developing and implementing care plans for complex analgesia interventions such as continuous morphine infusions, patient-controlled analgesia and epidural analgesia
- Developing guidelines on child observations, e.g. cardiovascular observations, pain assessment and sedation scores, and the frequency of recordings
- Developing an overall management strategy, such as an acute pain management algorithm (Figure 3.2e).

(Royal College of Anaesthetists 2000, 2001)

Acute pain teams are responsible for undertaking regular audits of the pain service enabling standards to be monitored and identification of future developments and areas for potential research (Lloyd-Thomas and Howard 1994; Goddard and Pickup 1996; Sherwood 1998). An

Essential care

The principles of good practice in managing acute pain in children include:

- Communicating effectively with children and asking them how they feel and how much pain they have
- Listening to children and understanding their fears and anxieties such as avoiding the use of injections
- Observing children and recognizing both physiological and behavioural indicators of pain
- Ensuring effective education of the child and family (both verbal and written) regarding pain and offering realistic choices
- Involving children in choice of assessment tool
- Ensuring a range of pain management strategies are available
- Ensuring clear and concise documentation, evaluating the effectiveness of treatments
- Involving the family in care and respecting their wishes.

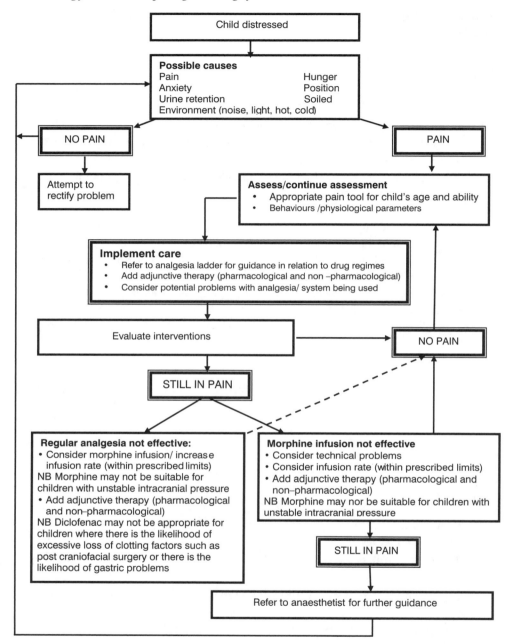

Figure 3.2e Example of an acute postoperative pain management algorithm

effective pain team is important but improving pain management for the child does not have to be a complex process and should be the responsibility of all healthcare professionals.

3.3 Wound care

The vast majority of surgical incisions following a neurosurgical procedure are closed at the time of surgery. In wounds where there has been considerable bacterial contamination, for example a large abscess, traumatic injury with an open wound or extensive tissue loss, it may not be possible to close the wound (Dealey 1999). While this is a possibility following neurosurgery, it is unlikely and therefore will not be discussed.

Management of primary closed wounds

The primary aim of wound closure is to restore the physical integrity of the damaged tissue and regain normal function with minimum disruption as quickly as possible (Hollander and Singer 1999). A second consideration is the aesthetic appearance of the wound. Primary closure is achieved by bringing the wound edges together in apposition and adequately securing the edges, so that the natural healing process can occur (Bruns *et al.* 1998; Vuolo 2006). The surface of the wound will usually be sealed within 48 hours (Dealey 1999). The effectiveness of primary closure will depend upon the right choice and correct application of closure materials (Heath 1998). The ideal wound closure technique should be easily and rapidly applied, be painless, of low risk to the healthcare professional using the technique, be inexpensive and result in minimal scarring with a low infection rate (Hollander and Singer 1999). Staples or clips are often used to close neurosurgery incisions because they are quick and easy to apply, cost effective, have a low risk of tissue reactivity, low risk of infection and a low risk of needle stick injury (Osmond *et al.* 1995; Bruns *et al.* 1998; Hollander and Singer 1999; Bernard *et al.* 2001; Tritle *et al.* 2001; Vuolo 2006). Traditional sutures are a suitable alternative. Tissue adhesives such as cyanoacrylate are becoming popular if the position of the incision in the scalp makes it difficult to place staples, or if staple removal in the child is anticipated to be especially difficult. Tissue adhesives can also improve cosmetic outcome (Vuolo 2006). If wounds are not closed effectively, the tensile strength of the wound may not be sufficient to maintain its integrity, with the potential for the wound to dehisce.

The management of primary closed wounds is relatively straightforward. There will be slight differences depending upon type of closure, wound depth, position of the wound and the individual child's and family's needs. The initial dressing is applied in theatre and therefore the type of dressing is usually determined by the surgeon's preference. In practice this usually consists of an island dressing such as a low-adherent dressing or a film dressing (Dealey 1999). The purpose of a wound dressing is to provide protection and maintain an ideal wound environment (Casey 1999). In addition, consideration should be given to the child's stage of development (particularly if accidental removal is to be minimized in the young child), the

Points to consider

The main types of wound dressings are:

- Woven dressings such as dry gauze and paraffin impregnated gauze. They are inappropriate for direct contact with the wound because they adhere to the wound and cause trauma to healing tissue on removal and do not promote a moist wound environment. They are usually used as absorbent medium for secondary dressing
- Film dressings are permeable to water vapour and oxygen, impermeable to water and micro-organisms. They ensure a moist environment, are convenient and allow for observation of the wound and are suitable for wounds that have been primary closed and where there is not expected to be an exudate. They can be used as a secondary dressing to provide a waterproof surface
- Hydrocolloids are highly absorbent and when wet form a gel which maintains a moist surface. They aid healing by gentle debriding action and are impermeable to water and bacteria. There are many forms such as wafers, gels and powders or in a combination with other dressings
- Hydrogels are composed of gel, which when in contact with a wound releases water. They are mainly used to rehydrate wounds, debride and clean sloughy or necrotic wounds.

(Russell 2002; Casey 2001)

preferences of the child and family and the frequency of dressing changes. The latter aspects are particularly important if parents are expected to continue wound care and dressing changes following discharge.

A film dressing allows for early inspection of the wound, whereas a low-adherent dressing will absorb any minor postoperative oozing. From a psychological point of view some children may prefer to view the wound site, while others may not. Unless there is any indication to do so, such as excessive oozing, or exudate, which may indicate either haemorrhage or infection respectively, there is no need to change the dressing daily. Routine swabbing with normal saline, is an outdated practice, and potentially exposes the wound to environmental contaminants, traumatizing fragile granulating tissue (Dealey 1999; Gould 2001). Unnecessary practices cause additional distress to the child and family. Once the wound surface has sealed (usually

Points to consider

Observations of the wound include:

- The colour of the wound and tissue in the surrounding area
- Blood loss and evidence of continued oozing
- Temperature of surrounding tissue
- The presence, colour and amount of any exudate on the wound surface and on the dressing
- Swelling.

by 48 hours), the dressing can be removed and does not need to be replaced. Removal of the dressing is the ideal opportunity to assess the wound for any abnormalities and ensure that the healing process is continuing appropriately.

Removal of the dressing should consider the psychological needs of the child, the assessment of pain likely to be experienced, the provision of analgesia and appropriate preparation and support of the child and family prior to, during and after the procedure. It is important that the first dressing change is not traumatic, particularly if it is anticipated that there will be regular dressing changes over a long period. Preparation should be appropriate for the age and stage of development of the child, and the type of procedure being performed (Casey 1999). For the young child preparation through the use of play and the involvement of a play therapist is invaluable (Chandler 1994; Ellerton and Merriam 1994).

In general, normal hygiene routines can be maintained once the dressing has been removed. The sutures or staples should be checked to ensure they are intact and the entry sites examined for any signs of inflammation. The application of a dressing if sutures or staples have been inserted should be considered because of the potential to catch on clothing or be pulled by the inquisitive young child. Drying of the wound can be prevented by the application of white petrolatum (Hollander and Singer 1999).

The timing of the removal of sutures or staples is a balance between providing the wound edges with support and achieving a good cosmetic result (Castille 1998). Generally, sutures and staples should be removed at about 7–10 days postoperatively, when epithelialization has occurred. Sutures or staples are usually left in place longer, up to 14 days, for wounds in the posterior fossa. This provides more time for the dura to heal sufficiently, minimizing the risk of cerebrospinal fluid leakage. Staff removing sutures or clips should be familiar with the appropriate procedures in their area of work.

Best practice recommendations

Good practice guidelines for ward-based care of surgical incision wounds include:

- Wound assessment should identify factors which may delay wound healing. Assessment should ensure early detection of wound infection and be an ongoing process
- Surgical wound incisions should only be cleaned if indicated, for example to remove material which may delay healing or for patient comfort
- If cleaning is required warmed normal saline should be used to irrigate the wound
- Surgical wounds should be cleaned using aseptic techniques
- Adequate analgesia should be administered to the child prior to changing the wound dressing
- The dressing should be semi-permeable and provide absorbency with low adherence
- Documentation should provide a systematic framework for organizing and evaluating care – be clear, accurate, relevant and up to date.

(Birchall and Taylor 2003)

Factors affecting wound healing

A range of factors affect wound healing and should be considered in the care of the child following surgery:

- Age – normal development of the dermis, which thickens during the first year of life, has the potential to assist wound healing in children (Morison *et al.* 1997). In addition, children will not have the systemic diseases associated with adults, in particular cardiovascular disease and complications of diabetes, which may compromise circulation and therefore tissue perfusion.
- Wound environment – cells function best at body temperature and in high humidity. Therefore, a warm and moist environment will encourage wound healing. Although a moist wound promotes healing, excessive moisture or bathing in large amounts of fluid delays healing by causing maceration of the granulation tissue and surrounding skin (Casey 1999). Swabbing wounds with gauze and cotton wool, for example to clean a wound, will damage the surface of the wound and delay healing (Parker 2000; Towler 2001)
- Presence of infection delays wound healing – systemic infection reduces the availability of white cells for wound healing (Dealey 1999). Infection in the actual wound prolongs the inflammatory stage of healing, thereby compromising the healing process (Dealey 1999). In addition, the toxins produced by many bacteria impair normal cell function (White *et al.* 2002). Infection may cause dehiscence in a wound that has been primary closed.
- Nutrition and drugs – the physiological processes of wound healing are energy dependent and require a range of nutrients to sustain cellular actively (Dealey 1999). Vascular supply complications, for example with anaemia or diabetes may contribute to delayed healing (Vuolo 2006), although this is less common in children.
- Choice of wound dressing (Lait and Smith 1998).

Wounds complications

Wound dehiscence

Wound dehiscence refers to opening or splitting of the wound and can occur in any of the layers of the wound, together or independently. While very unlikely following neurosurgery, factors which contribute to wound dehiscence include: poor selection of suture material (Hollander and Singer 1999), inadequate primary closure, early removal of sutures and the presence of infection (Dealey 1999). Care will depend upon the extent of the wound breakdown; treatment is generally conservative, and wound healing is promoted through the appropriate dressing selection and by allowing the wound to heal by granulation (Dealey 1999). Infections must be treated appropriately. Re-suturing may be necessary.

Wound infection

Despite increased understanding about the spread of infection and standards in maintaining asepsis, postoperative wound infection remains a significant complication (Emmerson *et al.*

Essential care

Understanding and adhering to policies of universal infection control precautions are essential to minimize the risk of would infection:

- Appropriate hand washing
- Correct disposal of waste (including sharps) and linen
- Wearing gloves and a plastic apron whenever contact with blood or body fluids is anticipated.

(Gould 1997; Bolyard *et al.* 1998; Xavier 1999)

1996; Plowman *et al.* 1999; Reilly *et al.* 2001). Therefore, the prevention of infection needs to be a priority for all healthcare professionals and in all healthcare settings. The spread of bacteria via hands is well established and hand washing had been implicated as the single most important procedure in preventing the spread of infection (Bree-Williams and Waterman 1996; Gould 1997; Gould and Chamberlain 1997; Bolyard *et al.* 1998; Xavier 1999).

Maintaining a meticulous aseptic technique when undertaking wound care will minimize the risk of cross infection between patients. Asepsis is the prevention of microbial contamination of living tissue by excluding, removing or killing micro-organisms (Xavier 1999). The aim of performing an aseptic technique is to prevent the spread of infection to a susceptible patient, by direct or indirect means (Xavier 1999). This would include preventing the transmission of micro-organisms into a healthy wound (Bree-Williams and Waterman 1996). There is much confusion relating to the cleansing of wounds. Not all wounds require routine cleaning, however, infected and contaminated wounds will require cleaning to remove any debris that might hinder the healing process (Towler 2001).

Best practice recommendations

The current consensus in wound cleansing includes:

- Avoiding direct swabbing because of the trauma caused to the wound bed
- Irrigation with normal saline is the current method of choice

(Towler 2001).

The four cardinal signs and symptoms of infection are redness in the tissue surrounding the wound, heat, pain and swelling. A systemic rise in temperature may be the first sign if infection develops in deeper tissues. Other indicators, which may indicate the presence of a wound infection, include (Cutting and Harding 1994; Gould 2001):

- Wound healing is not progressing at the expected rate
- Discharge/increased exudate or changes in the exudate such as colour, smell and texture
- Discolouration of the wound bed
- Cellulitis
- Granulation tissue which remains friable and continues to bleed
- Unexpected pain, tenderness or throbbing

- Puckering at the base of the wound
- Breakdown of a previously healthy wound

Most wounds are colonized with bacteria (Dealey 1999). Although a wound swab is necessary to determine type of bacteria, it does not prove an infection is present. Laboratory findings should be combined with a clinical evaluation of the wound, with treatment only commencing if there are clinical indications that an infection is present (Dealey 1999; Gould 2001). The bacteria most commonly associated with postoperative wound infections are staphylococci, gram-negative rods and streptococci (Gould 2001). Many bacteria that have the potential to cause wound infections are part of the normal flora of healthy individuals, including healthcare workers. In addition gram-negative bacteria thrive in warm damp environments where there is little organic material (Gould 2001). It is therefore essential that universal precautions such as keeping the environment clean and well ventilated, appropriately storing equipment, and meticulous hand hygiene are maintained.

The management of an infected wound will include a combination of systemic antibiotics, the use of topical agents and choosing the most appropriate dressing. The treatment options will depend upon causative organisms and assessment of the wound, in particular type of exudates. The management of resistant strains of organisms such as methicillin-resistant *Staphylococcus aureus* (MRSA) is particularly difficult and it is vital these infections are managed appropriately. Controlling the spread of MRSA is vital because treatments are expensive and, in severe cases, is associated with poor recovery rates (Morrison and Stolarek 2000). Local guidelines and policies regarding the management of MRSA should include the principles outlined in the guidelines from the British Society for Antimicrobial Chemotherapy, the Hospital Infection Society and the Infection Control Nurses Association (1998).

Discharge

With the increasingly-short hospital stay, education relating to early wound management and the recognition of signs of inflammation are vital. Although standardized wound care instructions

Essential care

On discharge the child and family will require detailed instructions relation to the care of the wound including:

- Pain management
- When to remove dressings (if this is not done prior to discharge or by the community nurse)
- Descriptions of signs and symptoms of inflammation
- Information on nutrition
- Bathing/showering instructions; showering is preferable, patting the wound dry, avoiding excessive rubbing, not using talcum powder
- Application of moisturisers/white petrolatum
- Details of where and when sutures/clips are removed
- Who to contact with any concerns, including contacts for nights and weekends.

Key messages from this chapter

- Children and families should be treated as individuals; care should consider the child's age, cognitive ability, usual care requirements, social, religious and emotional care needs, and family's wishes
- Effective communication between healthcare professionals across departments is essential
- Parents and children need to be prepared for the hospital experience
- The ward and theatre environments should be child friendly and suitably equipped to care for children
- Parents should be allowed to escort their child to theatre, one parent should be permitted to stay with their child in the anaesthetic room until they are unconscious, then allowed to rejoin the child in the recovery room
- Healthcare professionals should use a suitable pain assessment tool to ensure the child receives adequate analgesia
- Measures to prevent wound infection should be taken
- Prior to discharge, community teams should be advised about ongoing care needs of the child at home. Parents must feel confident in taking their child home and be competent in carrying out any specific care the child requires on discharge. Parents should be informed of follow-up arrangements and know who to contact if they have any worries or causes for concern.

Web resources

National Institute for Health and Clinical Excellence
provides national guidance on the promotion of good health and the prevention and treatment of ill health, and produces guidance relating to: public health (promoting good health and the prevention of ill health for those working in all healthcare sectors), health technologies (guidance on the use of new and existing medicines, treatments and procedures), and clinical practice guidance (appropriate treatment and care of people with specific diseases and conditions)
www.nice.org.uk
Scottish Intercollegiate Guidelines Network
develops and disseminates national clinical guidelines, derived from systematic reviews of the scientific evidence, to ensure practice is based on current evidence.
www.sign.ac.uk
National Library for Health
provides a range of health related resources
www.library.nhs.uk

may assist in improving compliance to care and aid in understanding, information must be tailored to each child's needs (Casey 1999; Hollander and Singer 1999).

References

Age of Legal Capacity (Scotland) Act (1991) section 1(1)b, section 2(4), and section 3(3)e.

American Society of Anesthesiologists (ASA) Task Force (1999) Practice guidelines for preoperative fasting and the use of pharmacological agents to reduce the risks of pulmonary aspiration: application to healthy patients undergoing elective procedures. *Anesthesiology* **90** (3): 896–905.

American Society of Anesthesiologists (ASA) (2002) Practice advisory for preanesthesia evaluation. *Anesthesiology* **96** (2): 485–96.

Association of Anaesthetists of Great Britain and Ireland (2001) *Preoperative Assessment. The Role of the Anaesthetist.* AAGBI, London.

Bailey R, Caldwell C (1997) Preparing parents for going home. *Paediatric Nursing* **9** (4): 15–17.

Baker C, Wong D (1987) QUEST: a process of pain assessment in children. *Orthopaedic Nursing* **6** (1): 11–21.

Bernard L, Friedlander SF, Eichenfield LF *et al.* (2001) A prospective comparison of octyl cyanoacrylate tissue adhesive (Dermabond) and suture material for the closure of excisional wounds in children and adolescents. *Archives of Dermatology* **137** (9): 1177–80.

Bieri D, Reeve RA, Champion GD, Addicoat L, Zeigler JB (1990) The Faces Pain Scale for the self-assessment of the severity of pain experienced by children: development, initial validation and preliminary investigation for ratio scale properties. *Pain* **41**: 139–50.

Birchall L, Taylor S (2003) Surgical wound benchmark tool and best practice guidelines. *British Journal of Nursing* **12** (17): 1013–23.

Bolyard EA, Tablan OC, Williams WW *et al.* (1998) Guidelines for infection control in healthcare personnel, 1998. *Infection Control and Hospital Epidemiology* **19**: 407–63.

Bradford R, Singer J (1991) Support and information for parents. *Paediatric Nursing* **3** (4): 18–20.

Bray RJ, Beeton C, Hinton W, Seviour JA (1986) Plasma morphine levels produced by continuous infusion in children. *Anaesthesia* **41**: 753–5.

Bree-Williams FJ, Waterman H (1996) An examination of nurses' practices while performing aseptic technique for wound dressings. *Journal of Advanced Nursing* **23**(1): 48–56.

Briggs M (1997) Principles of closed surgical wound care. *Journal of Wound Care* **6** (6): 288–92.

British Medical Association (2001) *Consent, Rights and Choices in Health Care for Children and Young People.* BMJ Publishing Group, London.

British Medical Association (2006) *British National Formulary for Children.* BMJ Publishing Group, London.

British Society for Antimicrobial Chemotherapy, the Hospital Infection Society and the Infection Control Nurses Association (1998) *Revised Guidelines for the control of methicillin-resistant* Staphylococcus aureus *Infections in Hospital. Journal of Infection Control* **39** (4): 253–90.

Broadbent C (2000) The pharmacology of acute pain. *Nursing Times* **96** (26): 39–41.

Brown K, De Lima J, McEwan A *et al.* (2000) Development and diseases in childhood. In Sumner E, Hatch DJ (eds) *Paediatric Anaesthesia*, 2nd edn. Arnold, London.

Brown V (1995) Parents in recovery: parental and staff attitudes. *Paediatric Nursing* **7** (7): 17–19.

Brown V (1997) The child in theatre: should parents be involved? *British Journal of Theatre Nursing* **7** (8): 5–7.

Bruns TB, Robinson BS, Smith RJ *et al.* (1998) A new tissue adhesive for laceration repair in children. *The Journal of Pediatrics* **132** (6): 1067–70.

Buckingham S (1993) Managing pain in children. Pain scales for toddlers. *Nursing Standard* **7** (Suppl 25): 12–13.

Burns LS (1997) Advances in pediatric anesthesia. *Nursing Clinics of North America* **32** (1): 45–71.

Burr S (1993) Managing pain in children. Myths in practice. *Nursing Standard* **7** (Suppl 25): 4–5.

Byrne A, Morton J, Salmon P (2001) Defending against patients' pain. A qualitative analysis of nurses' responses to children's postoperative pain. *Journal of Psychosomatic Research* **50**: 69–76.

Carter B (1994) *Child and Infant Pain, Principles of Nursing Care and Management.* Chapman and Hall, London.

Carter B, Lambrenos K, Thursfield J (2002a) A pain workshop: an approach to eliciting the views of young people with chronic pain. *Journal of Clinical Nursing* **11** (6): 753–62.

Carter B, McArthur E, Cunliffe M (2002b) Dealing with uncertainty: parental assessment of pain in their children with profound special needs. *Journal of Advanced Nursing* **38** (5): 449–57.

Casey A (1988) A partnership with child and family. *Senior Nurse* **8** (4): 8–9.

Casey G (1999) Wound management in children. *Paediatric Nursing* **11** (6): 39–44.

Casey G (2001) Wound dressings. *Paediatric Nursing* **13** (4): 39–42.

Castille K (1998) Suturing. *Nursing Standard* **12** (41): 41-48.

Chameides L, Hazinski MF (1997) *Pediatric Advanced Life Support.* American Heart Association, Texas.

Chandler K (1994) Play preparation for surgery. *Surgical Nurse* **7** (4): 14–16.

Chandler T (2000) Oxygen saturation monitoring. *Paediatric Nursing* **12** (8): 37–42.

Chandler T (2001) Oxygen administration. *Paediataric Nursing* **13** (8): 37–42.

Children's Forum of the Royal College of Surgeons (2007) *Surgery for Children – Delivering a First Class Service.* Royal College of Surgeons, London.

Cohen MM, Cameron CB, Duncan PG (1990) Pediatric anesthesia morbidity and mortality in the perioperative period. *Anesthesia and Analgesia* **70**: 160–7.

Cowan T (1998) Perioperative nursing. *Professional Nurse* **14** (1): 68–9.

Cummings EA, Reid GJ, Finley GA, McGrath PJ, Ritchie JA (1996) Prevalence and source of pain management in pediatric inpatients. *Pain* **68**: 25–31.

Cutting K, Harding KG (1994) Criteria for identifying wound infection. *Journal of Wound Care* **3** (4): 198–201.

Day T, Wainwright S, Wilson-Barnett J (2001) An evaluation of a teaching intervention to improve the practice of endotracheal suctioning in intensive care units. *Journal of Clinical Nursing* **10**: 682–96.

Day T, Farnell S, Haynes S, Wainwright S, Wilson-Barnett J (2002) Tracheal suctioning: an exploration of nurses' knowledge and competence in acute and high dependency ward areas. *Journal of Advanced Nursing* **39** (1): 35–45.

Dealey C (1999) *The Care of Wounds: A Guide for Nurses*, 2nd edn. Blackwell Science, London.

Department of Health (1989) *The Children Act.* HMSO, London.

Department of Health (2001) *The Reference Guide to Consent for Examination or Treatment.* Stationery Office, London.

Department of Health (2004) *National Service Framework for Children, Young People and Maternity Services: Change for Children – Every Child Matters.* Stationery Office, London.

Eland J (1981) Minimizing pain associated with pre-kindergarten intramuscular injections. *Issues in Comprehensive Pediatric Nursing* **5**: 361–72.

Eland J (1990) Pain in children. *Nursing Clinics of North America* **24** (40): 871–4.

Ellerton ML, Merriam C (1994) Preparing children and families psychologically for day surgery: an evaluation. *Journal of Advanced Nursing* **19**(6): 1057–62.

Emerson BM, Wrigley, SR, Newton M (1998) Preoperative fasting for paediatric anaesthesia. A survey of current practice. *Anaesthesia* **53** (4): 326–30.

Emmerson AM, Enstone JE, Griffin M, Kelsey MC, Smyth ET (1996) The second national prevalence survey of infection in hospitals: overview and results. *Journal of Hospital Infection* **32**: 175–90.

Family Law and Reform Act (1969), sub-section **8** and **22**(2).

Ferrari LR, Rooney FM, Rockoff MA (1999) Preoperative fasting practices in pediatrics. *Anesthesiology* **90** (4): 978–80.

Fetzer SJ (2002) Reducing venipuncture and intravenous insertion pain with eutectic mixture of local anesthetic. A meta-analysis. *Nursing Research* **51** (2): 119–24.

Fina DK, Lopas LJ, Stagnone JH, Santucci PR (1997) Parental participation in the postanesthesia care unit: fourteen years of progress at one hospital. *Journal of Perianesthesia Nursing* **12** (3): 152–62.

Fitzgerald M, Howard F (2003) The neurobiological basis of pediatric pain. In Schechter NL, Berde CB, Yaster M (eds) *Pain in Infants, Children and Adolescents.* Lippincott Williams and Wilkins, Philadelphia, PA.

Frayling IM, Addison GM, Chattergee K, Meakin G *et al.* (1990) Methaemoglobinaemia in children treated with prilocaine-lignocaine cream. *British Medical Journal* **301**: 153–4.

Gillick v. West Norfolk and Wisbech Area Health Authority (1985) All England Report **402**.

Goddard JM, Pickup SE (1996) Postoperative pain in children. Combing audit and a clinical nurse specialist to improve management. *Anaesthesia* **51**: 533–6.

Gould D (1997) *Hand Care Monitoring Standards. Hygienic Hand Decontamination.* Macmillan Magazines, London.

Gould D (2001) Clean surgical wounds: prevention of infection. *Nursing Standard* **15** (49): 45–52.

Gould D, Chamberlain A (1997) The use of a ward-based educational teaching package to enhance nurses' compliance with infection control policies. *Journal of Clinical Nursing* **6** (1): 55–67.

Hackeling T, Triana R, John O, Shockley W (1998) Emergency care of patients with tracheostomies: a 7-year review. *American Journal of Emergency Medicine* **16**: 681–5.

Heath S (1998) *Perioperative Care of the Child.* Quay Books, Salisbury.

Hickey JV (2003) Management of patients undergoing neurosurgical procedures. In Hickey JV (ed.) *The Clinical Practice of Neurological and Neurosurgical Nursing,* 5th edn. Lippincott, Philadelphia.

Hogg C (1994) *Setting Standards for Children Undergoing Surgery.* Action for Sick Children, London.

Hogg C, Cooper C (2004) *Meeting the Needs of Children and Young People Undergoing Surgery.* Action for Sick Children. London.

Hollander JE, Singer AJ (1999) Laceration management. *Annals of Emergency Medicine* **34** (3): 356–67.

Horwitz J, Chwals W, Doski J *et al.* (1998) Pediatric wound infections: a prospective multicentre study. *Annals of Surgery* **227** (4): 553–8.

Howard R, Lloyd-Thomas A (2000) Pain management in children. In Sumner E, Hatch DJ (eds) *Paediatric Anaesthesia,* 2nd ed. Arnold, London.

Hunt A, Mastroyannopoulou K, Goldman A *et al.* (2003) Not knowing – the problem of pain in children with severe neurological impairment. *International Journal of Nursing Studies* **40**: 171–83.

Imrie MM, Hall GM (1990) Body temperature and anaesthesia. *British Journal of Anaesthesia* **64**: 346–54.

International Association for the Study of Pain (1992). *Management of Acute pain: A Practical Guide.* IASP Press, Seattle.

Ireland L, Rushforth H (1998) Day care – in whose best interests? *Paediatric Nursing* **10** (5): 15–19.

Jackson KL (1995) The state we're in. *Child Health* **3** (1): 14–17.

Kankkunen P, Päivi K, Vehviläinen-Julkunen K, Pietilä AM, Halonen P (2003) Parents' use of nonpharmacological methods to alleviate children's postoperative pain at home. *Journal of Advanced Nursing* **41** (4): 367–75.

Kapadia FN, Bajan KB, Rajie KV (2000) Airway accidents in intubated intensive care unit patients: an epidemiological study. *Critical Care Medicine* **28**: 659–64.

Lait ME, Smith LN (1998) Wound management: a literature review. *Journal of Clinical Nursing* **7** (1): 11–17.

Lerman J (1992) Surgical and patient factors involved in postoperative nausea and vomiting. *British Journal of Anaesthesia* **69**: 24S–32S.

Lloyd-Thomas AR, Howard RF (1994) A pain service for children. *Paediatric Anaesthesia* **4**: 3–15.

Maikler VE (1998) Pharmacological pain management in children: a review of intervention research. *Journal of Pediatric Nursing* **13** (1): 3–14.

Mangram AJ, Horan TC, Pearson ML, Silver LC, Jarvis WR (1999) Guideline for prevention of surgical site infection. *American Journal of Infection Control* **27** (2): 97–132.

Mather L, Mackie J (1983) The incidence of postoperative pain in children. *Pain* **15**: 271–82.

McCaffery M (1968) *Nursing Practice Theories Relating to Cognition, Bodily Pain, and Man–Environment Interactions.* Lippincott, Los Angeles, CA.

McQuay HJ (1992) Pre-emptive analgesia. *British Journal of Anaesthesia* **69**: 1–3.

Meakin G, Murat I (2000) Immediate preoperative preparation. In Sumner E, Hatch DJ (eds) *Paediatric Anaesthesia*, 2nd edition. Arnold, London.

Mirakhur RK (1991) Preanaesthetic medication; a survey of current usage. *Journal of the Royal Society of Medicine* **84**: 481–3.

Moriarty A (1998) The pharmacological management of acute pain. In Twycross A, Moriarty A, Betts T (eds) *Paediatric Pain Management. A Multi-Disciplinary Approach*. Radcliffe, Oxford.

Morison M, Moffat C, Bridel-Nixon J *et al.* (1997) *A Color Guide to the Nursing Management of Chronic Wounds*. 2nd edn. Mosby, London.

Morrison L, Stolarek I (2000) Does MRSA affect patient outcomes in the elderly? A retrospective pilot study. *Journal of Hospital Infection* **45** (2): 169–71.

Munro J, Booth A, Nicholl J (1997) Routine preoperative testing: a systematic review of the evidence. *Health Technology Assessment* **1** (12): i–iv; 1–62.

Nash PL, O'Malley M (1997) Streamlining the perioperative process. *Nursing Clinics of North America* **32** (1): 141–51.

National Confidential Enquiry into Perioperative Deaths (1999) *Extremes of Age*. NCEPOD, London.

National Prescribing Centre (2000) The use of oral analgesics in primary care. *MeReC Bulletin* **11** (1): 1–4.

Newell P (1991) *The United Nations Convention and Children's Rights in the UK*. National Children's Bureau, London.

Noble RR, Micheli AJ, Hensley MA, McKay N (1997) Special considerations for the pediatric perioperative patient. A developmental approach. *Nursing Clinics of North America* **32** (10): 1–16.

Norman J, Jones PL (1990) Complications of the use of EMLA. *British Journal of Anaesthesia* **64**: 403–6.

Nursing and Midwifery Council (2007) *Guidelines for Keeping Records and Record Keeping*. NMC, London.

Olsson G (2000) Monitoring in paediatric anaesthesia. In Sumner E, Hatch DJ (eds) *Paediatric Anaesthesia*, 2nd edn. Arnold, London.

Osmond MH, Klassen TP, Quinn JV (1995) Economic comparison of a tissue adhesive and suturing in the repair of pediatric facial lacerations. *The Journal of Pediatrics* **126** (6): 892–5.

Parker L (2000) Applying the principles of infection control to wound care. *British Journal of Nursing* **9** (7): 398–404.

Phillips S, Daborn A K, Hatch J (1994) Preoperative fasting for paediatric anaesthesia. *British Journal of Anaesthesia* **73**: 529–36.

Plowman R, Graves N, Griffin M *et al.* (1999) *The Socioeconomic Burden of Hospital Acquired Infection*. Health Protection Agency, London.

Pölkki T, Pietilä AM, Vehviläinen-Julkunen K, Laukkala H, Ryhänen P (2002) Parental views on participation in their child's pain relief measures and recommendations to health care providers. *Journal of Pediatric Nursing.* **17** (4): 270–7.

Ratcliffe JM (1998) Recognition and management of shock. *Current Paediatrics* **8**: 1–5.

Re: E (a minor) Wardship; medical treatment (1993) Family Law Reform **386**.

Re: W (a minor) Medical treatment: a courts jurisdiction (1992) 3 Weekly Law Report **758**.

Reilly J, Baird D, Hill R (2001) The importance of definitions and methods in surgical wound infection audit. *Journal of Hospital Infection* **47** (1): 64–6.

Resuscitation Council (UK) (2005) *Resuscitation Guidelines 2005*. Resuscitation Council Publications, London.

Roberts GC (2005) Post-craniotomy analgesia: current practices in British neurosurgical centres – a survey of post-craniotomy analgesic practices. *European Journal of Anaesthesiology* **22**: 328–32.

Rømsing J, Walther-Larsen S (1997) Perioperative use of nonsteroidal anti-inflammatory drugs in children: analgesia efficacy and bleeding. *Anaesthesia* **52** (7): 673–83.

Royal College of Anaesthetists (2000) *Raising the Standard*. RCoA, London.

Royal College of Anaesthetists (2001) *Guidance on the Provision of Paediatric Anaesthetic Services*. RCoA, London.

Royal College of Nursing (1999) *Clinical Practice Guidelines: The Recognition and Assessment of Acute Pain in Children.* RCN, London.

Royal College of Nursing (2005) *Perioperative Fasting in Adults and Children – An RCN Guideline for the Multidisciplinary Team. Clinical Practice Guidelines.* RCN, London.

Royal College of Paediatrics and Child Health (1997) *Prevention and Control of Pain in Children – A Manual for Health Care Professionals.* BMJ, London.

Rushforth H, Bliss A, Burge D, Glasper EA (2000) A pilot randomised controlled trial of medical versus nurse clerking for minor surgery. *Archives of Disease in Childhood* **83** (3): 223–6.

Russell L (2002) Understanding of wound healing and how dressings help. In White R, Harding K (eds) *Trends in Wound Care.* Quay Books, Salisbury.

Sanders MK, Michel MZ (2002) Acute pain services – how effective are we? *Anaesthesia* **57** (9): 927–8.

Schofield P (1995) Using pain assessment tools to help patents. *Professional Nurse* **10** (11): 703–6.

Sethi AK, Chatterji C, Bhargava SK, Narang P, Tyagi A (1999) Safe pre-operative fasting times after milk or clear fluid in children. A preliminary study using real-time ultrasound. *Anaesthesia* **54** (1): 51–9.

Sherwood P (1998) Auditing paediatric pain management. *Paediatric pain* **10** (6): 15–7.

Simons J, Franck L, Roberson E (2001) Parent involvement in children's pain care: views of parents and nurses. *Journal of Advanced Nursing* **36** (4): 591–9.

Smalley A (1999) Needle phobia. *Paediatric Nursing* **11** (2): 17–20.

Smith AF, Vallance H, Slater RM (1997) Shorter postoperative fluid fasts reduce postoperative emesis. *British Medical Journal* **314** (7092): 1486.

Smith J, Dearmun A (2006) Improving care for children requiring surgery and their families. *Paediatric Nursing* **18** (9): 30–3.

Splinter WM, Schreiner MS (1999) Preoperative fasting in children. *Anesthesia and Analgesia* **89**: 80–9.

Stevens B, Koren G (1998) Evidence-based pain management for infants. *Current Opinion in Pediatrics* **10** (2): 203–7.

Steward DJ (1982) Preterm infants are more prone to complications following minor surgery than are term infants. *Anesthesiology* **56**: 304–6.

Tait AR, Malviya S, Veopel-Lewis T *et al.* (2001) Risk factors for perioperative adverse events in children with upper respiratory tract infections. *Anaesthesia* **95** (2): 299–306.

Taylor A (1998) Pain assessment in children. In Twycross A, Moriarty A, Betts T (ed.) *Paediatric Pain Management. A Multi-Disciplinary Approach.* Radcliffe, Oxford.

Thibault M, Girard F, Moumdjian R *et al.* (2007) Craniotomy site influences postoperative pain following neurosurgical procedures: a retrospective study. *Canadian Journal of Anaesthesiology* **54** (7): 544–8.

Thompson KL, Varni JW (1986) A developmental cognitive-biobehavioral approach to pediatric pain assessment. *Pain* **25**: 283–66.

Towler J (2001) Cleansing traumatic wounds with swabs, water or saline. *Journal of Wound Care* **10** (6): 231–4.

Tritle N, Haller J, Gray S (2001) Aesthetic comparison of wound closure techniques in a porcine model. *Laryngoscope* **111** (11): 1949–51.

Twycross A (1998a) Perceptions about paediatric pain. In Twycross A, Moriarty A, Betts T ed. *Paediatric Pain Management. A Multi-Disciplinary Approach.* Radcliffe, Oxford.

Twycross A (1998b) Non-drug methods of pain control. In Twycross A, Moriarty A, Betts T (eds) *Paediatric Pain Management. A Multi-Disciplinary Approach.* Radcliffe, Oxford.

Twycross A (2002) Managing pain in children: an observational study. *NT Research* **7** (3): 164–78.

Twycross A, Mayfield C, Savory J (1999) Pain management for children with special needs: a neglected area? *Paediatric Nursing* **11** (6): 43–45.

Unruh A, McGrath P, Cunningham SJ, Humphreys P (1983) Children's drawings of their pain. *Pain* **17**: 385–92.

Urschitz MS, Wolff J, Von Einem V *et al.* (2003) Reference values for nocturnal home pulse oximetry during sleep in primary school children. *Chest* **121** (1): 96–101.

Vuolo JC (2006) Assessment and management of surgical wounds in clinical practice. *Nursing Standard* **20** (52): 46–56.

Walco GA, Cassidy RC, Schechter NL (1994) Pain, hurt and harm: the ethics of pain control in infants and children. *New England Journal of Medicine* **331** (8): 541–4.

Walker I, Lockie J (2000) Basic techniques for anaesthesia. In Sumner E, Hatch DJ (eds) *Paediatric Anaesthesia*, 2nd ed. Arnold, London.

Watcha M (2000) The immediate recovery period. In Sumner E, Hatch DJ (eds) *Paediatric Anaesthesia*, 2nd ed. Arnold, London.

Welborn LG, Ramirez N, Oh TH *et al.* (1986) Postanesthetic apnea and periodic breathing in infants. *Anesthesiology* **65**: 658–61.

White R, Cooper R, Kingsley A (2002) A topical issue: the use of antibacterials in wound pathogen control. In White R, Harding K (eds) *Trends in Wound Care*. Quay Books, Bath.

Wise J (1999) Perioperative nursing. *Professional Nurse* **15** (1): 59–60.

Wolf AR, Stoddart PA, Murphy PJ, Sasada M *et al.* (2002) Rapid skin anaesthesia using high velocity lignocaine particles: a prospective placebo controlled trial. *Archives of Disease in Childhood* **86** (3): 309–12.

Wong D, Baker C (1988) Pain in children: comparison of assessment scales. *Pediatric Nursing* **14** (1): 9–17.

Wood CJ (1998) Endotracheal suctioning: a literature review. *Intensive and Critical Care Nursing* **14**: 124–36.

Woodgate R, Kristjanson LJ (1995) Young children's behavioural responses to acute pain: strategies for getting better. *Journal of Advanced Nursing* **22** (2): 243–9.

Xavier G (1999) Asepsis. *Nursing Standard* **13** (36): 49–53.

Yaster M, Deshpande JK (1988) Management of pediatric pain with opiod analgesics. *Pediatrics* **113**: 421–9.

Zeitz K, McCutcheon H (2002) Policies that drive the nursing practice of postoperative observations. *International Journal of Nursing Studies* **39**: 831–9.

4   Hydrocephalus

Hydrocephalus means excessive fluid within the cranial cavity. However, in a medical context, hydrocephalus is defined as a disturbance of cerebrospinal fluid (CSF) circulation causing the accumulation of intraventricular CSF, resulting in progressive ventricular dilatation (Mori *et al.* 1995). Hydrocephalus is virtually always due to an increase in the resistance of CSF flow within the CSF circulatory pathways resulting in an increase in CSF pressure, with the exception of rare disorders of excessive CSF production, for example as a result of a brain tumour.

An understanding of hydrocephalus is important for all healthcare professionals working within a neurosurgical environment because children admitted with hydrocephalus form a major part of the workload. Healthcare professionals must be able to recognize and act promptly when a child with hydrocephalus presents with acute raised intracranial pressure, outlined in Chapter 2, Section 3, and meet the long-term needs of the child and family. This chapter will provide an overview of the pathophysiology, epidemiology and classification, presentation and treatment options for children with hydrocephalus. Cerebrospinal fluid shunt management will be discussed in depth because healthcare professionals must understand the principles of shunts and their complications if appropriate care and support is to be provided for the child and family.

At the end of reading this chapter you will be able to:

Learning outcomes

- Appreciate the diverse needs of children who have hydrocephalus
- Describe in depth the care required for the child and family, where the child has a ventricular shunt
- Recognize the signs and symptoms of acute shunt failure.

4.1 Pathophysiology

CSF is produced in the choroid plexus primarily located in the lateral ventricles. From here CSF flows through the foramen of Monro to the third ventricle and continues via the aqueduct of Sylvius to the fourth ventricle. CSF leaves the fourth ventricle via the two foramina of Luschka and the foramen of Magendie, where it circulates within the subarachnoid space around the brain and spinal cord. CSF is reabsorbed into the blood stream via capillaries on the surface of the cerebral hemispheres (Chapter 1, Figure 1.5a). The lateral ventricles are deep within the cerebral hemispheres below the corpus callosum and above the thalamus, the third ventricle is situated at the junction of the midbrain and forebrain and the fourth ventricle is located between the brain stem and the cerebellum (Chapter 1, Figure 1.4a). Ventricular enlargement causes compression and destruction of adjacent brain structures, cerebral oedema, raised intracranial pressure and ultimately affects brain functioning (Fletcher *et al.* 1996; Del Bigio 1993).

Points to consider

The effect ventricular dilation has on the intracranial pressure will depend on the compliance of the skull and the speed of the increase.

In newborn babies and infants the skull is expandable because the skull sutures have not fused. A rise in CSF levels within the ventricles will cause an increase in head size to accommodate the ventricular enlargement. There will be a rapid decrease in pressure after treatment; the final intraventricular pressure will be relatively low and the ventricles will be large compared to children without hydrocephalus (Brett and Harding 1997). Expansion of skull sutures compensates for the increased ventricular size and prevents acute rises in intracranial pressure. In older children and adolescents, where the skull sutures have fused, there will be slow ventricular enlargement, relatively small final ventricular size, and relatively high intraventricular pressure after treatment (Brett and Harding 1997). Raised intracranial pressure with a high intraventricular pressure can develop in older children with very small increases in CSF levels and minimal ventricular dilation.

Although hydrocephalus is often viewed as a disorder of CSF imbalance, it is becoming increasingly recognized that there are disruptions to both the grey and white matters within the brain, particularly in the periventricular region (Fletcher *et al.* 1996; Del Bigio 1993). White matter changes include axonal damage and demyelination of the nerve fibres. Grey matter changes include disorganization of neurons and dendrite deterioration. In addition there may be associated brain malformations and primary neuronal damage that has occurred during the embryonic stages of development. The varied pathology of hydrocephalus may account for diversity of cognitive and visuomotor problems that may occur in children with hydrocephalus.

4.2 Incidence, classification and aetiology

Incidence

The overall incidence of hydrocephalus is 0.2–4.2 per 1000 births (Ingalls *et al.* 1954; Edwards 1958; Blackburn and Fineman 1994; Carey *et al.* 1994). The true incidence is difficult to establish because of different data collection methods, differing inclusion and exclusion criteria in the range of conditions that may result in hydrocephalus, and variations in the age ranges between studies.

The prevalence of hydrocephalus is an important consideration because it is a long-term condition with 75 per cent of children requiring a permanent shunt that diverts excess CSF fluid from the ventricles into another body cavity (Fernell and Hagberg 1998; Chumas *et al.* 2001). The crude mean prevalence rate for infantile hydrocephalus had been estimated to be 0.6 per 1000 births (Fernell *et al.* 1994; Fernell and Hagberg 1998), which may be declining due to improvements in neonatal care (Fernell and Hagberg 1998). However, these studies excluded neural tube defects and brain tumours, which can be associated with the development of hydrocephalus.

Classification

There have been several systems of classifying hydrocephalus including:

- Communicating hydrocephalus, where the blockage of CSF flow occurs outside the ventricular system, and non-communicating hydrocephalus where the blockage of CSF flow occurs within the ventricular system.
- Congenital and acquired hydrocephalus (Brett and Harding 1997).

The traditional classifications may not reflect the diversity of conditions that may cause hydrocephalus, or provide a link between the cause and potential outcomes. Mori *et al.* (1995) have attempted to classify non-tumoural hydrocephalus in children and adults to establish if any links exist between the classification of hydrocephalus and eventual outcomes.

Points to consider

Three major groups of hydrocephalus were identified:

- Congenital hydrocephalus divided into fetal, infantile and hydrocephalus associated with encephalocele or myelomeningocele
- Idiopathic adult hydrocephalus
- Secondary hydrocephalus divided into post-haemorrhagic hydrocephalus of the neonate, post-meningitic hydrocephalus, post-subarachnoid haemorrhage and post-traumatic hydrocephalus.

(Mori *et al.* 1995)

Congenital hydrocephalus is by far the largest group accounting for 50 per cent of all cases, followed by hydrocephalus occurring as a consequence of intraventricular haemorrhage (10 per cent), and as a complication of meningitis (7 per cent) (Mori *et al.* 1995).

Aetiology

Hydrocephalus comprises a highly diverse group of disorders that have little in common except an increase in the volume of CSF within the intracranial fluid spaces. The causes of hydrocephalus relating to the altered pathophysiology and the age of the child are summarized in Figures 4.2a and 4.2b respectively.

Congenital hydrocephalus

The most common cause of congenital hydrocephalus is aqueduct stenosis, accounting for about 15 per cent of all cases, usually occurring sporadically within families (Brett and Harding 1997). Aqueduct stenosis can be the result of a range of anatomical abnormalities at the aqueduct of Sylvius. For example the single aqueduct may not have formed properly and consists of many

Altered pathophysiology	Examples
Over secretion of CSF	• Papilloma of the choroid plexus
Obstruction of CSF pathways: Intraventricular blockage	• Inflammation, intraventricular haemorrhage
Foramen of Monro	• Tumours such as astrocytomas
Third ventricle	• Tumours such as craniopharyngioma • Aqueduct stenosis
Fourth ventricle	• Tumours and cysts, congenital malformations such as Arnold-Chiari and Dandy Walker • Haematomas, membranous obstruction of the foramen of Magendie
Extraventricular blockage	• Inflammation, tumours
Deficient reabsorption	• Venous hypertension • Compression of venous sinuses • Absence of villi • Increases venous pressure for example vein of Galen malformation
Unknown mechanisms	• Spinal cord tumours • Guillain-Barré syndrome • High CSF protein levels

Figure 4.2a Causes of hydrocephalus relating to altered pathophysiology

Age group	Cause
Fetal	• Myelomenigocele, encephalocele • Holoprosencehaly, corpus callosum agenesis • Chromosomal abnormalities • Prenatal haemorrhage • Prenatal infections such as toxoplasmosis • Prenatal tumours • Congenital malformation such as aqueduct stenosis
Infants	• Congenital malformation such as aqueduct stenosis • Dandy-Walker syndrome and related malformations, and Arnold-Chiari malformations • Late manifestations of prenatal causes • Intraventricular haemorrhage in the premature infant • Meningitis • Tumours and cysts • Vascular anomalies for example aneurysm of vein of Galen
Childhood	• Late manifestations of infant causes • Tumours such as posterior fossa tumour • Meningitis • Traumatic brain injury

Figure 4.2b Causes of hydrocephalus according to age

small channels or there may be a membrane across the aqueduct. The result is blockage or reduced CSF flow between the third and fourth ventricles.

The Arnold-Chiari malformation, which may also be referred to simply as Chiari malformation, is a complex deformity of the craniocerebral structures and is often associated with hydrocephalus and myelomeningiocele (Brett and Harding 1997). The malformation can range from mild forms where there is downward displacement of the medulla oblongata and cerebellar tonsils through the foramen magnum, to severe forms where there is downward herniation of the cerebellum hemispheres that causes a corresponding upward herniation of the vermix (midline portion) of the cerebellum and distortion of the brainstem. Distortion of the brainstem can potentially block the flow of CSF resulting in the development of hydrocephalus.

Dandy-Walker syndrome is characterized by a small, hypoplastic cerebella and a greatly distended fourth ventricle, and is often associated with facial and cardiovascular abnormalities. In 70 per cent of cases there will be hydrocephalus, cerebellar ataxia and mental retardation (Brett and Harding 1997).

Secondary causes of hydrocephalus

An important cause of secondary hydrocephalus is post-haemorrhagic hydrocephalus of the neonate, with 30–50 per cent of infants born under 1500grams at risk of intraventricular haemorrhage (Pikus *et al.* 1997). The overall prevalence of infantile hydrocephalus is 0.55–0.6 per 1000 live births (Fernell *et al.* 1994; Fernell and Hagberg 1998). However, the prevalence of hydrocephalus increases as the gestational age of the infant decreases, with the prevalence in infants born less than 32 weeks gestation between 13.7–25.4 per 1000 births (Fernell *et al.* 1994; Fernell and Hagberg 1998). This higher prevalence rate has been directly attributed to the susceptibility of pre-term infants to intraventricular haemorrhages (Fernell and Hagberg 1998). The fluctuations in prevalence of hydrocephalus in the young neonate is probably due to advances in neonatal care, which have improved the survival rates of very pre-term infants, but has the potential to both increase and decrease neurological sequelae. The initial increase in neurological problems is probably the result of a decrease in the gestational survival age but then improves as experience and technology of caring for the younger neonate expands (Meadow *et al.* 2004). Depending upon the severity of the bleed, intraventricular haemorrhages can cause a blockage within the ventricles and secondary obstruction due to permanent scar damage.

Other secondary causes of hydrocephalus in childhood include post-meningitis, post-subarachnoid haemorrhage and post-traumatic brain injury, which can result in adhesions between the epithelial linings of the CSF spaces that obstruct the flow of CSF. Tumours, depending upon their anatomical position within the brain and size, have the potential to obstruct the flow of CSF. Posterior fossa tumours are an important cause of hydrocephalus in older children. Rare causes of hydrocephalus include arteriovenous malformations, obstruction of venous sinuses, craniosynostosis, hypersecretion of CSF, intrauterine infectious diseases, prenatal haemorrhage and congenital tumours.

4.3   Clinical presentation, diagnosis and management options

The age hydrocephalus develops is important because of the differing presentation between the infant and older child (Kirkpatrick *et al.* 1989). Furthermore, the causes of hydrocephalus are different across the age span and age may influence management options and functional outcomes (Figure 4.2b) (Mori *et al.* 1995). The presentation and diagnosis in infants and older children will be outlined separately.

Clinical presentation and diagnosis

Fetal hydrocephalus

Fetal hydrocephalus can be diagnosed as early as the 13th week of gestation by ultrasound scan, where the size of the lateral ventricle is compared with the whole of the brain. However, diagnosis is not usually confirmed until the 20th–22nd week of pregnancy because of greater accuracy of ultrasound as a diagnostic tool at this gestational age. Dilated ventricles are not necessarily specific to hydrocephalus, therefore amniocentesis is advocated to assist in ensuring an accurate diagnosis is made. Amniocentesis is performed to obtain samples of amniotic fluid, which is tested for alpha-fetoprotein levels and to identify chromosomal abnormalities. If severe brain malformations are suspected termination may be offered. However, the timing of amniocentesis is often difficult due to the gestational period when tests results are more reliable. The overall prognosis of fetal hydrocephalus is poor with children often having multiple long-term neurological impairments and learning difficulties (Mori *et al.* 1996). Many pregnancies result in spontaneous abortions or stillbirths (Kirkinen *et al.* 1996).

Infantile hydrocephalus

An infant's skull bones remain separated at the suture sites. Unless there is a rapid increase in intracranial volume, any increase in intracranial contents, such as an increase in ventricle size, will result in an expansion of head size, preventing the intracranial pressure rising. Until compensatory mechanisms fail the infant with hydrocephalus will not present with the classic signs and symptoms of raised intracranial pressure (Chapter 2, Section 3). However, the signs of a rapidly increasing head circumference, tense anterior fontanelle, spayed skull sutures, scalp vein distension, loss of upward gaze and neck rigidity should make the diagnosis of hydrocephalus relatively straight forward in this age group (Kirkpatrick *et al.* 1989). Vomiting and irritability are important additional symptoms. It is worth noting that it has been estimated that up to 50 per cent of infants with hydrocephalus will be asymptomatic (Kirkpatrick *et al.* 1989). Table 4.3a provides a summary of the presentation of hydrocephalus in children.

It is more common for infants to develop a very slowly evolving hydrocephalus, sometimes referred to as occult hydrocephalus, rather than an acute expansion of the ventricles. Diagnosis is made following systematic serial measurements of the head circumference, with computerized tomography (CT) scanning confirming the diagnosis.

Hydrocephalus in older children

Unlike the infant, the skull in the older child cannot expand easily to compensate for the increased ventricular size resulting in signs of acute raised intracranial pressure. The older child is more likely to present with the classic signs of acute raised intracranial pressure: headache, pappilloedema and vomiting (Table 4.3a). CT or magnetic resonance imaging (MRI) scanning will be necessary to establish the cause of the raised intracranial pressure. However, imaging is a static investigation and cannot indicate the degree of raised intracranial pressure and direct pressure monitoring may be necessary to identify the extent of raised intracranial pressure (Kirkpatrick *et al.* 1989).

Table 4.3a Clinical presentation of hydrocephalus in infants and children

Infants less than 2 years of age	Children over 2 years of age
Symptoms of raised intracranial pressure are usually a late sign	More likely to have signs of raised intracranial pressure, vomiting, headache, pappiloedema and there may be altered levels of consciousness
Increasing head size	There may be slight increases in head size because up to about 12 years of age raised ICP may result in splaying of the cranial sutures
The anterior fontanelle will usually be large and tense even when the infant is in the sitting position and there will be splaying of the cranial sutures	
The infant often has a characteristic appearance with a small face in comparison to head size and the eyes have a typical sun setting appearance where the sclera is not visible below the iris due to difficulty in the ability to gaze upward Nystagmus may present	Visual problems such as strabismus, nystagmus
Poor feeding, vomiting	Vomiting, poor appetite
Lethargy and irritability	Lethargy, behavioural changes, altered school performance
Developmental delay	Ataxia

Management options

The management of hydrocephalus will depend on the cause and severity of the CSF obstruction. Very rarely hydrocephalus can arrest of its own accord. However, treatment must be balanced with the potential risk of compromising normal brain development.

Conservative management of hydrocephalus

The range of conservative treatments available for the management of hydrocephalus includes:

- Compressive head wrapping (Meyer *et al.* 1973; Epstein *et al.* 1974; Porter 1975).
- Regular CSF removal, for example lumbar punctures or ventricular taps (Ventriculomegaly Trial Group 1990).
- Diuretics (frusemide, acetazolomide), which decrease CFS production (Shinnar *et al.* 1985; International PHVD Drug Trial Group 1998; Kennedy *et al.* 2001).
- Intraventricular fibrinolytic therapy (streptokinase, recombinant tissue plasminogen activator) for hydrocephalus that occurs as a result of intraventricular haemorrhage (Whitelaw *et al.* 1992; Whitelaw *et al.* 1996).

Conservative management is rarely a long-term option for the treatment of hydrocephalus and is generally reserved for the premature infant post-intraventricular haemorrhage. In these acutely sick infants shunts are difficult to place and are more susceptible to shunt complications, particularity infections and blockages, necessitating repeated revisions (Pikus *et al.* 1997). Unfortunately there is little evidence to support the effectiveness of conservative treatments for hydrocephalus (Ventriculomegaly Trial Group 1990; Whitelaw *et al.* 1996; Kennedy *et al.* 2001). The majority of children who commence conservative treatment eventually require the insertion of a shunt (Ventriculomegaly Trial Group 1990; Whitelaw *et al.* 1996; Kennedy *et al.* 2001). Furthermore, the potential risk of CSF infection is significant due to the frequency and invasive nature of many of the procedures (Ventriculomegaly Trial Group 1990). Ventricular taps have the additional potential complication of puncture porencephaly (Chumas *et al.* 2001). The use of diuretics has been associated with increased neurological morbidity (International PHVD Drug Trial Group 1998).

Surgical management of hydrocephalus

The two main surgical procedures used to treat hydrocephalus are: endoscopic third ventriculostomy, where an opening is made through the third ventricle; and chiasmatic cistern facilitating cerebrospinal fluid drainage, and the insertion of a ventricular shunt system. The vast majority of children with hydrocephalus are managed by the surgical insertion of a ventricular shunt (Fernell and Hagberg 1998; Chumas *et al.* 2001). Ventricular shunts are discussed in Section 4.

Endoscopic third ventriculostomy has an advantage in that unlike ventricular shunts there is no need for a permanent implant (Cinalli *et al.* 1998). Early attempts at ventriculostomies resulted in mortality rates of 54 per cent (Laurence and Coates 1962). However, improvements in optical technology have made endoscopic third ventriculostomy a reasonable alternative to shunts for children with obstructive hydrocephalus. Current mortality rates are lower than 1.5 per cent and success, in terms of achieving a patent CSF pathway, is between 58–76 per cent (Cinalli *et al.* 1998; Hopf *et al.* 1999; Fukuhara *et al.* 2000; Gorayeb *et al.* 2004). Unfortunately, to achieve a successful outcome 20 per cent of children will undergo more than one procedure (Cinalli *et al.* 1998). Successful outcome appears to relate to the underlying cause of the hydrocephalus and age of the patient (Cinalli *et al.* 1998; Hopf *et al.* 1999; Fukuhara *et al.* 2000; Gorayeb *et al.* 2004). Failure rates are higher in children less than 1 year of age (Cinalli *et al.* 1998; Hopf *et al.* 1999; Gorayeb *et al.* 2004).

Endoscopic third ventriculostomy is only appropriate for hydrocephalus that occurs as a result of direct obstruction of the third ventricle primarily as a result of aqueduct stenosis, toxoplasmosis, tumours of the midbrain and posterior fossa, and Chiari malformations (Cinalli *et al.* 1998; Hopf *et al.* 1999; Fukuhara *et al.* 2000; Gorayeb *et al.* 2004). Successful outcome is linked to the underlying condition causing the hydrocephalus with a reported 95 per cent success rate for tumours, 55–80 per cent for aqueduct stenosis and 45 per cent for Chiari malformations (Cinalli *et al.* 1998; Hopf *et al.* 1999; Fukuhara *et al.* 2000; Gorayeb *et al.* 2004). However, it is not always easy to determine which children will benefit because of associated problems that may contribute to the development of hydrocephalus, such as poor CSF absorption (Siomin *et al.* 2002).

Complications of endoscopic third ventriculostomy are primarily a result of intra-operative haemorrhage and postoperative meningitis, which occur in 5–11 per cent of procedures (Cinalli *et al.* 1998; Hopf *et al.* 1999; Fukuhara *et al.* 2000; Gorayeb *et al.* 2004). There do not appear to be any studies that evaluate the morbidity following endoscopic third ventriculostomy in terms of the child's long-term neurological functioning. Despite the variable success rate of endoscopic third ventriculostomy, it is a potential option for obstructive hydrocephalus and, if successful, negates the need for a shunt. In children where the endoscopic third ventriculostomy has failed a shunt is required to manage the hydrocephalus.

Points to consider

In general, no specific preoperative care is required for the child undergoing ventriculostomy. However, it is vitally important that the child and family fully understand the potential risks of the procedure and that failure may result in the child requiring further surgery and potential shunt insertion. In the immediate postoperative period it is usual practice for the child to be nursed upright to encourage CSF drainage and maintain the patency of the new opening. Postoperative observations, including a detailed neurological assessment, are essential to detect haemorrhage and infection. Follow up is vital to monitor the success of the procedure.

External causes that cause pressure in the ventricles

Hydrocephalus caused by external pressure, for example the presence of a tumour or haematoma, which blocks the CSF pathways, will initially and, where possible, be treated by removal of the lesion to restore CSF circulation. However, immediate postoperative oedema and later postoperative complications such as the development of scar tissue and adhesions can result in a secondary blockage of the CSF pathways, necessitating the insertion of a shunt. If tumour resection is not immediately advisable or there is a sudden acute raise in intracranial pressure caused by compression of CSF pathways, a shunt or an external ventricular drain may be the first treatment option (Vernon-Levett and Geller 1997).

Fetal surgery

There have been recent developments in the surgical treatment of hydrocephalus in the fetal period. Procedures such as ventriculoamniotic shunting have the potential to prevent ventricular dilation. However, in general fetal surgery is new and remains experimental (Manning *et al.* 1986; Sutton *et al.* 2001).

4.4 Ventricular shunts

Shunts were developed in the late 1950s as a method of managing hydrocephalus because of the poor outcome for these children if left untreated. Ventricular shunting operations aim to divert CSF from the ventricles to another body cavity. This is achieved by inserting a catheter into the ventricles, known as the proximal catheter, via a burr hole usually made in the temporal bone of the skull, just behind the ear. The proximal catheter is attached to a unidirectional valve. The valve is placed outside the skull just under the skin. The valve is attached to a second catheter, known as the distal catheter. The other end of this second catheter is placed into a body cavity such as the peritoneum (ventriculoperitoneal shunts) or the left atrium (ventriculoatrial shunts) (Figure 4.4a). Ventriculoatrial shunts were initially the preferred technique (Pudenz *et al.* 1957; Spitz 1959), however, higher mortality rates and life-threatening complications such as bacteraemia, nephritis, pulmonary emboli and cardiac tamponade with ventriculoatrial shunts has resulted in the peritoneum being the preferred site for distal catheter placement (Forrest and Cooper 1968; Keucher and Mealey 1979). Furthermore ventriculoperitoneal shunts are technically easier to insert, catheters can be of sufficient length to allow for growth and there is

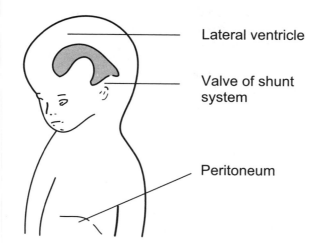

Lateral ventricle

Valve of shunt system

Peritoneum

Figure 4.4a Position of a ventriculoperitoneal shunts

good absorption of CSF across the peritoneum. Potentially shunts can be placed in the pleural space or lumbar subarachnoid space, but these sites are rarely used.

Shunt designs

Since the original designs in the 1950s (Pudenz 1981), there has been a myriad of developments in intraventricular shunt systems, particularly shunt valves. Currently valve designs include silicone rubber slit valves, silicone rubber diaphragm valves, silicone rubber mitre valves and metallic spring ball valves. However, all valves operate on the same principle; the valve has a threshold pressure below which the valve remains closed and above which the valve opens allowing CSF to flow through the shunt system. Different valve systems have different resistant pressures. In general, standard valve classifications are based upon their opening pressures: low pressure ($5cmH_2O$) medium pressure ($10cmH_2O$) and high pressure ($15mmH_2O$) valves (Drake and Kestle 1996). In addition to the range of valve designs, valves and catheters are available in different sizes.

A functional problem with the design of shunt valves is CSF flow increases when the child is upright due to the effects of gravity resulting in over-drainage of the ventricles (Pudenz and Foltz 1991). This occurs because when in an upright posture a larger pressure differential exists between the head and abdomen, resulting in CSF flowing at a higher rate than when a child is lying flat. Two shunt systems particularly advocated for use in children to overcome problems of over-drainage are the Orbis-Sigma valve (Cordis Corporation) and the Delta valve (Medtronic PS Medical) (Drake *et al.* 1998). The Orbis-Sigma valve has a flexible diaphragm and operates on a flow pressure system, which differs from traditional valves. The valve has a piston system which is capable, to some extent, of regulating CSF flow across different pressure gradients. The Delta valve is a standard valve with an inbuilt anti-siphon device. A relatively new concept in shunt design is programmable pressure valves, where the pressure setting of the valve can be adjusted non-invasively by applying the programmer (a device that records the pressure with the valve and alters the valve setting by magnetic impulses). The advantage of the programmable valve is that precise pressure adjustments can be made to suit individual needs, reducing the potential problems of under- or over-drainage (Yamashita *et al.* 1999). However, these types of shunts may not be suitable for all causes of hydrocephalus.

Despite the range of shunts available and the need for a trouble-free system, there has only been one clinical trail to date which compares the efficacy of shunt systems (Chumas *et al.* 2001). Unfortunately, Drake *et al.*'s (1998) randomized controlled trial of shunt valve designs for use in children with hydrocephalus could not recommend any one design. The choice of valve depends on many factors such as the age of child, the intracranial pressure and the predicted final intraventricular pressure, but ultimately is the surgeon's preference.

Complications of shunts

A trouble free shunt is a desirable but currently elusive goal and, unfortunately, once inserted a shunt is a permanent implant and prone to complications (Chumas *et al.* 2001). The complication rate for shunts is between 45–50 per cent (Piatt and Carson 1993; Drake *et al.* 1998; Tuli *et al.* 2004) with 70 per cent of children requiring at least one revision during their lifetime (Drake *et al.* 1998). Forty percent of shunt malfunctions occur during the first year following insertion and a further 14 per cent during the second year following insertion (Drake *et al.* 1998). The mortality rate for shunt-related deaths remains high at approximately 12 per cent within 10 years of insertion (Tuli *et al.* 2004).

Points to consider

Shunt malfunction results in the child requiring hospitalization and surgery to revise the shunt to prevent severe neurological complications or death occurring (Rekate 1991). Shunt malfunction is a major issue for children with hydrocephalus.

Shunt complications can be broadly divided into three groups: infection, mechanical failure and functional problems (Table 4.4a). The most common causes of shunt failure are mechanical obstruction (72–84 per cent), infection (16–18 per cent) and over-drainage (8 per cent) (Piatt and Carson 1993; Drake *et al.* 1998).

A range of factors have been investigated in an attempt to establish possible factors that may contribute to shunt malfunction including:

- The age of the child.
- The child's underlying condition.
- The length of time following insertion of the shunt.
- Type of shunt system.
- Position of the shunt reservoir.
- Surgeon experience and case load.
- The use of perioperative antibiotics and rigid infection control procedures within the theatre environment.

> (Piatt and Carson 1993; Drake *et al.* 1998; Tuli *et al.* 2000; Cochrane and Kestle 2003;Choksey and Malik 2004; Enger *et al.* 2004; Smith *et al.* 2004)

The younger the age of the child (particularly infants under 6 months of age) at the time of the initial shunt placement, the greater the risk of shunt malfunction (Piatt and Carson 1993; Drake *et al.* 1998; Tuli *et al.* 2000). Children under 1 year of age have a 20 per cent greater chance of shunt failure malfunction following initial insertion of the shunt compared with children over

Table 4.4a Main complications of ventricular shunts

Complication	Examples
Infection causes colonisation of the shunt system which becomes blocked with bacteria debris	Meningitis Wound infection Peritonitis (ventriculoperitoneal shunts) Septicaemia (ventriculoatrial shunts)
Mechanical failure can result in malfunction or blockage of system	Proximal obstruction: the catheter becomes lodged in tissue such as choroid plexus, brain tissue
	Distal obstruction: the development of intra-abdominal cysts, CSF ascites
	Catheter misplacement: intracranial, intra-abdominal, intravascular
	Fractures and disconnections of the catheter Migration of catheter into hollow viscera such as bladder or inguinal canal
Functional failure	Over drainage
	Under drainage
	Miscellaneous problems affection shunt functioning: *Intracranial hypotension* *Post-shunt pericerebal collections* *Slit ventricle syndrome*

1 year (Tuli *et al.* 2000). Shunt malfunction is more likely to occur in children where infection or intraventricular haemorrhage is the cause of the hydrocephalus and again more likely to occur in the neonate (Piatt and Carson 1993). Neurosurgeons with a high caseload of children with hydrocephalus, and working within large neurosurgical centres appear to have a lower mortality rate and lower shunt infection rate compared to neurosurgeons with a low caseload and working in small centres (Cochrane and Kestle 2003; Smith *et al.* 2004,).

There is a wide variance in reported incidence of infections of shunts, from 0.5–18 per cent (Piatt and Carson 1993; Drake *et al.* 1998; Vinchon *et al.* 2002; Choksey and Malik 2004; Enger *et al.* 2004). The lower rate was attributed to the adoption of strict infection control protocols and the administration of prophylactic antibiotics periopertaively, resulting in infection rates of 0.5 per cent (Choksey and Malik 2004).

Recognizing and managing shunt malfunctions in children

Shunt failure results in progressive hydrocephalus and consequently raised intracranial pressure (Kirkpatrick *et al.* 1989).

Points to consider

The classic signs of raised intracranial pressure, headache, vomiting and paplioedema, may not always be present in children with shunt failure (Kirkpatrick *et al.* 1989). Detecting shunt malfunction in children is not an easy task as many of the signs and symptoms are common to general childhood illnesses.

Some children may be relatively symptom free but the shunt may be failing, while other children may present with symptoms for only 24 hours before raised intracranial pressure develops to a critical life-threatening level (Kirkpatrick *et al.* 1989; Iskandar *et al.* 1998; Garton *et al.* 2001; Barnes *et al.* 2002).

Points to consider

Understanding the signs and symptoms of shunt malfunction is an essential aspect of caring for children with hydrocephalus.

Headache, vomiting and drowsiness are the classic symptoms of shunt malfunction but are the same presenting symptoms of many childhood disorders particularly viral infections (Watkins *et al.* 1994; Barnes *et al.* 2002). Consequently between 40–60 per cent of children who present with a potential shunt malfunction ultimately have an alternative diagnosis such as gastroenteritis, otitis media, tonsillitis, low-pressure headache, chest infections, migraine and urinary tract infections (Watkins *et al.* 1994; Barnes *et al.* 2002).

Points to consider

The signs and symptoms of shunt malfunction include:

- Headache
- Vomiting
- Drowsiness or lethargy
- Decreased levels of consciousness
- Irritability
- Bulging fontanelle in the infant
- Loss of developmental milestones
- Behavioural changes
- Strabismus
- Neck retraction
- Distended neck veins.

(Kirkpatrick *et al.* 1989; Garton *et al.* 2001)

Loss of consciousness and erythema around the shunt site are 100 per cent predictive of shunt malfunction (Garton *et al.* 2001). The presence of drowsiness, headache and vomiting together are very likely to be predictive of shunt malfunction (Barnes *et al.* 2002). The variability, unreliability, unusual nature and lack of symptoms in some children ultimately require the child to undergo imaging (shunt X-Ray series and CT scanning), and in some children a percutaneous manometry tap will be required to assist in the diagnosis of a shunt malfunction (Watkins *et al.* 1994; Iskandar *et al.* 1998). CT scan is the investigation of choice and is relatively accurate, in that positive scans have a 100 per cent accuracy in detecting shunt malfunction, but there can be false negatives where there is no change in ventricular size but the shunt is blocked (Watkins *et al.* 1994). Therefore it is particularly important to monitored children with a negative scan but who have presenting signs and symptoms of a shunt malfunction. A percutaneous manometry tap, which measures CSF pressure and flow, can assist in diagnosing shunt malfunction, but may not detect proximal catheter blockage or over drainage of the shunt (Watkins *et al.* 1994). However, investigations are not without risks, CT scanning in children often requires sedation and the frequency of scans in some children has the potential to expose these children to excessive amounts of radiation. Shunt tapping is an invasive procedure and has the risk of introducing bacteria into the shunt system which will rapidly multiply in the CSF leading to the development of an infection.

Essential care

A child presenting with acute raised intracranial pressure because of shunt malfunction requires emergency surgery to replace the shunt and re-establish the CSF flow.

If the shunt malfunction is due to a blockage in the shunt system because of colonization with bacteria, the infection must be treated prior to reinsertion of a new shunt system. To maintain the flow of CSF the child will require insertion of an external ventricular drain. The incidence of infection in shunts is between 0.5 and 18 per cent (Piatt and Carson 1993; Drake *et al.* 1998; Vinchon *et al.* 2002; Choksey and Malik 2004; Enger *et al.* 2004). Shunt infections are a significant complication of shunts because of the cost of treating children, the need for added surgical procedures and prolonged hospitalization. Management of the child with an infected shunt is described in Section 4.5.

Functional problems of shunts such as over and under drainage are not always easy to manage. The child may present with a range of general problems but headaches are a particular feature. Under and over drainage of the shunt valve may require surgery to change the valve for one of a different pressure. Subdural haematomas are a potential complication of over drainage.

4.5 Principles of caring for a child requiring insertion or revision of a ventricular shunt

In general, there are few specific perioperative requirements for the child requiring neurosurgery. *Chapter 3* provides details of the perioperative requirements for the child requiring neurosurgery. The specific perioperative care of the child requiring insertion or revision of a ventricular shunt is outlined below. Care of an infected shunt is also discussed.

Preoperative care

Preoperative care will depend primarily on the clinical presentation of the child. A child admitted acutely with raised intracranial pressure, due to a rapidly increasing ventricular size, will require care to be focused on monitoring the child's neurological state and being alert to the immediate dangers of raised intracranial pressure with its potential life-threatening consequences (Chapter 2, Section 3). In addition to performing neurological observations care will be primarily aimed at preparing the child for investigations, primarily CT scanning, and surgery in an organized and structured manner, while offering support to the child and family. The administration of a sedative, if necessary prior to CT scanning, will necessitate increased monitoring of the child because of the compounding effects on an already raised intracranial pressure (Coté *et al.* 2000; Lawson 2000). The child who has been vomiting as a result of increased intracranial pressure will require the insertion of a cannula, measurement of electrolytes and the commencement of intravenous fluids to correct dehydration.

For the infant and child having planned surgery, the emphasis of care will be much more directed towards preparing and supporting the child and family for the procedure. Parents will need information and support to assist them to come to terms with the child's diagnosis. It is necessary to foster an environment which allows the parents to participate and become actively involved in their child's care. Parents will have many questions relating to their child's immediate needs and the long-term impact of living with a child with hydrocephalus. It is important their questions are answered openly and honestly and it may not be possible to give definitive answers because of the uncertain nature of the condition. The Association for Spina Bifida and Hydrocephalus (ASBAH) offer an effective support network and a range of information for children and their families. Parents should be offered contact details for the local ASBAH advisor.

Postoperative care

In addition to the general principles of caring for the child post-neurosurgery, the nurse must ensure care is appropriate for the age of the child and the procedure the child has undergone. The premature infant will be at particular risk of respiratory problems and cardiac instability post-anaesthesia (National Confidential Enquiry into Perioperative Deaths 1999) and will require appropriate monitoring.

The specific immediate potential postoperative complications following insertion of a shunt include intraventricular haemorrhage, blockage of the shunt and subdural haemorrhage as a result of rapid over drainage of the ventricles. The signs of rapid over drainage of the ventricles include: headaches, irritability and pallor, and in the neonate and young infant, a depressed fontanelle. If over drainage is suspected lay the child flat, undertake a rapid assessment of the child to identify if a life-threatening situation has developed and contact the neurosurgeon. Neonates and young infants should be monitored for respiratory depression, which is a potential consequence of rapid ventricular decompression (May 2001). Neurological assessment of the child is vital to detect and manage postoperative complications promptly.

Positioning of the child is an important consideration and will be influenced by the type of shunt inserted; nursing staff must ensure they have clear postoperative instructions. It may be necessary to nurse the child upright in a sitting position but the child must be monitored for signs of over drainage of the ventricles. There is no specific care relating to the shunt once inserted, avoiding lying on the shunt site may prevent skin breakdown particularly in the immediate postoperative period. The practice of routine palpation of the shunt is an outdated practice and there is no evidence to suggest it is of any value (Piatt 1992).

Unless there are associated problems, re-establishing normal routines such as feeding can commence as soon as the child has recovered from the anaesthetic. Until feeding is re-established, intravenous fluids will be required to maintain hydration. The position of the child in theatre and tunnelling of the distal catheter can cause considerable neck discomfort. Pain assessment is important and the child should be given regular analgesia. The usual methods of wound closure are sutures or staples, which are usually removed seven days postoperatively. There may be abdominal sutures following insertion of a ventriculoperitoneal shunt. These are usually subcutaneous and therefore do not require removal. A protective wound dressing is usually applied in theatre but can be removed once the wound surface has sealed, usually by 48 hours. Following removal of the dressing it is not usually necessary to replace it and the child can have a bath and hair washed as normal.

Management of the child with a infected shunt

Standard treatment of infected shunts involves externalization of the ventricular catheter, removal of the shunt valve, which acts as a reservoir for bacteria, and administration of intraventricular antibiotics (Kulkarni *et al.* 2002). Antibiotic therapy usually consists of intrathecal vancomycin and oral or intravenous rifampicin because the most common infective organisms are coagulase-negative *Staphylococcus* and *Staphylococcus aureus* (Kulkarni *et al.* 2002). Modification of antibiotics may be required, depending upon the results of the culture and sensitivity of CSF samples.

An external ventricular drainage (EVD) system is inserted and set up in the operating department under general anaesthesia because the conditions are sterile and the induction of a general anaesthetic prevents distress for the child. A catheter is inserted into one of the lateral ventricles via a burr hole and brought out to the surface through the skull and skin where it is sutured in place. There are a range of EVD systems available but all have similar principles. The systems all have several components: self-sealing injection port, collection chamber, pressure scale mounting port and drainage bag (Figure 4.4b). The ventricular catheter is attached to a flow chamber that allows for drainage and measurement of CSF, and a drainage bag ensures the system remains closed. Occasionally the child's existing shunt catheter is externalized and connected to the EVD system. The system operates by gravity with the flow of CSF dependant on the height of the flow chamber.

The flow chamber is connected to a mounting panel which has pressure scale markings and a zero marker. It is vital that the position of the system is maintained at the appropriate level. Both the flow chamber and mounting panel have adjustable heights which enable the position of the flow chamber to be modified. To ensure there is consistency in positioning of the flow chamber, a zero reference point is needed (Woodward *et al.* 2002). This is usually the midpoint of the ear because this is approximately in line with the lateral ventricles. It is important that the reference point is ascertained with a spirit level to ensure correct position of the drain (Woodward *et al.* 2002).

The actual level the flow chamber requires setting will be prescribed by the neurosurgeon because it will be individual to each child and will depend on the pressure of the CSF measured during surgery and the child's clinical picture. Typical intracranial pressure values are 5–15mmHg, but may be slightly lower in infants (Chitnavis and Polkey 1998; Bullock *et al.* 2000). Once the zero reference point on the child is aligned with the reference point on the mounting chamber, the base of the adjustable flow chamber should be positioned against the prescribed pressure setting. This allows CSF to only flow through the system when the pressure is greater than the prescribed pressure setting.

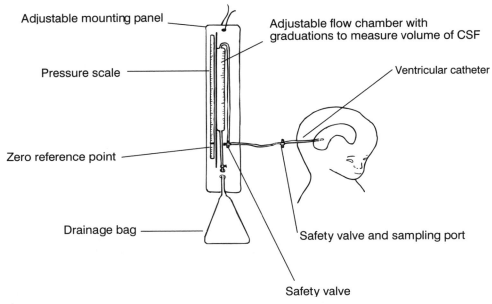

Figure 4.4b External ventricular drainage system

Care of an EVD and monitoring of CSF flow is an important aspect of managing the child with an infected shunt (Woodward *et al.* 2002). The neurosurgeon will provide a guide as to the expected hourly rate of CSF drainage.

Essential care

If the child is suddenly raised above the prescribed position of the system there is a potential for rapid siphoning of CSF from the ventricles into the collecting chamber, with potentially serious neurological consequences.
If the child is positioned below the prescribed position of the system CSF will not drain from the ventricles into the collecting chamber.

The child will require a detailed neurological assessment, usually hourly, to detect signs and symptoms of under or over drainage of the system. Potential complications of an EVD include over or under drainage of CSF, blockage of the system and re-infection or secondary infection. If the system is blocked it may be possible to aspirate/flush the system but this should only be undertaken by an experienced nurse or doctor competent to undertake the procedure. Immediate action is required if the system becomes disconnected. Nurses must be alert to any indication that the system is under or over draining or is blocked.

Best practice recommendations

The principles of caring for a child with an EVD include:

- Assessing the position and patency of the EVD hourly, ensuring the safety valves are open and all tubing is secured
- Checking the zero reference point hourly
- Ensuring the flow chamber is never lower then the reference point, which can result in rapid siphoning of CSF. If the child requires moving then the safety valves should be temporarily closed and reopened when the child is repositioned and the zero reference point reassessed
- The family, and child where appropriate, will require education and support regarding the purpose of the EVD and the necessity to ensure correct positioning of the EVD is maintained
- After measuring and recording the CSF output, empty the flow chamber into the collecting bag hourly and if necessary adjust the flow chamber, within prescribed limits, to ensure there are no excessive variations in the amount of CSF drained each hour
- Reporting excessive variations in CSF volumes or failure of the catheter to drain. CSF is produced at a rate of about 10–20mls/hr
- The drainage bag should be changed when it is three-quarters full, using aseptic technique principles, because over full bags impair drainage
- Observing the insertion site for signs of infection
- Monitoring the colour and clarity of CSF
- Ensuring that any procedures, for example drug administration and CSF sampling which break the closed EVD system, are performed aseptically
- The EVD tubing must be clearly labelled to prevent accidental administration of intravenous drugs into the system.

(Woodward *et al.* 2002)

Essential care

Accidental disconnection of any parts of the system requires prompt action. Leakage of CSF must be prevented by clamping the ventricular catheter. If any parts of the system become disconnected, cover any tubing still connected to the child with a sterile towel or dressing. The EVD system will require changing aseptically. If the ventricular catheter has become totally dislodged then firm pressure must be applied over the wound. The neurosurgeons must be contacted immediately and a decision made relating to re-establishing the EVD system. The child may require repeat surgery.

Points to consider

Signs of under drainage of CSF include:

- Headaches
- Vomiting
- Irritability
- Lethargy
- In infants there will be a tense bulging fontanelle

Signs of over drainage of CSF include:

- Headaches
- Irritability
- Pallor
- In infants there will be a sunken fontanelle.

If sudden over drainage has occurred turn the system off, lay the child flat, undertake a rapid assessment of the child to identify if a life-threatening situation has developed and contact the neurosurgeon.

Policies and procedures should be available in units which care for children with EVD relating to changing the drainage system, unblocking the system if blocked, taking CSF samples and the administration of intrathecal drugs. This is usually in the domain of the doctors, and must follow strict aseptic technique as per hospital policies. CSF sampling and drug administering should be undertaken via the port nearest to the patient. For drug administration it is usual practice to remove a recipient amount of CSF to compensate for the drug fluid volume administered. Saline will need to be inserted into the port after the drug is administered to ensure the drug reaches the ventricles. It is usual practice to close the safety valves for a period of time, usually one hour, following the administration of intrathecal drugs. This prevents the drugs draining into the EVD system and allows for the drugs to circulate within the ventricles. External drainage of CSF depletes the body's normal sodium content, therefore monitoring the child's urea and electrolytes is important. The child will require oral sodium supplements which should be adjusted as appropriate, depending on the amount of CSF drained and plasma sodium levels.

Usually the wound site is covered with a clear occlusive dressing and only changed if it becomes loose or contaminated using a strict aseptic technique. The site should be observed for any signs of redness or swelling that might indicate a wound infection. Leakage of CSF around the site should be reported. An absorbent dry dressing should be firmly applied. If leakage is presented the site may require suturing.

The presence of an EVD results in constraints for the child. These constraints will be further compounded in the child who requires elbow splints to prevent the ventricular catheter being accidentally dislodged. Restrictions to normal activities can be particularly frustrating for the young and active child. The play specialist has a vital role in ensuring the child has appropriate and stimulating activities and ensuring there is family involvement in play and education therapies. Once CSF cultures are negative, there is reduction of the CSF white cell count and the child shows signs of clinical improvement, a new shunt system can be inserted.

Discharge planning and long-term care needs

Discharge planning must involve all the multidisciplinary team and consider the overall needs of the child and potential problems associated with hydrocephalus and its treatments. The child's long-term care needs will depend upon the presence of associated neurological deficits and concomitant conditions (Section 4.6). The child and family will require detailed verbal and written advice regarding detecting signs and symptoms of shunt failure. Parents will require emergency contact details; many units have access to 'an open door policy' (Barnes *et al.* 2002). Prior to discharge it is important to ensure parents and main carers understand the complications of shunts, are aware when and where to obtain healthcare advice and have all the relevant contact details in the event their child becomes unwell (May 2001). There must be effective liaison between the hospital and community team to ensure continuing support following discharge. If the child and family have not already had contact with ASBAH, parents should be given information about the organization and contact information.

4.6 Long- term outcomes and ongoing care needs of a child with hydrocephalus

The mortality rate for untreated hydrocephalus has been estimated to be between 49–80 per cent (Laurence and Coates 1962; Yashon *et al.* 1965). The morbidity of untreated hydrocephalus in regards to the functional outcome appears mixed, with 68 per cent of children having a physical disability and 27 per cent an intelligence quotient below 50 (Laurence and Coates 1962; Yashon *et al.* 1965). These early studies suggest that the outcome for children surviving untreated hydrocephalus is poor and justifies the widespread use of shunts to treat hydrocephalus, despite the potential complications. The mortality rate of children with shunted hydrocephalus is between 4–16 per cent (Casey *et al.* 1997; Fernell and Hagberg 1998; Iskandar *et al.* 1998). There appears to be a paucity of research relating to the long-term outcomes for children with shunted hydrocephalus (Chumas *et al.* 2001). The major difficulties in studying the long-term outcomes of hydrocephalus are distinguishing the effects of treatments and raised intracranial pressure from the underlying brain pathology and underlying aetiology (Del Bigio 1993; Chumas *et al.* 2001; Heinsbergen *et al.* 2002).

Points to consider

Factors which influence the outcome of hydrocephalus include the:

- Underlying aetiology
- Degree of primary brain damage and associated brain malformations
- Degree and duration of ventricular dilation and raised intracranial pressure
- Timing of treatments
- Complications of treatments.

Overall, 40–60 per cent of children with hydrocephalus will have neurological deficits such as physical, cognitive and behavioural difficulties (Casey *et al.* 1997; Hoppe-Hirsch *et al.* 1998). The majority of children with hydrocephalus will attend mainstream school (Casey *et al.* 1997). However, many children will have complex and often subtle learning difficulties, such as recognition memory, prose recall and visuoconstructive memory, and affected serial learning, communication (both verbal and nonverbal), visuospatial perception and visual dexterity (Fletcher *et al.* 1996; Scott *et al.* 1998).

Hydrocephalus that occurs as a result of intraventricular haemorrhage appears to have the worst outcomes in relation to both physical disabilities and intellectual functions, with the extent of the intraventricular haemorrhage a significant prognostic factor (Pikus *et al.* 1997). The outcomes in terms of impairments for children with hydrocephalus due to intraventricular haemorrhage indicate 31 per cent of children will have cerebral palsy, 31 per cent a learning disability, 25 per cent epilepsy and 13 per cent severe visual problems (Fernell and Hagberg 1998). Unfortunately these figures are proportionally higher in babies born before 32 weeks of gestation.

The child's long-term care needs will depend upon the presence of associated neurological deficits and additional conditions. Assessment of mental and cognitive abilities, hearing and visual problems, memory, speech and language difficulties, and musculoskeletal problems are essential if the child with hydrocephalus is to receive appropriate health, social and education input to ensure the child's full potential is reached. Repeated hospitalization can be disruptive and many families are anxious about potential shunt blockages. However, it is important that the family encourage and allow the child opportunities to develop. The transition to adulthood can be difficult, and there may be concerns about independent living, employment and contributing fully within society, relationships and sexuality. It is important that the child and family are offered individualized and appropriate support.

Key messages from this chapter

- Hydrocephalus is a disturbance of CSF circulation causing the accumulation of intraventricular CSF, resulting in progressive ventricular dilatation
- Hydrocephalus is a diverse group of disorders and in children the main causes are congenital hydrocephalus, intraventricular haemorrhage and as a complication of meningitis
- The vast majority of children with hydrocephalus are managed by the surgical insertion of a ventricular shunt
- Shunt malfunction is a major issue for children with hydrocephalus. Shunt complications can be as a result of infection, mechanical failure and functional problems
- Some children with hydrocephalus will have neurological deficits such as physical, cognitive and behavioural difficulties
- The majority of children with hydrocephalus will attend mainstream school but many children will have complex and often subtle learning difficulties.

Web resources

Association for Spina Bifida and Hydrocephalus (ASBAH)
is the leading UK registered charity providing information and advice about spina bifida
and hydrocephalus to individuals, families and carers.
www.asbah.org.uk
Scope
provides support for people with disabilities.
www.scope.org.uk

References

Barnes NP, Jones SJ, Hayward RD, Harkness WJ, Thompson D (2002) Ventriculoperitoneal shunt blockage: what are the best predictive clinical indicators? *Archives of Diseases in Childhood* **87**: 198–201.

Blackburn BL, Fineman RM (1994) Epidemiology of congenital hydrocephalus in Utah 1940–1979: report of an iatrogenically related 'epidemic'. *American Journal of Medical Genetics* **52**: 123–9.

Brett EM, Harding BN (1997) Hydrocephalus and congenital anomalies of the nervous system other than myelomeningocele. In Brett EM (ed.) *Paediatric Neurology*, 3rd edn. Churchill Livingstone, London.

Bullock R, Chestnut RM, Clifton G *et al.* (2000) Guidelines for the management of severe traumatic brain injury. *Journal of Neurotrauma* **17** (6/7): 451–553.

Carey CM, Tullous MW, Walker ML (1994) Hydrocephalus, etiologic, pathological effects, diagnosis and natural history. In Check WR (ed.) *Pediatric Neurosurgery: Surgery of the Developing Nervous System*, 3rd edn. W.B. Saunders, Philadelphia, PA.

Casey AT, Kimmings EJ, Kleinlugtebeld AD *et al.* (1997). The long-term outlook for hydrocephalus in childhood. A ten-year cohort study of 155 patients. *Pediatric Neurosurgery* **27**: 63–70.

Chitnavis BC, Polkey CE (1998) Intracranial pressure monitoring. *Care of the Critically Ill Child* **14** (3): 80–4.

Choksey MS, Malik IA (2004) Zero tolerance to shunt infections: can it be achieved? *Journal of Neurology, Neurosurgery and Psychiatry* **75** (1): 87–91.

Chumas P, Tyagi A, Livingston J (2001) Hydrocephalus – what's new? *Archives of Disease in Childhood. Fetal and Neonatal Edition* **85** (3): 149–54.

Cochrane DD, Kestle JR (2003) The influence of surgical operative experience on the duration of first ventriculoperitoneal shunt function and infection. *Pediatric Neurosurgery* **38** (6): 295–301.

Coté CJ, Notterman DA, Karl HW, Weinberg JA, McCloskey C (2000) Adverse sedation events in pediatrics: a critical incident analysis of contributing factors. *Pediatrics* **105**: 805–14.

Cinalli G, Salazar C, Mallucci C *et al.* (1998) The role of third ventriculostomy in the management of shunt malfunction. *Neurosurgery* **43** (6): 1323–7.

Del Bigio MR (1993) Neuropathological changes caused by hydrocephalus. *Acta Neuropathologica* **85**: 573–85.

Drake JM, Kestle J (1996) Determining the best cerebrospinal fluid shunt valve design: the pediatric valve design trial. *Neurosurgery* **38** (3): 604–7.

Drake JM, Kestle JR, Milner R *et al.* (1998) Randomized trial of cerebrospinal fluid shunt valve design in pediatric hydrocephalus. *Neurosurgery* **43** (2): 294–305.

Edwards JH (1958) Congenital malformations of the central nervous system in Scotland. *British Journal Preventive & Social Medicine* **12**: 115–30.

Enger PØ, Svendsen F, Wester K (2004) CSF shunt infections in children: experiences from a population-based study. *Acta Neurochirurgica (Wien)* **145** (4): 243–8.

Epstein F, Wald A, Hochwald GM (1974) Intracranial pressure during head wrapping in treatment of neonatal hydrocephalus. *Pediatrics* **54**: 786–90.

Fernell E, Hagberg (1998) Infantile hydrocephalus: declining prevalence in preterm infants. *Acta Paediatrica* **87**: 392–6.

Fernell E, Hagberg G, Hagberg B (1994) Infantile hydrocephalus epidemiology: an indicator of enhanced survival. *Archives of Diseases in Childhood, Fetal and Neonatal Edition* **70**: 123–8.

Fletcher JM, McCauley S, Brandt ME *et al.* (1996) Regional brain tissue composition in children with hydrocephalus: relationship with cognitive development. *Archives of Neurology* **53** (6): 549–57.

Forrest DM, Cooper DGW (1968) Complications of ventriculo-artial shunts: a review of 455 cases. *Journal of Neurosurgery* **29**: 506–12.

Fukuhara T, Vorster S, Luciano M (2000) Risk factors for failure of endoscopic third ventriculostomy for obstructive hydrocephalus. *Neurosurgery* **46** (5): 1100–11.

Garton HJ, Kestle JR, Drake JM (2001) Predicting shunt failure on the basis of clinical symptoms and signs in children. *Journal of Neurosurgery* **94**: 202–10.

Gorayeb RP, Cavalheiro S, Zymberg ST (2004) Endoscopic third ventriculostomy in children younger than 1 year of age. *Journal of Neurosurgery* **100** (Suppl 5 Pediatrics): 427–9.

Heinsbergen I, Rotteveel J, Roeleveld N, Grotenhuis A (2002) Outcome in shunted hydrocephalic children. *European Journal of Paediatric Neurology* **6**: 99–107.

Hopf NJ, Grunert P, Fries G, Resch KD, Perneczky A (1999) Endoscopic third ventriculostomy: outcome analysis of 100 consecutive procedures. *Neurosurgery* **44** (4): 795–804.

Hoppe–Hirsch E, Laroussinie F, Brunet L *et al.* (1998) Late outcome of the surgical treatment of hydrocephalus. *Child's Nervous System* **14**: 97–9.

Ingalls TH, Pugh TF, MacMahon B (1954) Incidence of anencephalus, spina bifida and hydrocephalus related to birth rank and maternal age. *British Journal of Preventive & Social Medicine* **8** (1): 17–23.

Iskandar BJ, Tubbs S, Mapstone TB *et al.* (1998) Death in shunted hydrocephalic children in the 1990s. *Pediatric Neurosurgery* **28**: 173–6.

International PHVD Drug Trial Group (1998) International randomised controlled trial of acetazolamide and furosemide in posthaemorrhagic ventricular dilation in infancy. *Lancet* **352**: 433–40.

Kennedy CR, Ayers S, Campbell MJ *et al.* (2001). Randomized controlled trial of acetazolamide and furosemide in posthemorrhagic ventricular dilation in infancy: follow up at 1 year. *Pediatrics* **108** (3): 597–607.

Keucher TR, Mealey J (1979) Long–term results after ventriculoartial and ventriculoperitoneal shunting for infantile hydrocephalus. *Journal of Neurosurgery* **50**: 179–86.

Kirkinen P, Serlo W, Jouppila P, Ryyanen M, Martikainen A (1996) Long-term outcome of fetal hydrocephaly. *Journal of Child Neurology* **11**: 189–92.

Kirkpatrick M, Engleman H, Minns RA (1989) Symptoms and signs of progressive hydrocephalus. *Archives of Disease in Childhood* **64**: 124–8.

Kulkarni AV, Rabin D, Lambert-Pasculli M, Drake JM (2002) Repeated cerebrospinal fluid shunt infections in children. *Pediatric Neurosurgery* **35** (2): 66–71.

Lawson GR (2000) Controversy: Sedation of children for magnetic resonance imaging. *Archives of Disease in Childhood* **82**: 150–4.

Laurence KM, Coates S (1962) The natural history of hydrocephalus. Detailed analysis of 182 unoperated cases. *Archives of Diseases in Childhood* **37**: 345–62.

Manning FA, Harrison MR, Rodeck C (1986) Catheter shunts of fetal hydrocephalus. Report of the International Fetal Surgery Registry. *New England Journal of Medicine* **315**: 336–40.

May L (2001) Hydrocephalus. In May L (ed.) *Paediatric Neurosurgery: A Handbook for the Multidisciplinary Team*. Whurr Publishers, London.

Meadow W, Lee G, Lin K, Lantos J (2004) Changes in mortality for extremely low birth weight infants in the 1990s: implications for treatment decisions and resource use. *Pediatrics* **113** (5): 1223–39.

Meyer H, Price BE, Reubel CD (1973) Complications arising from head wrapping for the treatment of hydrocephalus. *Pediatrics* **52**: 867–8.

Mori K, Shimada J, Kurisaka M, Sato K, Watanabe K (1995) Classification of hydrocephalus and outcome of treatment. *Brain and Development* **17**: 338–4.

National Confidential Enquiry into Perioperative Deaths (1999) *Extremes of Age*. NCEPOD, London.

Piatt JH (1992) Physical examination of patients with cerebrospinal fluid shunts: is there useful information in pumping the shunt? *Pediatrics* **89**: 470–3.

Piatt JH, Carlson CV (1993) A search for determinants of cerebrospinal fluid shunt survival: a retrospective analysis of a 14-year institutional experience. *Pediatric Neurosurgery* **19**: 233–42.

Pikus HJ, Levy ML, Gans W, Mendel E, McComb JG (1997) Outcome, cost analysis and long-term follow up in preterm infants with massive grade IV germinal matrix haemorrhage and progressive hydrocephalus. *Neurosurgery* **40** (5): 983–9.

Porter FN (1975) Hydrocephalus treated by compressive head wrapping. *Archives of Disease in Childhood* **50**: 816–8.

Pudenz RH (1981) The surgical treatment of hydrocephalus – an historical overview. *Surgical Neurology* **15**: 15–26.

Pudenz RH, Foltz EL (1991) Hydrocephalus: over drainage by ventricular shunts. A review and recommendations. *Surgical Neurology* **35**: 200–2.

Pudenz RH, Russell FE, Hurd AH, Shelden CH (1957) Ventriculo-auriculostomy; a technique for shunting cerebrospinal fluid into the right auricle; preliminary report. *Journal of Neurosurgery* **14:** 171–9.

Rekate HL (1991) Shunt revision: complications and their prevention. *Pediatric Neurosurgery* **17**: 155–62.

Scott MA, Fletcher JM, Brookshire BL *et al.* (1998) Memory functions in children with early hydrocephalus. *Neuropsychology* **12** (4): 578–89.

Shinnar S, Gammon K, Bergman EW, Epstein M, Freeman JM (1985) Management of hydrocephalus in infancy: use of acetazolamide and furosemide to avoid cerebrospinal fluid shunts. *Journal of Pediatrics* **107**: 31–7.

Siomin V, Cinalli G, Grotenhuis A *et al.* (2002) Endoscopic third ventriculostomy in patients with cerebrospinal fluid infection and/or hemorrhage. *Journal of Neurosurgery* **97** (3): 519–24.

Smith ER, Butler WE, Barker FG (2004) In-hospital mortality rates after ventriculoperitoneal shunt procedures in the United States, 1998 to 2000: relation to hospital and surgeon volume of care. *Journal of Neurosurgery* **92** (Suppl 2 Pediatrics): 90–7.

Spitz EB (1959) Neurosurgery in the prevention of exogenous mental retardation. *Pediatric Clinics of North America* **6**, 1215–35.

Sutton LN, Sun P, Adzick NS (2001) Fetal neurosurgery. *Neurosurgery* **27**: 124–44.

Tuli S, Drake J, Lawless J, Wigg M, Lamberti-Pasculli M (2000) Risk factors for repeated cerebrospinal shunt failures in pediatric patients with hydrocephalus. *Journal of Neurosurgery* **92** (1): 31–8.

Tuli S, Tuli J, Drake J, Spears J (2004) Predictors of death in pediatric patients requiring cerebrospinal fluid shunts. *Journal of Neurosurgery* **100** (Suppl 5 Pediatrics): 442–6.

Ventriculomegaly Trial Group (1990) Randomised trial of early tapping in neonatal posthaemorrhagic ventricular dilatation. *Archives of Disease in Childhood* **65**: 3–10.

Vernon-Levett P, Geller M (1997) Posterior fossa tumors in children: a case study. *AACN Clinical Issues* **8** (2): 214–26.

Vinchon M, Lemaitre MP, Vallee L, Dhellemmes P (2002) Late shunt infections: incidence, pathogenesis and therapeutic implication. *Neuropediatrics* **33** (4): 167–73.

Watkins L, Hayward R, Andar U, Harkness W (1994) The diagnosis of blocked cerebrospinal fluid shunts: a prospective study of referral to a paediatric neurosurgical unit. *Child's Nervous System* **10**: 87–90.

Whitelaw A, Saliba E, Fellman V *et al.* (1996) Phase I study of intraventricular recombinant tissue plasminogen activator for treatment of posthaemorrhagic hydrocephalus. *Archives of Disease in Childhood* **75** (1): F20–6.

Whitelaw A, Rivers R, Creighton L, Gaffney P (1992) Low dose intraventricular fibrinolytic treatment to prevent posthaemorrhagic hydrocephalus. *Archives of Disease in Childhood* **67**: 10–4.

Woodward S, Addison C, Shah S *et al.* (2002) Benchmarking best practice for external ventricular drainage. *British Journal of Nursing* **11** (1): 47–53.

Yashon D, Jane JA, Sugar O (1965) The course of severe untreated infantile hydrocephalus. Prognostic significance of the cerebral mantle. *Journal of Neurosurgery* **23**: 509–16.

Yamashita N, Kamiya K, Yamada K (1999) Experience with a programmable valve shunt system. *Journal of Neurosurgery* **91**: 26–31

5   Traumatic brain injury

The clinical presentation and final outcome of mild, moderate or severe injury in traumatic brain injury (TBI) primarily depends on the severity of and distribution of the brain damage and the child's age (Johnson and Rose 1996). Minor injuries account for more than 75 per cent of TBI (Durkin *et al.* 1998) with the outcome generally very good (Satz *et al.* 1997). The survival rate following severe TBI has increased as a result of technological advances such as computerized tomography (CT) scanning (Hirsch *et al.* 2002), changes in medical management including an increased use of intracranial pressure and cerebral function monitoring (Tilford *et al.* 2001), and a more systematic approach to the initial assessment and early management following TBI (National Institute for Health and Clinical Excellence (NICE) 2003, 2007). However, severe TBI has the potential to cause significant morbidity including physical, cognitive and emotional disabilities (Mahoney *et al.* 1983). The focus of this chapter is primarily severe TBI and will provide an overview of the factors which predispose children to TBI, outline the types of injury and the management of children following TBI. It may be useful to revisit Chapter 2, Section 3 – normal and raised intracranial pressure – because of the links with the acute management of TBI, and Chapter 2, Section 8 – the principles of rehabilitation.

At the end of reading this chapter you will be able to:

Learning outcomes

- Outline the causes of TBI in children
- Describe the principles of managing a child who has sustained a TBI
- Understand the need for an interdisciplinary approach when caring for the child and family, where the child has sustained a TBI
- Appreciate the impact TBI has on the child and family.

5.1 Classification, incidence and aetiology

Classification

Traumatic brain injury, head injury or craniocerebral trauma can be defined as an insult to the brain, not of a degenerative or congenital nature, caused by an external force that results in a diminished or altered state of consciousness (Kraus *et al.* 1987; Brain Injury Association of America 2004). Minor TBI is usually defined as a brief loss of consciousness, no abnormal neurological signs, a Glasgow Coma Score (GCS) above 13, and transient symptoms such as dizziness, confusion, headaches and vomiting (Satz *et al.* 1997).

Points to consider

Severe TBI is defined as a GCS of less than 8 (Bullock et al. 2000, NICE 2003). Severe TBI results in unconsciousness which is potentially life threatening because vital functions are compromised and there is an inability to maintain the airway.

Incidence

In 2002, 2 per cent of deaths in children in the UK between 0–14 years of age were the result of a TBI (Office of National Statistics 2004). It has been estimated that 1 million people in the UK attend hospital each year as a result of a TBI (McMillan and Greenwood 1993). For every 100,000 of the population, 10–15 people will sustain a severe head injury, 15–20 a moderate head injury and 250–300 people a mild head injury. The death rate following TBI is approximately 9 in 1000 injuries (McMillan and Greenwood 1993). There has been a dramatic increase in the number of hospital admissions of children with a TBI over the last 30 years, from approximately 4 per cent in the 1970s to 14 per cent in the 1990s, primarily due to increased road traffic use (Mahoney *et al.* 1983; Kraus *et al.* 1987; McMillan and Greenwood 1993). Although there has been a marked improvement in the survival following TBI, there is an associated health impact on the child and family with many children having resultant deficits (Parslow *et al.* 2005).

Points to consider

Traumatic brain injury:

- The leading cause of mortality and morbidity in childhood
- Accounts for a quarter to one-third of accidental deaths in childhood
- Results in the highest number of both minor and major injuries in children under 1 year of age
- Is the leading cause of accidental injury in adolescents.

(Mahoney *et al.* 1983; Kraus *et al.* 1987; Durkin *et al.* 1998; Parslow *et al.* 2005)

Aetiology

Although there are slight variations between studies the causes of TBI are primarily:

- Road traffic accidents which cause the greatest severity of injury and account for approximately 40–60 per cent of head injuries, with the majority resulting from a child pedestrian being hit by a moving car.
- Falls, accounting for 20–30 per cent of head injuries, although severe head trauma is rare in home accidents.

- Assaults, accounting for approximately 10 per cent of head injuries, with non-accidental injury the most common cause of severe head injury under 1 year.
- Other causes of TBI include sports accidents, falling objects and firearm accidents.
                                        (Henry *et al.* 1992; Durkin *et al.* 1998; Parslow *et al.* 2005)

Associated factors

There are a range of factors that contribute to TBI occurring in children including:

- Increased risk in boys; the ratio of girls versus boys who sustain a head injury is approximately 2:1. This increases with age and is related to greater risk-taking in boys. In addition boys develop cognitive functions relating to distance and spatial awareness later than girls.
- TBI incidence peaks in the spring and summer seasons, and between 2pm and 10pm, when children are more likely to play outside.
- Other variables that influence a child's vulnerability to TBI include the presence of visual or hearing deficits, learning deficits, low socioeconomic status, urban residence and previous head injury.
                              (Kraus *et al.* 1987; Henry *et al.* 1992; Durkin *et al.* 1998; Parslow *et al.* 2005)

5.2 Pathophysiology and clinical presentation

Pathophysiology

There are several ways of describing the pathophysiology of TBI (Table 5.2a) including (Graham 2000):

- Primary damage versus secondary damage.
- Focal damage versus diffuse damage.
- Direct injury versus acceleration–deceleration injury.

The pathophysiology outlined below will describe primary and secondary damage in TBI.

Table 5.2a Ways of describing the pathophysiology of traumatic brain injury

Primary damage	*Secondary damage*
Scalp injuries	Ischaemia
Skull fractures	Swelling/oedema
Surface contusions and lacerations	Infections
Intracranial haematomas	Raised intracranial pressure
Diffuse axonal injury	
Focal damage	*Diffuse damage*
Scalp injuries	Ischaemia
Skull fractures	Swelling/oedema
Surface contusions and lacerations	Infections
Intracranial haematoma	Axonal injury
Raised intracranial pressure	
Direct injuries	*Acceleration/deceleration injuries*
Scalp injuries	Tearing of veins within meninges and subdural
Skull fractures	haematomas
Surface contusions, lacerations and intracranial	Acute vascular injury
haematoma	Diffuse axonal injury pressure
	Intracranial haematoma

Source: adapted from Graham 2000

Primary brain damage

Primary brain damage occurs at the time of injury and is a result of direct mechanical force that can cause scalp injuries, skull fractures, brain surface contusions and lacerations, tearing of blood vessels, intracranial haematomas and diffuse axonal injury. The type of damage will depend on the mechanism of how the injury occurs and the anatomic structures involved. TBI occurs mainly as a result of two mechanisms: direct injury, where a force is applied to the head, with the intensity and duration of the mechanical pressure determining the degree of initial damage; and rapid acceleration–deceleration forces. Acceleration–deceleration injuries occur as a result of unrestricted brain movement within the skull. Acceleration injuries are sustained when the head is struck by a moving object and deceleration injuries are sustained when the head hits a stationary object. If the head is rocked back and forth or rotated, the brain must follow the movement of the skull resulting in an acceleration–deceleration, also known as coup–countercoup, injury. Damage to brain tissues and blood vessels occurs because the inside of the skull has sharp bony ridges, against which the brain collides, damaging brain cells and blood vessels.

Local lesions such as scalp lacerations and bruising may not be significant in isolation but may contribute to the overall damage and can help identify associated injuries. Localized contusion or tissue bruising may result in surface haemorrhages. These often occur on the crest of the gyri of the cerebral cortex, and although they may produce dramatic focal neurological signs at the time of injury, overall progress tends to be good. However, local contusions with associated swelling and subdural bleeding may act as a mass lesion and cause intracranial pressure to rise. Scarring from contusions can result in post-trauma epilepsy. If the initial injury results in widespread contusions deep within the brain, intracranial haemorrhage and haematoma formation are likely to develop, and without prompt treatment can be catastrophic (Graham 2000).

Skull fractures are usually associated with more severe injuries (Graham 2000). However, the flexibility of the skull in infants and young children may result in severe underlying brain injury occurring without the presence of a skull fracture. Skull fractures can occur with or without damage to the brain and can be either open or closed, with an open fracture classified as a fracture where there is a tear in the dura mater. Crushing injuries often result in extensive skull fractures with little underlying brain damage (Graham 2000). Open fractures and compound fractures, where there is an associated scalp laceration, are a potential source of infection. The majority of skull fractures are linear. Depressed skull fractures occur when the fragments of the fracture are displaced inwards and are associated with post-trauma epilepsy. Basal skull fractures are particularly important due to the danger of secondary CSF infection and potential cranial nerve damage. In cases of non-accidental injuries occipital fractures are often a result of the back of the head being struck against a hard surface.

Diffuse axonal damage can occur when there is generalized damage throughout the brain that results in degeneration of the white matter. Widespread axonal damage is more likely to occur after high acceleration and deceleration injuries which result in sheared, stretched, twisted and torn nerve fibres. However, mild injuries can also produce widespread damage throughout the brain. Rotational injuries will add to the shearing effect within the brain substance, particularly in areas where structures are more mobile, such as the proximal brain stem and corpus callosum. Rotational injuries are particularly common as a result of non-accidental shaking and road traffic accidents where the child is a pedestrian and the impact of the car causes the child to rotate as they fall to the ground. Infants have softer skulls and shallower convolutions than adults, which are thought to add to the considerable damage done by shearing forces on the young brain. This can cause severe disruption of the grey–white matter demarcation. The mechanism and progression of diffuse axonal injury is unclear (Graham 2000).

Points to consider

Hypoxia can occur at the time of injury because of choking or aspiration, haemorrhage or as a consequence of loss of consciousness, which may result in an inability to maintain the airway or sustain sufficient respiratory effort. Hypoxia contributes to secondary brain damage.

Secondary brain damage

The causes of secondary brain damage are cerebral oedema, vascular injury, seizures and infections. Superimposed secondary brain damage occurs after the initial impact and is a consequence of both the intracranial and systemic responses to injury, resulting in cerebral hypoxia, systemic hypotension and raised intracranial pressure.

Points to consider

Hypoxia and hypotension are particularly associated with a poor prognosis (Chapter 2, Section 3 provides an overview of cerebro-haemodynamics) (Prabhakaran *et al.* 2004).

The predominant stimulus for cerebral autoregulation of blood flow is cerebral perfusion pressure (CPP), which indirectly influences the intracranial pressure (ICP) (Prabhakaran *et al.* 2004). Severe hypotension following TBI decreases the CPP and causes hypoxia resulting in vasodilation in an attempt to increase oxygenation of the brain by improving the cerebral blood flow. This results in an increase in cerebral blood volume which causes an increase in ICP (Prabhakaran *et al.* 2004). This rise in ICP causes the CPP to fall further and a cycle is initiated where normal cerebral haemodynamic autoregulatory measures fail (Chapter 2, Section 3, Figure 2.3c).

Following severe TBI there is an inability of normal physiological mechanisms to maintain the blood–brain barrier resulting in vasodilation and diffuse swelling. Oedema occurs as a result of vascular damage, hypoxia and retention of fluids within the extracellular spaces (Graham 2000). Peak swelling occurs 24–48 hours after the injury. A rise in $PaCO_2$ will compound the situation and further increase tissue swelling. Diffuse brain swelling can result in widespread ischaemic brain damage (Graham 2000). More than 90 per cent of children with fatal head injuries show pathological evidence of diffuse hypoxic-ischaemia damage and may have hippocampal damage due to brain compression, secondary to raised intracranial pressure (Crouchman 1998).

Points to consider

Cerebral oedema results in a rise in intracranial pressure that becomes self-perpetuating and there is loss of the normal mechanisms that maintain the intracranial pressure within acceptable limits (Chapter 2, Section 3, Figure 2.3c).

Haemorrhage can occur directly into the substance of the brain as a result of diffuse intra-cerebral haemorrhage or can result in the formation of a haematoma. In extradural haematomas, blood collects in the space between the skull and the dura. Symptoms such as deterioration in conscious levels usually develop within 12 hours following the injury and death can occur if not treated promptly.

Points to consider

In subdural haematoma, blood collects between the dura and the underlying brain, which may be acute, subacute or chronic. If blood collects slowly in the subdural space there may be a delay from the time of injury to the presentation of symptoms.

Other secondary complications of severe TBI include seizures and brain abscess, and less commonly areocele or hydrocephalus may develop. The neurons within the brain can respond to injury by becoming overexcited, resulting in seizure activity. Seizures occur mainly within the first 24–48 hours after injury. Brain abscess is a potential consequence of a compound depressed fracture or penetrating head injury. Abscess formation can be minimized through early surgical debridement of the wound. Meningitis can occur secondary to basal skull fractures with dural tearing in the paransal sinus or middle ear. This can be suspected from the pattern of bruising around the eyes and the development of rhinorrhea or otorrhea. Meningitis in this context is invariably due to pneumococcus.

Clinical presentation

Minor head injuries result in transient symptoms such as concussion, dizziness, confusion, headaches and vomiting (Satz *et al.* 1997). Concussion is usually described as a temporary loss of neurological function with no apparent structural damage. In minor head injury the period of unconsciousness is usually brief.

Severe TBI results in unconsciousness that can potentially compromise vital functions including an ability to maintain the airway. If unconsciousness is prolonged following the initial injury there will be decreased responsiveness, dilated pupils and decreased response to light, abnormal motor activity, headaches, nausea and vomiting. A rise in blood pressure with a compensatory bradycardia, apnoea and progressively elevated ICP are indications of imminent catastrophe (Hazinski *et al.* 1999).

Points to consider

TBI is potentially life threatening. The severity of the initial injury and the ability to minimize secondary brain damage will influence the outcome. Children who have sustained a major TBI must be transferred to a children's trauma unit (Adelson *et al.* 2003).

5.3 Management of a child following traumatic brain injury

The management of TBI will be considered in three stages: the initial management and stabilization; the principles of managing raised intracranial pressure; and rehabilitation. The general principles of rehabilitation are outlined in *Chapter 2, Section 8*, therefore only the specific stages and impact of TBI will be outlined.

Initial management and stabilisation

Minor head injury is common in children (Satz *et al.* 1997). Admission to hospital is not always necessary following minor head injury but is often a precaution if there has been a seizure, a skull fracture, an unstable GCS, the cause is suggestive of more serious injuries, the cause is suspicious or symptoms such as vomiting require additional management from healthcare professionals (NICE 2007).

Best practice recommendations

The National Institute of Health and Clinical Excellence (2007) guidelines relating to the triage, assessment and management of head injuries in infants, children and adults outlines the initial priorities of care as:

- Assessment and stabilization of the airway, breathing and circulation
- Assessment of neurological status
- Ascertaining the degree of the injury to initiate appropriate levels of care.

Points to consider

All children who have a GCS less than 13, depressed or basal skull fractures, post-traumatic seizures or focal neurological deficits usually require a CT scan and admission to hospital (NICE 2007). The focus of care must be the detection of neurological changes by undertaking a thorough neurological assessment and ongoing observations (Chapter 2, Section 2).

The child and family will require appropriate support and detailed discharge advice. Discharge information following minor TBI must be provided to the child and family of all children who have attended accident and emergency or have had a brief period of hospitalization.

Best practice recommendations

The NICE (2007) guidelines provide suggestions about the content of written guidelines following discharge from a minor TBI, which include:

Return to hospital as soon as possible if your child:
- Becomes unconscious
- Is confused
- Is drowsy outside their normal sleeping routines
- Is difficult to wake
- Does not respond as normal

- Has loss of balance or problems walking, or not moving as normal
- Complains of headache
- Has problems with their eyes or eyesight
- Vomits
- Fits
- Has any fluid draining from their ears or nose
- Has any blood draining from their ears

Do not worry if your child:
- Has an occasional headache
- Feels sick but does not vomit
- Feels irritable or bad tempered
- Has a poor appetite
- Has difficulty in sleeping

It is advisable:
- To have access to a telephone for emergencies
- To keep your child quiet and allow plenty of rest
- To avoid contact sport for three weeks
- Not to give your child any sleeping pills
- Not to leave your child alone for the first 48 hours
- To keep your child away from school until they have fully recovered

Points to consider

All children with a GCS less than 8, after stabilization, must be transferred to a tertiary paediatric intensive care facility (NICE 2007). A CT scan is important to establish early management options, particularly the need for surgical interventions (Hirsch 2002). Any indication of cervical spine injury will necessitate spinal X-rays and appropriate protection of the cervical spine until disproved (NICE 2007). The cervical spine is protected by applying a hard collar, ensuring effective log rolling procedures when positioning the child and the use of a spinal board during transfers between departments (Advanced Paediatric Life Support 2002).

Principles of managing acute raised intracranial pressure

In the ward environment the management of a child with the potential of developing acute raised intracranial pressure (RICP) must be aimed at detecting and acting upon changes in the child's neurological state promptly. This includes understanding and interpreting neurological assessments (Chapter 2, Section 2), and applying the underlying knowledge of the reasons RICP may develop to each individual child. Children with alterations in neurological status, fluctuations in conscious levels and who are unable to maintain an airway should be cared for in a paediatric intensive care unit, where there are staff experienced in caring for children with acute neurological impairments.

Essential care

Elective intubation and ventilation are essential in the child who has sustained a major TBI if:

- GCS is less than 8 or there is significant deterioration of conscious levels
- There is loss of protective reflexes
- There is ventilatory insufficiency, hypoxaemia or hypercarbia
- Seizures are difficult to control.

(NICE 2007

Points to consider

The prime objectives when caring for a child with a severe TBI are to minimize secondary insults and manage hypoxia and cerebral ischaemia effectively (Prabhakaran *et al.* 2004).

The management of hypoxia is based on the need to maintain an adequate CPP to prevent cerebral ischaemia which will lead to tissue necrosis. It has been suggested that to avoid 'plateau waves', where there are periods of extremely high ICP resulting in low cerebral perfusion, the CPP needs to be maintained above the threshold of 60mmHg. Therefore CPP levels of 70–80mmHg are more desirable if ischaemia is to be avoided (Rosner and Daughton 1990). However, maintaining a CPP above 60mmHg when the ICP is extremely high (CPP = MAP – ICP) can be difficult in the paediatric setting (Chapter 2, Section 3). There is a lack of research that conclusively demonstrates the outcome of CPP treatment regimens in children, which may account for the variable practices, particularly ICP and electroencephalography (EEG) monitoring (Tasker 2000; Tilford *et al.* 2001; Adelson *et al.* 2003). The majority of treatment modalities and their effectiveness have been extrapolated from adult studies (Bullock *et al.* 2000; Adelson *et al.* 2003; Prabhakaran *et al.* 2004).

Best practice recommendations

There are evidence-based guidelines relating to the management of TBI in both children and adults (Bullock *et al.* 2000; Adelson *et al.* 2003). The principles within these guidelines include:

- Ventilate and maintain oxygenation, aim for a $PaCO_2$ between 30–35mmHg and PaO_2 between 90–100mmHg. Hyperventilation is not a recommended treatment for TBI but may be of value for brief periods where the $PaCO_2$ is elevated and there is associated acute neurological deterioration, such as acute rises in ICP
- Minimizing the brain's metabolic needs and preventing activities which normally produce transient rises in ICP by providing adequate sedation, analgesia and paralysis. No specific evidence is currently available relating to the best sedative, analgesia or neuromuscular blocking agent in the management of head injury. Choice will

depend on local guidelines and practices. The use of sedation, analgesia and paralysis will limit the ability to perform full neurological assessments

- Maintaining an adequate systemic mean arterial pressure, above 75mmHg for children over 10 years of age and above 65mmHg for those less than 10 years of age to ensure an adequate CPP.
  - This is achieved by appropriate fluid resuscitation and the administration of inotropic drugs. An inotrope is an agent which alters the force or energy of muscular contractions. This group of drugs is useful for resuscitation of seriously ill patients, and for the treatment of hypotension in intensive care settings. In theses situations inotropes such as dopamine or dobutamine are administered by continuous infusion. Fluid resuscitation must be judicious due to the potential of increasing cerebral oedema if over hydration occurs
- Maintaining CPP above 60mmHg for children over 10 years of age and above 50mmHg for those less than 10 years of age. Maintaining an adequate mean arterial pressure will require the use of inotropic support
- Maintaining normal electrolyte balance with precise fluid management
- Monitoring and recording ICP levels and wave patterns, identify 'plateau' waves early (Figure 2.3b). ICP above 20mmHg will require active treatment such as diuretic therapy. Mannitol 20% is the diuretic of choice and the usual dose is 0.25–0.5g/kg. Monitor serum osmolarity with mannitol use and maintain a level of less than 320mOmols/L
- Decompression surgery may be indicated if the child has an extremely high ICP and high blood pressure due to medical interventions due to generalized cerebral oedema but the child's brain is likely to recover
- Optimizing cerebral venous return by maintaining the head at an angle of 30° and position the head in the midline to prevent constriction of the blood vessels
- Maintain normothermia
- Monitor EEG to detect seizure activity and ensure prompt treatment of seizures.

Surgery will be indicated if there is a localised mass, haemorrhage or the ICP is significant necessitating the removal of a bone flap to reduce the intracranial pressure. It has been estimated that 30 per cent of children who sustain a major TBI will require emergency neurosurgery (Tasker *et al.* 2006). Regional paediatric transfer teams experienced in the transfer of critically ill children should undertake the transfer of children with major TBI from local to specialty services (SIGN 2000, Adelson *et al.* 2003; NICE 2007). This requires coordination between services if the recommended 4 hour time frame is to be achieved (DH 1997). However, in remote areas there may be a tension between the time taken to mobilize regional paediatric transfer teams and the ability to meet the 4 hour timeframe (Tasker *et al.* 2006). Local guidelines, taking into account geographical constraints, must be in place to ensure these children are transfer to a regional neurosurgical centre safely and timely.

In adult patients, there is ongoing debate as to the value of inducing moderate hypothermia as a treatment option following severe TBI (Alderson *et al.* 2005). In children there is some evidence to suggest that moderate hypothermia may improve intracranial hypertension (Biswas *et al.*

2002). The aim of inducing moderate hypothermia is to minimize secondary damage by reducing oxygen demands, cerebral ischaemia and tissue injury in the brain. Using a cooling blanket the child's temperature is reduced to 5°C lower than normal body temperature for the first 24–48 hours after injury. Re-warming must be undertaken gradually, aiming for a maximum 1°C increased per hour (Biswas *et al.* 2002). However, inducing moderate hypothermia as a treatment option is experimental and at present there is limited evidence that supports cooling as an effective treatment option.

The child who is ventilated, paralysed and sedated is dependent upon healthcare professionals to minimize complications of immobility. Unfortunately for the child with an RICP, many activities, particularly nursing, aimed at reducing potential complications of enforced immobility have the potential to further increase ICP. Care must be directed towards avoiding complications of immobility while minimizing the risk of secondary insults, this often involves limiting external stimuli.

Points to consider

In the brain-injured child consideration needs to be given to nursing procedures that may increase ICP including:

- Avoiding extreme flexion, which will impair venous drainage (Williams and Coyne 1993). Log roll the child and maintain the head in a neutral position
- Preventing abnormal tone and posture, which can increase ICP, by avoiding placing the child supine and promoting the use of side lying (Palmer and Wyness 1988). If the supine position cannot be avoided support the knee and elbow joints to minimize extensor tone; ensure physiotherapists and occupational therapists are available to assess and recommend aids for positioning
- Turning and, in particular, rapid repositioning can have dramatic effects on the ICP (Boortz-Marx 1985; Rising 1993; Jones 1994). Ensure the child is turned slowly, monitor the effect repositioning has on ICP levels and the time it takes for the ICP to stabilize, which will influence the frequency of repositioning. It may be necessary to consider bolus sedation prior to repositioning
- Endotracheal suctioning can dramatically increase the ICP (Rudy *et al.* 1991; Crosby and Parsons 1992; Paratz and Burns 1993). However, maintaining a patent airway and reducing respiratory complications are essential in preventing atelectasis, which may result in hypoxia and consequently impact on cerebral perfusion
- The decision to perform suction must be based upon clinical signs and include increasing ventilation pressures, a deterioration in arterial blood gases and oxygen saturation levels, and the presence of secretions in the bronchial tree. The effect suction has on ICP can be limited by only passing the catheter twice during each suction procedure to minimize distress and limiting suction to 10 seconds each catheter insertion to avoid hypoxia (Rudy *et al.* 1991; Crosby and Parsons 1992)
- Noxious stimuli, e.g. painful procedures, loud noises (Muwaswes 1985) and frequent care or clustering care together with insufficient rest periods (Rising 1993) have been reported to cause increases to ICP. Noxious stimuli should be minimized by allowing at least 1 hour rest between procedures to enable the ICP to stabilize

- Including family members in care. Their presence and the effect of gentle touch have not been demonstrated to increase ICP (Walleck 1983; Treloar *et al.* 1991). It is vitally important that the family become involved in the care of their child at an early stage.

Once the child is stable and no longer requires intensive care facilities the child is usually transferred to a high dependency area or a ward experienced in caring for the neurologically compromised child. The principles of caring for the child who is unconscious are described in Chapter 2, Section 6. It must be noted that increased metabolic demands, up to 140 per cent greater than normal, and nitrogen losses are significant following TBI, requiring particular attention when managing the child's nutritional state (Bullock *et al.* 2000; Adelson *et al.* 2003). Early enteral feeding is essential during the intensive period with continual assessment during the rehabilitation stage.

Stages of the recovery process

Singer (1996) has described four distinct phases through which a child and family progress following a child sustaining a TBI.

Phase 1

TBI is a sudden unwanted event and the initial impact of the injury is life threatening. There is immediate disruption to family life. At this stage the outcome of the injury is unpredictable.

Points to consider

The aim of care is to stabilize the child, prevent secondary ischaemic damage, begin the rehabilitation process and support the child and family.

Phase 2

Following stabilization the duration of life support systems and time in a coma is variable, with fluctuating responses and ongoing uncertainty. An agitated child is often challenging and may be distressing for parents. Often parents feel hopeless during this phase. Additional stresses occur as the family attempt to maintain some degree of normal family life.

Points to consider

The aim of care is to minimize complications for the child, encourage restorative synaptogenesis through structured rehabilitation and ongoing support for the family.

Phase 3

The child's level of awareness begins to return and there may be early motor and cognitive recovery. However, the family may find the fluctuation in progress difficult to interpret and understand. The full extent of injuries becomes more apparent and the enormity of the changes may become overwhelming.

Points to consider

The aim of care is to continue and adapt the rehabilitation programme in response to changing needs and ongoing support for the family.

Phase 4

Although there may be continued physical and cognitive recovery, emotional recovery can result in changes in personality and behaviours which can be difficult to cope with. Discharge from hospital is a stressful time for the family, transition to community care needs to be well planned if the child and family are to adjust to the effects of the injury (Chapter 2, Section 8). Issues relating to the future education and schooling of the child are major considerations, which require detailed assessment and advanced planning.

Points to consider

The aim of care is to ensure timely and appropriate discharge with community support systems in place. Children who have sustained a severe TBI will require continual assessment to monitor development because later milestones may not be achieved or the child may grow into deficits.

The family often desire detailed information about the recovery process and although the phases can be described, it must be stressed that each child is unique and these phases will vary greatly between children. The general psychological needs of the child and family, and principles of rehabilitation are outlined in Chapter 2, Sections 7 and 8 respectively.

Points to consider

It cannot be overstated that the family is central to the rehabilitation process for a child who has sustained a TBI because:

- All family members are directly affected by the injury, the family is the intermediary between the outside world and treatments
- The family provides continuity of care and takes responsibility for the child on discharge (Singer 1996).

It is therefore vital that parents understand the purpose and processes of rehabilitation, which are to maximize the child's potential and minimize disability, and are encouraged to become equal partners in decisions about the care of their child (Neumann 1995).

Each stage of the recovery process brings new challenges for the child and family. The family's response and ability to cope in the face of adversities will influence the achievement of the goals of rehabilitation, which must be realistic, and the successful reintegration of the child back into the community (Kepler 1996). Research relating to the needs of families with children who have sustained a TBI has identified that parents wanted more information relating to developing the child's cognitive abilities, to have their questions answered honestly, to be assured services are appropriate to the child's needs and to have a named professional that may be contacted for advice and ongoing support (Kepler 1996).

Unfortunately the needs of the family where a child has a TBI are not always met because care provision has primarily been developed to meet acute needs with little attention given to the long-term resources required to meet ongoing needs (Marks *et al.* 1993). Furthermore, the barriers between society, education and healthcare have not always facilitated the provision of seamless care for the child and family (DH 2004, Hawley *et al.* 2004). Deficiencies in service provision can be reduced by the development of specific TBI teams, where professionals have an understanding of the physical, cognitive and neurobehavioural sequelae following a TBI.

Role of the TBI team

The family will have many needs when a child has sustained a TBI including: gaining knowledge of TBI and the phases of recovery, the nursing care and therapies specific to the child's needs, support with behavioural problems, support with securing the best welfare services for the child, support with ensuring the child receives the most appropriate educational needs, respite care and counselling. One professional will not have all of the skills required to meet all of the needs of the child and family who has sustained a TBI. An effective team requires professionals that not only work towards the same goals but share the same approaches to treatment and accept roles will overlap (Neumann 1995).

Points to consider

The establishment of a TBI team can:

- Facilitate effective flow of information between healthcare professionals and with the family, which will ensure continuity of care
- Considers the child and family from a range of perspectives by recognising that physical, cognitive, and emotional problems do not occur in isolation and often overlap
- Facilitate the reinforcement of skills in a variety of environments. This is necessary because there is often poor memory and lack of ability to generalize skills learned
- Facilitate the development of expertise
- Act as a resource for the range of services and professionals who will come in contact with the child and family
- Develop links with adult teams, so that transition between child and adult services is smooth.

(Neumann 1995)

Points to consider

All members of the team must have an understanding of the challenges when caring for individuals with head injuries, and appreciate that:

- Although a vast number of children will return to normal, a significant number will have resultant disabilities with care needed for a considerable length of time
- The youth of the victims can result in disruption to future development with constantly changing needs, therefore professionals need to be responsive to these changes
- The burden of disability can include costs to individuals, families, employment opportunities, and society
- There will be a range of physical, cognitive and emotional problems. It is difficult to predict long-term outcomes, and therefore difficult to plan for future needs
- The family expectations, fears and anxieties must be addressed and the family's capabilities must be assessed
- Interagency working particularly between health, educational and social services is essential if all the child's needs are to be met.

(Neumann 1995)

5.4 Long-term care needs of the child who has sustained a TBI and the impact on the family

The outcome following minor head injury is favourable and in general there are no long-term cognitive and psychosocial effects (Satz *et al.* 1997). However, the results of the studies reviewed by Satz *et al.* (1997) suggest that the spectrum of injuries within the general classification of minor TBI are varied. The outcomes for children who have sustained 'major' minor head injury are more variable and include cognitive and behavioural difficulties (Satz *et al.* 1997). In light of the uncertain outcome for children grouped together as minor TBI ongoing monitoring to facilitate early identification of deficits is essential. Local guidelines must be in place to ensure these children receive appropriate follow up and systems for referral to regional TBI teams, where appropriate. The remainder of this section will focus on severe TBI. Severe TBI can result in physical deficits and discrete or complex cognitive and psychosocial functioning that impedes normal activities, future development, education and career opportunities, and the prospect of independent living (Johnson and Rose 1996). The main factors that affect the outcome of TBI are the mechanism and severity of injury, age, extent of secondary damage, disruption to normal development and predisposing factors such as prior learning disabilities (Crouchman 1998).

Factors that influence outcomes for the child who has sustained a TBI

There are a range of factors that influence the outcome for the child who has stained a TBI.

Mechanism and severity of injury

There is relatively little evidence relating to predicting the outcome of TBI because of the range of scoring tools available and difficulties in determining the severity of injury which have resulted in an inability to compare studies (Appleton 1998). The severity of TBI and probability of survival has been shown to be related to:

- The Glasgow Coma Scale – a GCS of 3–4 on admission to hospital is linked to higher morbidity and mortality rates (Kraus *et al.* 1987)
- The Abbreviated Injury Scale – this scale codes injuries from 1–6 for each of the five body parts but does not summate scores and therefore does not reflect the severity of multiple injuries (American Association for Automotive Medicine 1985). In head injury a score of 1 would equate to a minor injury where the child is concussed but awake on initial examination, 2 moderate injury where there is minimal loss of consciousness, 3 serious injury where there was cerebral contusion, 4 severe injury where there is subdural haematoma, a score of 5 is a critical injury where there was diffuse brain injury and a score of 6 would be an un-survivable injury due to laceration of the brain stem (Appleton 1998)
- The Injury Severity Score – developed from the abbreviated injury scale, but uses statistical summation that incorporates multiple injury scores and ranges from 1–75. It is often used to evaluate trauma outcome in accident and emergency (Baker *et al.* 1974). Severe trauma is usually assigned to a score of 16 or above
- The Trauma Score – a tool that uses the four parameters of systemic blood pressure, capillary refill, respiratory rate and GCS to assess the severity of the injury and can be used with the Injury Severity Score. Through statistical analysis a trauma injury severity score can be calculated and provide the quantifiable probability of survival (Boyd *et al.* 1987). The advantage is that the score can be adjusted for age
- Glasgow Outcome Scale – categorises levels of recovery as good, moderate disability, severe disability, persistent vegetative state and death (Wilson *et al.* 2000). The first three are subjective measures and therefore a relatively crude measure of outcome and the scale does not consider long-term developmental issues in children.

Other indicators of poor outcome include length of time in a coma, abnormal electrical activity and persistent elevated ICP levels.

Disruption to normal development: the concept of neuroplasticity

The traditional approach to neuroanatomy and physiology associates body functions with specific brain structures. This view would suggest that the brain has little capacity to grow and regain function once damage has occurred. Clinical observations of children who have made a dramatic recovery following severe TBI suggest that recovery does occur despite significant injuries (Kaplan 1988). Ongoing debates among neuroscientists and healthcare professionals relate to the processes which underpin brain recovery and whether brain damage of an equivalent extent is less impairing in children than in adults (Johnson and Rose 1996).

Evidence suggests that the brain functions as a 'plastic structure'; this malleability results in the brain being capable of returning to a similar form and function once altered (Kaplan 1988). Therefore, although the brain appears to be organized into discrete areas associated with specific function, these may not be fixed and latent areas could take on the function of damaged areas. Plasticity makes the brain particularly vulnerable to changes in the environment but this same plasticity may provide a means to advancing recovery following damage.

Traditionally it was thought that new synapses could not form in the mature brain. An example of normal plasticity occurs in the development of visual acuity. Lack of visual input to one or both eyes can result in permanent visual problems, even though all the structures may be anatomically correct. However, evidence from animal studies suggests that environment factors after birth influence the continued development of the central nervous system, for example highly stimulating environments increase; cortical thickness, glial cells, synaptic connections and dendrite branching (Kaplan 1988). In response to brain injury reactive synaptogenesis may participate in the recovery of function but it may also compete with the process and form aberrant connections. It is thought that early rehabilitation may initiate restorative synaptogenesis in preference to simply reactive proliferation (Kaplan 1988).

> **Points to consider**
>
> Recovery will be influenced by the ability of the neuron to survive, regenerate new axons and form new synaptic connections (Chapter 1, Section 9).

The concept that brain malleability and the ability to utilize latent areas of the brain are greater in children has resulted in the misconception that brain damage of an equivalent extent is less impairing in children than in adults (Johnson and Rose 1996). This, combined with the view that children recover from illness better than adults and the clinical condition on discharge as measured by tools such as the Glasgow Outcome Scale has led to the general belief that outcomes following TBI are more favourable in children. Furthermore, studies which have considered short-term outcomes following severe TBI have suggested that the majority of children, up to 70 per cent, have no long-term deficits (Mahoney *et al.* 1983). However, post-TBI the child may have long-term impairments in attention, memory and motivation which can result in a significant reduction in levels of interaction of the child with their environment (Rose *et al.* 1997). Cognitive, behavioural and psychological recovery and future development may not necessarily correlate with physical improvements and deficits in behaviour are more likely to appear as the child develops (Kraus *et al.* 1987; Johnson and Rose 1996). The child will require detailed ongoing assessment to monitor development as later milestones may not be achieved, or the child may grow into deficits.

> **Points to consider**
>
> The assumption that 'younger is better' in terms of long-term outcome following TBI could result in lack of appropriate care and follow up for these children.

Pre-existing deficits

A TBI sustained in children with the presence of existing neurological deficits has the potential to amply long-term deficits (Johnson and Rose 1996). Furthermore, children who are already under-achieving because of the effects of poor socioeconomic backgrounds may be more vulnerable to the subsequent effects of TBI (Johnson and Rose 1996).

Age at the time of injury

The brain develops in an organized manner, continuing after birth until late teens (Johnson and Rose 1996). The development of the brain will be altered from the time of the TBI. The mortality and morbidity of severe TBI is poorest in children under 1 year of age (Mahoney *et al.* 1983, Raimondi and Hirschauer 1994, Johnson and Rose 1996). Although not fully understood, the reasons could include:

- The greater susceptibility of the immature unmyelinated brain to the primary insult, particularly shearing injuries
- The maximum extrauterine brain growth occurs during the first two years of life and at this time the brain is most vulnerable to injury
- Poor ability to respond to secondary events in particular poor autoregulation of vascular perfusion
- The younger child has had less opportunity for learning and has fewer skills to build upon after the accident.

The impact of TBI on the child and family

Both the short- and long-term impact on the child and family following a child sustaining a significant TBI are substantial (Wade *et al.* 2006; Youngblut and Brooten 2006). For families of a child who has sustained a significant TBI the initial transition of care from hospital to home and reintegrating the child back into the family are enormous. Parents can experience significant psychological distress which relate to the child's appearance, the burden of child's behaviours and emotions, and the change in caring environment (losing the familiarity of the hospital setting and the constant presence of healthcare professionals) (Youngblut and Brooten 2006). Family functioning in the immediate weeks following discharge is variable, with those families displaying greater functioning, cohesion and family adaptability having the ability to develop effective support systems (Youngblut and Brooten 2006). Preparing the child and family for the transition from hospital to home care is essential, and is described in depth in Chapter 2, Section 8.

The long-term impact for the child following a TBI includes difficulties in performing daily living skills, poor communication skills, and general adaptation (Stancin *et al.* 2002). Overall, the health-related quality of life in mental and general health is poor for children who have suffered a severe TBI (Stancin *et al.* 2002). High-risk children are those who have pre-injury problems and children from socially disadvantaged families (Stancin *et al.* 2002). Often the child's cognitive development following a severe TBI remains static, or learning is slow to develop, with the differences between the child's abilities compared to their peers' increasing over time (Johnson and Rose 1996). This will disadvantage the young person when they reach an age when living independently or seeking employment becomes important.

In addition to long-term difficulties in performing usual activities of daily life for the child, TBI results in long-term adversities for the family (Stancin *et al.* 2002). There is evidence to suggest that parents of a child who has had a TBI exhibit high stress levels that are clinically significant and financial hardships that are related to the severity of the injury (Hawley *et al.* 2003). Identifying parents with high stress levels and providing appropriate information and follow up is essential if the family is to be offered appropriate support. For families of a child who has sustained a significant TBI the long-term burden placed on the family cannot be underestimated, and can have an impact for many years following the initial injury. For some children the need for parents to contribute to meeting the child's physical and psychosocial needs will be life long, while other children may improve over time. Parents experience persistent anxieties relating to their child's future and ability to function independently (Wade *et al.* 2006).

Key messages from this chapter

- Traumatic brain injury is the leading cause of mortality and morbidity in childhood, most commonly as a result of road traffic accidents
- Primary brain damage occurs at the time of injury
- Secondary brain damage such as cerebral oedema, vascular injury, seizures and infections occur as a consequence of the body's response to trauma
- The management of TBI occurs in three stages: the initial management and stabilization, the principles of managing raised intracranial pressure and rehabilitation
- Initial priorities of care are stabilization of the airway, breathing and circulation, assessment of neurological status and ascertaining the degree of the injury to initiate appropriate levels of care. The aim of care is to stabilize the child, prevent secondary ischaemic damage, begin the rehabilitation process and support the child and family
- The outcome following minor head injury is in general positive
- The outcome for children who have sustained 'major' minor head injury are variable and include cognitive and behavioural difficulties
- For some children meeting their physical and psychosocial needs will require life-long support

Web resources

National Institute for Health and Clinical Excellence
provides national guidance on the promotion of good health and the prevention and treatment of ill health, and produces guidance relating to: public health (promoting good health and the prevention of ill health for those working in the all healthcare sectors), health technologies (guidance on the use of new and existing medicines, treatments and procedures), and clinical practice guidance (appropriate treatment and care of people with specific diseases and conditions).
www.nice.org.uk

Child Brain Injury Trust
supports anyone in the UK affected by childhood acquired brain injury. They provide information, support and training to families and professionals.
www.cbituk.org

Contact a Family
Contact a Family is the only UK-wide charity providing advice, information and support to the parents of all disabled children, no matter what their health condition. It enables parents to get in contact with other families, on a local or national basis.
www.cafamily.org.uk

Scope
Scope provides support for people with disabilities.
www.scope.org.uk

References

Adelson PD, Bratton PD, Carney NA *et al.* (2003) Guidelines for the acute medical management of severe traumatic brain injury in infants, children and adolescents. *Pediatric Critical Care Medicine* **4** (3): 1–76.

Advanced Paediatric Life Support (2002) *Advanced Paediatric Life Support: The Practical Approach*, 3rd edn. BMJ Publications, London.

Alderson P, Gadkary C, Signorini DF (2005) Therapeutic hypothermia for head injury. **1**, The Cochrane Library.

American Association for Automotive Medicine (1985) *The Abbreviated Injury Scale 1985. Revision*. AAAM, Arlington Heights, IL.

Appleton R (1998) Epidemiology – incidence, causes and severity. In Appleton R, Baldwin T (eds) *Management of Brain-Injured Children*. Oxford University Press, New York.

Baker SP, O'Neill B, Haddon W, Long WB (1974) The injury severity score: a method for describing patients with multiple injuries and evaluating emergency care. *Journal of Trauma* **14**: 187–96.

Biswas AK, Bruce DA, Sklar FH, Bokovoy JL, Sommerauer JF (2002) Treatment of acute traumatic brain injury in children with moderate hypothermia improves intracranial hypertension. *Critical Care Medicine* **30** (12): 2742–51.

Boortz-Marx R (1985) Factors affecting intracranial pressure: a descriptive study. *Journal of Neurosurgical Nursing* **17** (2): 89–94.

Boyd CR, Tolson MA, Copes WS (1987) Evaluating trauma care: the TRISS method. Trauma Score and the Injury Severity Score. *Journal of Trauma* **27** (4): 370–8.

Brain Injury Association of America (2005) *Facts About Traumatic Brain Injury*. Fact Sheet. Available: www.biausa.org/elements/aboutbi/factsheets/factsaboutBI.8.29.05.pdf. Accessed February 2007.

Bullock R, Chestnut RM, Clifton G *et al.* (2000) Guidelines for the management of severe traumatic brain injury. *Journal of Neurotrauma* **17** (6/7): 451–553.

Crouchman M (1998) Traumatic brain injury. In Ward-Platt MP, Little RA (eds) *Injury in the Young Child*. Cambridge University Press, Cambridge.

Crosby LJ, Parsons LC (1992) Cerebrovascular response of closed head-injured patients to a standardized endotracheal tube suctioning and manual hyperventilation procedure. *Journal of Neuroscience Nursing* **24** (1): 40–9.

Department of Health (1997) *Paediatric Intensive Care: A Framework for the Future*. The Stationery Office, London.

Department of Health (2004) *National Service Framework for Children. Every Child Matters*. The Stationery Office, London.

Durkin M, Olsen S, Barlow B, Virella A, Connolly ES (1998) The epidemiology of urban pediatric neurological trauma: evaluation of, and implications for, injury prevention programs. *Neurosurgery* **42** (2): 300–10.

Graham DI (2000) Closed head injury. In Mason JK, Pudue BN (eds) *The Pathology of Trauma*. Arnold, New York.

Hawley CA, Ward AB, Magnay AR, Long J (2003) Parental stress and burden following traumatic brain injury amongst children and adolescents. *Brain Injury* **17** (1): 1–23.

Hawley CA, Ward AB, Magnay AR, Mychalkiw W (2004) Return to school after brain injury. *Archives of Disease in Childhood*. **89** (2): 136–42.

Hazinski MF, Headrick C, Bruce D (1999) Neurological disorders. In Hazinski MF (ed.) *Manual of Pediatric Critical Care*. Mosby, St Louis, MO.

Henry PC, Hauber RP, Rice M (1992) Factors associated with closed head injury in a pediatric population. *Journal of Neuroscience Nursing* **24** (6): 311–16.

Hirsch W, Schobess A, Eichler G *et al.* (2002) Severe head trauma in children: cranial computer tomography and clinical consequences. *Paediatric Anaesthesia* **12**: 337–44.

Johnson D, Rose D (1996) Brain injury in childhood – is younger better? *Disability Awareness* **13** (2): 1.

Jones B (1994) Effects of patient repositioning on intracranial pressure. *Australian Journal of Advanced Nursing* **12** (2): 32–9.

Kaplan MS (1988) Plasticity after brain lesions: contemporary concepts. *Archives Physical Medicine and Rehabilitation* **69**: 984–91.

Kepler KL (1996) The needs of families with children with ABI. In Singer GHS, Glang A, Williams JM (eds) *Children with Acquired Brain Injury*. Brookes Publishing, Baltimore.

Kraus JF, Fife D, Conroy C (1987) Pediatric brain injuries: the nature, clinical course and early outcomes in a defined United States' population. *Pediatrics* **79** (4): 501–7.

Mahoney WJ, D'Souza BJ, Haller JA *et al.* (1983) Long-term outcome of children with severe head trauma and prolonged coma. *Pediatrics* **71** (5): 756–62.

Marks M, Sliwinski M, Gordon WA (1993) An examination of the needs of families with a brain-injured child. *NeuroRehabilitation* **3** (3): 1–12.

McMillan TM, Greenwood RJ (1993) Models of rehabilitation programmes for the brain injured adult: services and suggestions for change in the UK. *Clinical Rehabilitation* **7**: 346–55.

Muwaswes M (1985) Increased intracranial pressure and its systemic effects. *Journal of Neurosurgical Nursing* **4**: 238–43.

National Institute for Health and Clinical Excellence (2003) *Head Injury. Triage, Assessment, Investigation and Early Management of Head Injury in Infants, Children and Adults*. NICE, London.

National Institute for Health and Clinical Excellence (2007) *Head Injury. Triage, Assessment, Investigation and Early Management of Head Injury in Infants, Children and Adults*, 2nd edn. NICE, London.

Neumann VC (1995) Principles and practices of treatment. In Chamberlain MA, Neumann VC, Tennant A (eds) *Traumatic Brain Injury Rehabilitation Services, Treatment and Outcomes*. Chapman and Hall Medical, London.

Office of National Statistics (2004). Childhood, infant, and perinatal mortality statistics. DH3, no. 45, ONS, London.

Palmer M, Wyness MA (1988) Positioning and handling: important considerations in the care of the severely head-injured patient. *Journal of Neuroscience Nursing* **20** (1): 42–8.

Paratz J, Burns Y (1993) The effect of respiratory physiotherapy on intracranial pressure, mean arterial pressure, cerebral perfusion pressure and end tidal carbon dioxide in ventilated neurosurgical patients. *Physiotherapy Theory and Practice* **9**: 3–11.

Parslow RC, Morris KP, Tasker RC *et al.* (2005) Epidemiology of traumatic brain injury in children receiving intensive care in the UK. *Archives of Disease in Childhood* **90**: 1182–7.

Prabhakaran P, Reddy AT, Oakes WJ *et al.* (2004) A pilot trial comparing cerebral perfusion pressure-targeted therapy to intracranial pressure-targeted therapy in children with severe traumatic brain injury. *Journal of Neurosurgery* **100** (5 Suppl Pediatrics): 454–9.

Raimondi AJ, Hirschauer J (1984) Head injury in the infant and toddler. Coma scoring and outcome scale *Child's Brain* **11**: 12–35.

Rising CJ (1993) The relationship of selected nursing activities to ICP. *Journal of Neuroscience Nursing* **25** (5): 302–8.

Rose FD, Johnson DA, Attree EA (1997) Rehabilitation of the head-injured child: basic research and new technology. *Pediatric Rehabilitation* **1**(1): 3–7.

Rosner MJ, Daughton S (1990) Cerebral perfusion pressure management in head injury. *Journal of Trauma* **30**: 933–40.

Rudy EB, Turner BS, Baun M, Stone KS, Brucia J (1991) Endotracheal suctioning in adults with head injury. *Heart & Lung* **20** (6): 667–4.

Satz P, Zaucha K, McCleary C *et al.* (1997) Mild head injury in children and adolescents: a review of studies (1970–1995). *Psychological Bulletin* **122** (2): 107–31.

Scottish Intercollegiate Guidelines Network (2000) *Early Management of Patients with a Head Injury*. SIGN, Edinburgh.

Singer GHS (1996) Constructing supports. In Singer GHS, Glang A, Williams JM (eds) *Children with Acquired Brain Injury*. Paul H Brookes Publishing, Baltimore.

Stancin T, Drotar D, Taylor HG *et al.* (2002) Health-related quality of life of children and adolescents after traumatic brain injury. *Pediatrics* **109** (2): 34–42.

Tasker RC, Morris KP, Forsyth RJ *et al.* (2006) Severe head injury in children: emergency access to neurosurgery in the United Kingdom. *Emergency Medicine Journal* **23**: 519–22.

Tasker RC (2000) Neurological critical care. *Current Opinion in Pediatrics* **12**: 222–6.

Tilford JM, Simpson PM, Yeh TS *et al.* (2001) Variation in therapy and outcome for pediatric head trauma patients. *Critical Care Medicine* **29** (5): 1056–61.

Treloar DM, Nalli BJ, Guin P, Gary R (1991) The effects of familiar and unfamiliar voice treatments on intracranial pressure in head-injured patients. *Journal of Neuroscience Nursing* **23** (5): 295–9.

Wade SL, Gerry Taylor H, Yeates KO *et al.* (2006) Long-term parental and family adaptation following pediatric brain injury. *Journal of Pediatric Psychology* **31** (10): 1072–83.

Walleck C (1983) The effects of purposeful touch on intracranial pressure. *Heart & Lung* **12**: 428–9.

Williams A, Coyne SM (1993) Effects of neck position on intracranial pressure. *American Journal of Critical Care* **2** (1): 68–71.

Wilson JT, Pettigrew LE, Teasdale GM (2000) Emotional and cognitive consequences of head injury in relation to the Glasgow outcome scale. *Journal of Neurology, Neurosurgery, Psychiatry* **69**: 204–9.

Youngblut JM, Brooten D (2006) Pediatric head trauma: parent, parent–child, and family functioning 2 weeks after hospital discharge. *Journal of Pediatric Psychology* **31** (6): 608–18.

6   Craniosynostosis

Craniosynostosis is a condition of premature fusion of the skull sutures affecting approximately 1 in 2,000 children (Child Neurology 2002). Although broadly defined as the premature fusion of one or more of the skull sutures, craniosynostosis can occur as part of a more complex syndrome in which the facial bones are also involved. If left untreated, craniosynostosis can result in increased intracranial pressure which occurs as the brain continues to grow and develop but is restricted because of abnormal skull growth. The child usually requires surgery to correct the deformity and resultant disfigurement, but also to relieve raised intracranial pressure and, where possible, prevent complications such as impaired vision, hearing and learning difficulties.

At the end of reading this chapter you will be able to:

Learning outcomes

- Outline the causes of craniosynostosis and the pathophysiology changes that occur as a result of premature fusion of the skull sutures
- Describe the nursing care of the child and family, where the child requires surgery to treat the craniosynostosis
- Discuss the long-term care needs of the child and family.

6.1 Classification, incidence and aetiology

Classification

The term craniosynostosis was first introduced in the 1850s to describe a premature fusion of one or more of the skull sutures (Virchow 1851). This is a broad definition and does not reflect the complexities of the condition. Although there are variations in the definition and classification of craniosynostosis, Hockley's (1993) definition appears to be well accepted: primary craniosynostosis is a congenital disorder with significant skull deformity, as a result of premature fusion of the cranial sutures, and can be subdivided into simple or complex craniosynostosis. Simple craniosynostosis is a synostosis of a single suture with no involvement of the facial skeleton. Complex craniosynostosis is a synostosis of one or more sutures with involvement of the facial skeleton, and includes the plethora of craniosynostotic syndromes.

Sixty-two syndromes have been identified where craniosynostosis is the predominant feature (Cohen and MacLean 2000) but it has been estimated that craniosynostosis may be a feature in more than 150 syndromes (Warren *et al.* 2001). The majority of these syndromes are genetic in origin, with Apert's and Crouzon's syndromes being the most well known. In addition, craniosynostosis can develop as a complication of diseases such as rickets, spherocytosis (diseased red blood cells), hypophosphatasia (an inherited absence of alkaline phosphatase, an enzyme essential in bone formation), hyperthyroidism and hypercalcaemia (excessive calcium in the blood), microcephaly and shunted hydrocephalus (Panchal and Uttchin 2003).

Incidence

The incidence of craniosynostosis varies within the literature and has been estimated to be between 1 in 1,000 to 1 in 3,000 births (Kershner and Claussen 1986; Hockley 1993; Sarnat and Menkes 2000; Johnston 2001; Warren *et al.* 2001; Child Neurology 2002; Lee *et al.* 2002). It has been estimated that 50 per cent of children with craniosynostosis have a related syndrome (Okkerse *et al.* 2004). Because of isolated clusters reported in England and North America during the 1990s, there have been concerns that craniosynostosis is increasing (Hunt 1993; Kirby *et al.* 1993; Suttaford 1993; Jones *et al.* 1997). Two large population studies carried out in North America support these concerns (Mynanthopolous 1977; Alderman *et al.* 1988). However, overall there is a lack of evidence to indicate a true increase. The reported increase may be due to increased awareness, improved diagnosis of the condition in children and incorrect diagnosis of positional skull deformities.

Aetiology

There is much speculation about the aetiology of craniosynostosis. Most cases are sporadic, with the cause of the defect largely unknown. There is evidence to support a genetic link because many of the craniosynostosis syndromes have a hereditary mode of inheritance (Boyadjiev 2007). Primary craniosynostosis may be due to a single gene defect with both autosomal dominant and autosomal recessive inheritance being implicated (Boyadjiev 2007). However, autosomal dominant transmission is thought to be the most common mode of inheritance with high penetrance; if a parent and child have craniosynostosis, or two siblings have craniosynostosis with unaffected parents, there is an increased risk that future children will be affected, although a different suture may be fused in affected individuals within the same family. Heterogenecity is further complicated by the fact that even though the gene responsible for craniosynostosis may be identical within the same family, it may not be the same gene in a different family with an identical mode of inheritance. Sagittal synostosis has been associated with an X-linked mode of inheritance because it is much more common in males.

There are few comprehensive studies that have investigated the epidemiology of craniosynostosis. One exception is the Colorado study which investigated factors that might be associated with the development of craniosynostosis (Alderman *et al.* 1988).

Points to consider

Craniosynostosis is more likely to occur in:

- Boys
- Multiple births
- Older maternal and/or paternal age
- Low birth-weight babies
- Caucasian ethnic group
- If there have been complications with labour.

There is a weak positive association between craniosynostosis and altitude, water basin and rural areas. The Colorado study supports a genetic mode of inheritance for craniosynostosis because links were found with increased maternal age and could be due to a greater likelihood of chromosomal mutations with an increase in maternal age. Maternal race was also identified as a factor with no cases of craniosynostosis identified in children with African mothers (Alderman *et al.* 1988). The association of craniosynostosis with multiple births supports the theory that fetal head constraints from early lightening may contribute to the development of skull defects.

Although not substantiated craniosynostosis has been linked with (Hockley 1993):

- Drug teratogenicity, particularly the anticonvulsant phenytoin
- Maternal excesses of vitamins A and D and ethanol
- Intrauterine compression
- Pesticides, lead and pollution

6.2 Pathophysiology, clinical presentation and diagnosis

Pathophysiology

The anatomy of the bones of the skull are described in Chapter 1, Section 7 and represented diagrammatically in Figure 1.7a. Eighty per cent of brain growth occurs during the first three years of life (May 1992). Under normal circumstances the skull enlarges in response to the growing brain, which reaches 50 per cent of adult size by six months of age and 98 per cent by the age of two years. To allow for this brain growth, the sutures do not normally fully close until late childhood. There are wide variations in the age at which closure of the sutures takes place. It is thought the metopic suture begins to close in the late prenatal period (Moos and Hide 1993). At about three months of age, the posterior fontanelle closes and at 20 months of age the anterior fontenelle closes. At about eight years, ossification of the craniobasal bones is complete. By age 12 years, the sutures usually cannot be separated if the intracranial pressure rises; however, they continue to be visible on radiography until about 30 years of age (Johnston 2001). Closure of a suture before the expected time inhibits normal perpendicular brain expansion. Compensatory growth occurs when the brain is forced to grow in a direction parallel to the fused suture resulting in an alteration of normal head shape (Johnston 2001).

The underlying cause of the pathophysiological changes in craniosynostosis are unknown (Panchal *et al.* 2001; Panchal and Uttchin 2003). However, animal models indicate a relationship between the expression of growth factors initiated by regional dura mater that influence changes in the bone growth of cranial sutures (Panchal and Uttchin 2003). The cause for initiation of growth factors is unknown (Panchal *et al.* 2001). One theory suggests that genetic abnormalities in the underlying cortex result in abnormal brain growth, which may be the trigger for the dural cells to express abnormal growth factors (Panchal *et al.* 2001).

There is a relationship between brain growth and maintaining the patency of the cranial sutures. In children with microcephaly, brain growth failure results in premature fusion of the sutures. In contrast, conditions such as hydrocephalus can result in continuation of suture patency to accommodate increased intracranial volume (Panchal and Uttchin 2003).

Points to consider

The distinction between microcephaly and primary craniosynostosis is an important consideration and must be made prior to treatment options being discussed with the child and family (Fenichel 1997).

Clinical presentation

In craniosynostosis the resultant skull shape depends on the specific suture or sutures that are fused (Figure 6.2a). The clinical features occur because normal skull bone growth is inhibited at the fused suture site but continues parallel to the fused suture (Sarnat and Menkes 2000). Bones remain small and underdeveloped at the site of fusion, while the unaffected bones enlarge to compensate, thus allowing brain growth (May 1992). Usually the first indication the child has craniosynostosis is an abnormal head shape that is detected within the first few weeks of life (Fenichel 1997). Occasionally there may be an indication that there is an abnormality of the skull sutures during routine ultrasound in the antenatal period (May 1992).

Points to consider

The child's clinical picture will depend on: the specific suture that has closed, the order in which they close (if more than one suture is involved), the age of the child when the suture closes and the success or failure of the other sutures to compensate.

Common types of craniosynostosis

Sagittal synostosis

Premature fusion of the sagittal suture is the most common form of craniosynostosis (Johnston 2001). It accounts for 60 per cent of all cases of craniosynostosis and is more common in boys than girls (Boltshauser *et al.* 2003). Premature fusion of the sagittal suture results in scaphocephaly, typified by a long, narrow head often associated with an expansion of the forehead (frontal bossing), biparietal pinching, occipital protuberance and a ridge at the sagittal suture site (Johnston 2001). Approximately 40 per cent of children with sagittal synostosis will have learning difficulties (Sarnat and Menkes 2000).

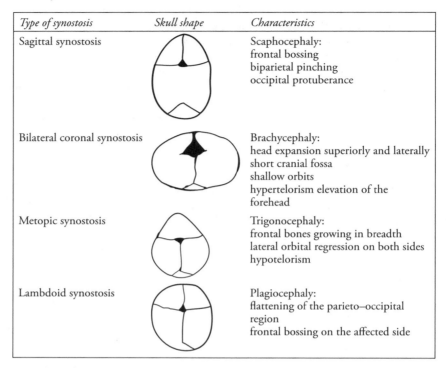

Type of synostosis	*Skull shape*	*Characteristics*
Sagittal synostosis		Scaphocephaly: frontal bossing biparietal pinching occipital protuberance
Bilateral coronal synostosis		Brachycephaly: head expansion superiorly and laterally short cranial fossa shallow orbits hypertelorism elevation of the forehead
Metopic synostosis		Trigonocephaly: frontal bones growing in breadth lateral orbital regression on both sides hypotelorism
Lambdoid synostosis		Plagiocephaly: flattening of the parieto–occipital region frontal bossing on the affected side

Figure 6.2a The different presentations of craniosynostosis

Coronal synostosis

Coronal synostosis is less common than sagittal synostosis, accounting for approximately 20 per cent of all cases of craniosynostosis and is more frequent in girls (Fenichel 1997). Coronal synostosis results in brachycephaly characterized by head expansion superiorly and laterally, a short cranial fossa, shallow orbits, hypertelorism (wide spacing between the eyes) and elevation of the forehead. Approximately 50 per cent of affected children with synostosis of both coronal sutures have learning difficulties (Sarnat and Menkes 2000).

Plagiocephaly

Premature fusion of one of the lambdoidal sutures or one of the coronal sutures results in plagiocephaly. The result is flattening of the parieto-occipital region and compensatory frontal bossing on the affected side (Moos and Hide 1993). There may be torsion of the skull base with ear asymmetry. It has been suggested that true plagiocephaly is rare, constituting 3–5 per cent of all cases of craniosynostosis (Mouradian 1998). True occipital plagiocephaly is often confused with positional deformities as a result of infant sleeping positions. These deformities have increased following the successful 'back to sleep' campaigns during the 1990s, which were aimed at reducing the mortality in children as a result of sudden infant death syndrome (Jones *et al.* 1997; Mouradian 1998). It is vital that positional deformities are differentiated from true synostosis because the former require no treatment or conservative management such as molding-helmet therapy, compared to true plagiocephaly which requires surgery to correct the deformity (Panchal *et al.* 2001; Panchal and Uttchin 2003).

Metopic synostosis

Premature fusion of the metopic suture results in metopic synostosis. There are two conflicting views of the timing of normal metopic suture fusion: fusion of the suture occurs in the second year of life (Huang *et al.* 1998); or fusion of the suture begins *in utero* and therefore the deformity could be present at birth (Moos and Hide 1993). Either way, the result is trigonocephaly, where the frontal bones grow in breadth with lateral orbital regression on both sides of the skull and hypotelorism (abnormally decreased space between the eyes). This results in a narrow triangular shaped head (Moos and Hide 1993). This type of synostosis accounts for about 10 per cent of all cases of craniosynostosis (May 1992).

Craniostenosis or oxycephaly

Craniostenosis, sometimes referred to as oxycephaly, is a result of premature closure of all the cranial sutures. Of all types of craniosynostosis, oxycephaly can produce the most severe central nervous system (CNS) involvement because total brain growth is restricted and increased intracranial pressure is likely. This may lead to impaired mental and motor functions, optic nerve atrophy and death. Divergent strabismus (muscle failure and nerve defects in the eyes causing them to move in separate directions), optic atrophy (wasting of the optic disc), anosmia (impairment of the sense of smell) and bilateral pyramidal tract signs can either occur as associated CNS anomalies or because of a lack of sufficient space to allow for expansion of the brain. Psychomotor difficulties can result from prolonged increased intracranial pressure, but more often are caused by associated cerebral malformations or concurrent hydrocephalus (Sarnat and Menkes 2000).

Common syndromes associated with craniosynostosis

1   Crouzon's syndrome, also referred to as craniofacial dysostosis, affects 1 in 60,000 live births (Hockley 1993) and is the combination of premature closure of any or all of the cranial sutures and maldevelopment of the facial bones (Fenichel 1997). The facial deformity is present at birth and, if left untreated, will become more pronounced during infancy. The skull is usually widened anteriorly as a result of premature closure of the coronal suture, causing the child to have an abnormally high forehead (Fenichel 1997). The child usually presents with hypertelorism and exophthalmos (bulging of the eye balls). The midface is usually underdeveloped and the child may have receded cheekbones and an underdeveloped lower jaw. Adding to the deformity is a beak-like nose, high arched palate and protuberant tongue. Hydrocephalus develops in a large proportion of children with Crouzon's syndrome, and is thought to be a result of intracranial venous hypertension or from the early closure of the lambdoid sutures causing raised intracranial pressure (Fenichel 1997). Children with Crouzon's syndrome often have normal intellect (Sarnat and Menkes 2000). Crouzon's syndrome is thought to be of autosomal dominant inheritance as a result of a genetic defect on chromosome 10 (Sarnat and Menkes 2000).

2   Acrocephalosyndactyly is a global term used for several different syndromes with the same basic combination of features. These include craniosynostosis, syndactyly (fusion of fingers and toes) and usually some degree of mental retardation. The four most common of the *acrocephalosyndactyly* syndromes are Apert's, Carpenter's, Chotzen and Pfeiffer syndromes.

a Apert's syndrome affects 1 in 10,000 live births (Hockley 1993) and is characterized by syndactyly and premature closure of the coronal sutures resulting in brachycephaly (Fenichel 1997) (Figure 6.2a). The head and facial configuration are similar to those seen in Crouzon's syndrome, but the face bones are usually affected less. Under-development of the upper jaw causes misalignment and crowding of the teeth. Approximately one-third of children with this syndrome have a cleft palate (Sarimski 2001). Most cases are sporadic, but autosomal dominant inheritance is suspected (Fenichel 1997) and like Crouzon's syndrome, Apert's syndrome has been linked to a defect on chromosome 10 (Sarimski 2001). Raised intracranial pressure is present in about 80 per cent of cases. Problems associated with Apert's syndrome could be as a result of concomitant brain malformations (Sarimski 2001). Only a small proportion of children with Apert's syndrome have normal intelligence; 50 per cent have difficulties relating to peers, which may be a result of psychosocial difficulties associated with the severe facial deformity, the children are often anxious when faced with having to interact in social situations and many have attention problems (Sarnat and Menkes 2000; Sarimski 2001).

b Carpenter's syndrome is thought to be transmitted by autosomal recessive inheritance patterns (Fenichel 1997). Although the underlying cause is unknown, there is evidence of genetic inheritance with siblings often affected (World Craniofacial Foundation (WCF) 2004). The child will have polydactyly (more than usual number of fingers or toes) as well as syndactyly. All of the cranial sutures close prematurely. The child may have malformation of the eyes, low set ears, short neck, small mandible and high arched narrow palate. The child is usually obese and, in boys, there will be hypogonadism (Fenichel 1997; WCF 2004). Approximately 75 per cent of children with Carpenter's syndrome have some degree of mental retardation, secondary to cerebral malformations, which can be identified on MRI scanning (Fenichel 1997).

c Chotzen syndrome is caused by an alteration of a gene located on chromosome 7, and has an autosomal dominant mode of inheritance (National Craniofacial Association (NCA) 2003a). It is characterized by fusion of the cranial sutures, which causes asymmetry of the head and face, low set frontal hairline, deviated nasal septum and ptosis (drooping of one or both upper eyelids). Fingers and toes are often shortened and syndactyly of the second and third fingers may be present. Intelligence is not usually impaired (Fenichel 1997; NCA 2003a).

d Pfeiffer syndrome is abnormal genes mapped to chromosomes 8 and 10 and has an autosomal dominant mode of inheritance (WCF 2004). The child will have craniosynostosis, and hypertelorism (wide set eyes) with ocular ptosis (bulging eyes due to shallow sockets). The thumbs and big toes are broad and short, and syndactyly is usually present (NCA 2003b).

Diagnosis

Craniosynostosis may be obvious at birth because the infant has an abnormally shaped head or face, but the deformity usually becomes more pronounced during rapid growth in early infancy (Hockley 1993). Diagnosis is usually made by visual inspection of the skull and palpation of the sutures (Fenichel 1997). The shape of the skull is indicative of the fused suture or sutures (Figure 6.2a). A prematurely closed suture will present on X-ray as a band of increased bone density at the site of the closure (Fenichel 1997). A computerized tomography (CT) scan is the definitive investigation and allows for a two-dimensional view of each suture and will reveal the degree of the increase in density of the bone at the site of the fused sutures (Panchal and Uttchin 2003).

A magnetic resonance imaging (MRI) scan may also be performed if there are indications of hydrocephalus or abnormalities of cortical architecture (Sarnat and Menkes 2000, Panchal and Uttchin 2003). Infants may present with acute problems, such as airway difficulties and choanal atresia, requiring immediate treatment such as oxygen via nasal prongs or the formation of a tracheostomy. Occasionally the child will present with signs and symptoms of raised intracranial pressure (Chapter 2, Section 3) and may require insertion of a ventricular peritoneal shunt prior to a craniectomy (May 1992).

6.3 Management of the child with craniosynostosis

The surgical management of craniofacial anomalies was pioneered in the late 1960s, with operative correction of the deformity now the treatment of choice (Moos and Hide 1993). The decision to operate is not easy in cases of single-suture synostosis because there are no long-term studies which identify that surgery improves functional outcomes (Polley *et al.* 1998; Arnaud *et al.* 2002; Boltshauser *et al.* 2003). Furthermore, in some cases, aesthetic appearance can become less obvious as the child grows (Boltshauser *et al.* 2003). However, surgery may prevent deterioration in neurological function (Panchal *et al.* 2001; Polley *et al.* 1998).

Points to consider

It is essential the family understand the indications and outcomes of surgery from the outset so that they can make an informed choice

Surgery can range from excision of the fused suture, for example in sagittal synostosis, to complex craniofacial surgery involving excision of the fused suture, cranial decompression, cranio-orbital reconstruction and reshaping of the skull and facial bones (Kershner and Claussen 1986; Polley *et al.* 1998). Although paediatric neuroscience is regarded as a specialist field of practice (Chumas *et al.* 2002; DH 2002), the complexities involved in craniofacial surgery have resulted in this type of surgery being further identified as a sub-specialty (Society of British Neurological Surgeons 2001; Child Neurology 2002).

Points to consider

Children requiring complex craniofacial surgery must be cared for within a designated centre, where there is an experienced team of healthcare professionals and suitable facilities to manage a child with the potential to be neurologically and haemodynamically unstable (Panchal and Uttchin 2003).

Several studies have been undertaken regarding the optimum age the child should undergo surgery, but in general the findings are inconclusive (Speltz *et al.* 1997; Kapp-Simon 1998; Panchal *et al.* 2001). It has been suggested that the optimal period for surgical correction is between three to six months of age, preferably within the first year of life to maximize subsequent mental and psychomotor development (MacKenzie 1990; Speltz *et al.* 1997; Kapp-Simon 1998; Johnston 2001; Panchal *et al.* 2001). Within this timeframe the deformity will not have progressed, the bones will be more malleable and the growing brain will promote a normal shape, resulting in greater cosmetic improvements. The psychological trauma for the family may be reduced if the surgery is performed at a young age (May 1992). Early treatment potentially minimizes later complications, such as visual, nasal, phonetic, dental problems, psychological dysfunctions and learning disabilities (Panchal and Uttchin 2003). If left untreated, skull deformities become permanent and there is increased risk of raised intracranial pressure developing (Moos and Hide 1993).

> **Points to consider**
>
> Correction of complex craniofacial syndromes requires surgery throughout childhood, with future procedures determined by alterations to craniofacial structures as the child grows (Panchal and Uttchin 2003).

The aim of surgery is to correct the deformity, improve the appearance of the head, allow normal growth of the brain and treat or prevent raised intracranial pressure (Cohen and Persing 1998). Linear crainectomy (excision of the fused suture) is effective for sagittal synostosis. Oesteotomies of the skull base are suitable for remaining types of synostosis as required to facilitate brain expansion. Craniofacial surgery for craniosynostosis involves the repositioning and reshaping of the skull and facial bones, as well as a range of soft tissue reconstructive techniques, such as canthoplasties, nasal reconstructions and facial cleft repairs (Kershner and Claussen 1986). The stages of surgery for complex craniofacial syndromes are usually (Panchal and Uttchin 2003):

1   Correction of the craniosynostosis (before 1 year of age).
2   Correction of syndactyly (1–2 years of age).
3   Correction of mid-face distortions (4–5 years of age).
4   Correction of hypertelorism (4–6 years of age).
5   Mandibular reconstruction once full maturity has been reached.

Preoperative care

Depending on the complexity of the abnormality the child may require supportive management prior to surgery, including respiratory, nutritional and visual assessments, with the initiation of appropriate interventions as necessary (May 2001). There is a need to involve a range of healthcare professionals and ensure effective interdisciplinary team-working if parents are to be supported appropriately. Genetic counselling is important to assist parents in understanding the reasons the condition may have occurred and to offer advice regarding future pregnancies. Difficulties of parents forming attachments to the child with facial abnormalities have been reported (Barden *et al.* 1989). Identifying families where difficulties occur and offering parents support are essential if a positive relationship is to be developed with their child.

Points to consider

Psychological assessment and support are a vital parts of the initial care of the child and family. A preoperative neurodevelopmental assessment is necessary to establish if there are any developmental problems prior to surgery which will aid in predicting the long-term outcomes of surgery and will enable clinicians to offer realistic expectations (Panchal and Uttchin 2003).

The general principles of caring for a child requiring neurosurgery are described in Chapter 3 and apply to the child undergoing surgery for craniosynostosis. The child will usually be admitted to the neurosurgical ward at least the day before the operation and will require a general assessment and a full blood count and group and cross match. The child will require a detailed assessment by an anaesthetist, particularly of the respiratory system to identify any potential difficulties in the administration of the anaesthetic or intubation. The family will have discussed all aspects of the surgery prior to admission but should be given opportunity to discuss any further concerns before the consent for operation is obtained. The parents should be given realistic expectations of the postoperative appearance of their child to avoid disappointment (Drew 1990). They need to be informed that the child's head shape may appear fairly normal immediately after surgery but significant postoperative swelling will occur within a few hours and the child may not be able to open his or her eyes. This swelling usually reaches a peak at about 2–3 days postoperatively. Parents should be reassured that although the swelling is uncomfortable, it is not usually painful and will resolve (Johnston 2001). Parents should be allowed to visit the postoperative care area if the child will not be returning to the admitting ward.

Postoperative care

The general principles of postoperative care described in Chapter 3 will apply to the child undergoing surgery for craniosynostosis. The child will be nursed in the high dependency area of the paediatric neurosurgical ward or on a paediatric intensive care unit usually for the first 24–48 hours after surgery (Panchal and Uttchin 2003). If there are any indications of breathing difficulties, or if surgery has been lengthy, the child will require elective ventilation in the initial postoperative period. The child will require detailed assessment of neurological functions because the potential risk of intracranial pressure increases as a result of generalized cerebral oedema and haemorrhage. The management of raised intracranial pressure is outlined in Chapter 5, Section 3.

In the young infant the amount of blood loss during surgery may be two or three times the circulating blood volume, and although this will have been replaced intra-operatively, it may be advisable to electively ventilate the infant until haemodynamically stable (MacKenzie 1990). The amount of blood loss and circulating fluid volumes must be regularly assessed through repeated blood sampling to monitor full blood count, haemoglobin levels, urea and electrolytes, clotting factors and serum osmolality. Maintaining fluid and electrolytes is a balance between ensuring adequate circulatory blood volume to maintain good cerebral perfusion and preventing over-hydration, which will add to cerebral oedema and blood loss at the capillary beds. The child should be nursed at a 45° head tilt to reduce cerebral oedema. Initially the child will require continual cardiac, arterial and central venous pressure (CVP) monitoring (May 1992). Management of type and amount of fluid will be specific to each child's needs, haemoglobin levels and urea and electrolyte profile. Colloids will be required to treat hypovolaemia and blood transfusion(s) will be indicated if the haemoglobin levels fall, usually when less than 9 g/dL. The child's fluid balance must be accurately recorded and monitored. Oral feeds may be introduced to non-ventilated infants as soon as the cough and gag reflexes have returned and once fully recovered from the anaesthetic. The child must be monitored for signs of haemorrhage including observing bandages and drains if present for excessive blood loss, changes in conscious levels, raised pulse, falling blood pressure and changes in peripheral perfusion (May 2001).

The child will require regular analgesia (Chapter 3, Section 2). Paracetamol and diclofenac are suitable analgesia which can be given at regular intervals. Opioid analgesics, such as codeine phosphate, should be used for moderate to severe pain. Morphine infusion can be used in the immediate postoperative period, however the child will require appropriate monitoring (MacKenzie 1990). Morphine can depress respirations, induce drowsiness and sleep, and cause the pupils to constrict due to its effect on the nucleus of the third cranial nerve, resulting in difficulty in accurately assessing the child's neurological status. Codeine phosphate and morphine are both opioids and should not be used in combination.

The child's temperature must be monitored postoperatively, as an elevated temperature could be an indication of wound infection. However, hyperpyrexia is common postoperatively, usually as a result of irritation of cerebral tissues by the presence of blood, but this usually subsides after the first 72 hours (Panchal and Uttchin 2003). Paracetamol, in additional to its analgesic properties, is an antipyretic but may mask the symptoms of infection.

In general, complications of surgery such as wound infection, wound dehiscence and cerebrospinal fluid leakage are low (Panchal and Uttchin 2003). Mortality and morbidity is associated with insufficient blood replacement in the intra-operative and immediate postoperative stages (Panchal and Uttchin 2003). Once the child is stable and no longer requires mechanical ventilation, usually within 24–48 hours, they should be transferred back to the paediatric neurosurgery ward. If there are no problematic events discharge is usually around 4–5 days post-surgery. A CT scan may be performed prior to discharge to record and determine skull symmetry but practice varies (Panchal and Uttchin 2003). Parents will require support in handling their child post-surgery and are advised not to lay them prone for one week.

Long-term follow up is essential to evaluate the outcome of the surgery, assess the need for further surgery and monitor the child's development. Head circumference should be monitored at follow-up appointments and as part of routine health surveillance to help detect signs of increased intracranial pressure, which may indicate the development of hydrocephalus (Hudgins *et al.* 1998). The ultimate aim of care is to support the child in achieving their full potential, including social interactions with other children, and to adapt into their socio-cultural environment. This will require input from a range of professionals across health, social and educational services.

6.4. Long-term care needs of a child with craniosynostosis

The extent of the child's long-term care needs and resultant deficits depends on a range of factors including: the presence of an associated syndrome; the severity of craniosynostosis; damaging effects of increased intracranial pressure; and repeated shunt infections if hydrocephalus is present. Physical problems include visual and hearing deficits, facial dysostosis and prognathism (Drew 1990). There is great variability in the level of cognitive and psychomotor function. However, for many of the children and their families, body image is a significant issue. Although it is uncommon for parents to reject their child at birth, the attitude of the midwife and other healthcare professionals is a significant factor in assisting parents to establish a positive relationship with the infant (MacKenzie 1990). Parents are likely to feel that people are staring at their child's unusual head shape and altered facial structure and this can result in parents feeling alone and isolated, with no-one else around them facing the same anxieties (Drew 1990). Parents may feel a sense of guilt and will require support for them to come to terms with their feelings (Drew 1990). Some parents may find support groups helpful, where they can meet other parents in a similar position, and this can reduce their sense of isolation (MacKenzie 1990).

Children with single-suture synostosis may have minor learning difficulties and developmental delay, particularly motor functioning (Kapp-Simon 1998, Panchal *et al.* 2001). Fortunately these deficits may not be functionally important with the majority of children maintaining normal levels of schooling and are usually psychologically well adjusted (Boltshauser *et al.* 2003). Syndromic craniosynostosis is a heterogeneous group, resulting in a wide range of neurological deficits and more complex difficulties compared with single-suture synostosis (Arnaud *et al.* 2002). These children may require a range of support systems to achieve their maximum potential.

The diversity of the long-term outcomes for children requires an individualized and family-centred approach to care, based upon the child's assessment and specific needs. The team of professionals involved may include a neurosurgeon and plastic surgeon, ophthalmologist, ear-nose-throat surgeon, orthodontist, faciomaxillary surgeon, psychologist, geneticist, teachers, nurses, physiotherapists, occupational therapists, speech therapists, educationalists and social workers. The team must work together to ensure there is a seamless care delivery package. The family must be an integral part of the team. The nurse plays a vital role in this team, aiding communication and coordination of care. Educational assessment may result in the child requiring additional support (Drew 1990). The follow-up care for children with craniosynostosis will vary depending on the extent of the individual child's needs; for children with complex needs, follow-up care is life-long.

Key messages from this chapter

- Craniosynostosis is a condition of premature fusion of the skull sutures with the resultant skull shape being depending on the specific suture, or sutures, that are fused
- Craniosynostosis is more likely to occur in: boys, multiple births, older parents, low birth weight babies, Caucasian ethnic groups, and if there have been complications with labour
- Fusion of the sagittal suture is the most common form of craniosynostosis
- It is vital that positional deformities are differentiated from true synostosis
- It is essential the family understand the indications and outcomes of surgery from the outset, so that they can make an informed choice
- Surgery can range from excision of the fused suture to complex craniofacial surgery
- Long-term problems include visual and hearing deficits, facial dysostosis and prognathism and there is great variability in the level of cognitive and psychomotor function
- For many of the children and their families, body image is a significant issue.

Web resources

Child-Neuro UK
provides a range of information relating to craniosynostosis
www.child-neuro.org.uk
Contact a Family
is the only UK-wide charity providing advice, information and support to the parents of all disabled children, no matter what their health condition. It enables parents to get in contact with other families on a local and national basis.
www.cafamily.org.uk/index.html
Faces
The National Craniofacial Association in the US has a wide range of information relating to craniofacial deformities.
www.faces-cranio.org
Headlines
A British based support group for parents of children with craniosynostosis
www.headlines.org.uk
Cranio Kids
Created as a caring and educational environment where families can find support, friendships, and fun.
www.craniokids.org

References

Alderman BW, Lammer EJ, Joshua SC *et al.* (1988) An epidemiologic study of craniosynostosis: risk indicators for the occurrence of craniosynostosis in Colorado. *American Journal of Epidemiology* **128** (2): 431–8.

Arnaud E, Meneses P, Lajeunie E *et al.* (2002) Postoperative mental and morphological outcome for nonsyndromic brachycephaly. *Plastic and Reconstructive Surgery* **110** (1): 6–12.

Barden RC, Ford ME, Jenson AG, Rogers-Salyer M, Salyer KE (1989) Effects of craniofacial deformity in infancy on the quality of mother-infant interactions. *Child Development* **60** (4): 819–24.

Boltshauser E, Ludwig S, Dietrich S, Landolt MA (2003) Sagittal craniosynostosis: cognitive development, behaviour, and quality of life in unoperated children. *Neuropediatrics* **34** (6): 293–300.

Boyadjiev SA (2007) Genetic analysis of non-syndromic craniosynostosis. *Orthodontics & Craniofacial Research* **10** (3): 129–37.

Child Neurology (2002) Craniosynostosis. Fact sheet. Available: www.child-neuro.org.uk/neurotext/93.html. Accessed October 2007.

Chumas P, Hardy D, Hockley A *et al.* (2002) Safe paediatric neurosurgery 2001. *British Journal of Neurosurgery* **16** (3): 208–10.

Cohen MM (1979) Craniosynostosis and syndromes with craniosynostosis: incidence, genetics, penetrance, variability, and new syndrome updating. *Birth Defects* **15** (5B): 13–63.

Cohen SR, Persing JA (1998) Intracranial pressure in single-suture craniosynostosis. *Cleft Palate–Craniofacial Journal* **35** (3): 194–6.

Cohen MM, MacLean RE (2000) *Craniosynostosis: Diagnosis, Evaluation and Management,* 2nd edn. Oxford University Press, New York

Department of Health (2002) *Specialised Services for Children – Definition No. 23*. Available: www.dh.gov. uk/en/Managingyourorganisation/Commissioning/Commissioningspecialisedservices/Specialised servicesdefinition/DH_4001699. Accessed February 2008.

Drew A (1990) A parent's perspective. *Paediatric Nursing* **2** (6): 22–4.

Fenichel GM (1997) Disorders of cranial volume and shape. In Fenichel GM (ed.) *Clinical Pediatric Neurology. A Signs and Symptoms Approach*, 3rd edn. W.B. Saunders, Philadelphia, PA.

Hockley AD (1993) Craniosynostosis. *Lancet* **342**: 189–90.

Huang MH, Mouradian WE, Cohen SR, Gruss (1998) The differential diagnosis of abnormal head shapes: separating craniosynostosis from positional deformities and normal variants. *Cleft Palate–Craniofacial Journal* **35** (3): 204–11.

Hudgins RJ, Cohen SR, Burstein FD, Boydston WR (1998) Multiple suture synostosis and increased intracranial pressure following repair of single suture, nonsyndromal craniosynostosis. *Cleft Palate– Craniofacial Journal* **35** (2): 167–72.

Hunt L (1993) 'Second group of skull deformity babies found'. *The Independent*. July 7: 2.

Johnston SA (2001) Calvarial vault remodelling for sagittal synostosis. *AORN Journal* **74** (5): 632–47.

Jones BM, Hayward R, Evans R, Britto J (1997) Occipital plagiocephaly: an epidemic of craniosynostosis? *British Medical Journal* **315** (7110): 693–4.

Kapp-Simon KA (1998) Mental development and learning disorders in children with single suture craniosynostosis. *Cleft Palate–Craniofacial Journal* **35** (3): 197–203.

Kershner DD, Claussen JA (1986) Craniofacial reconstruction. Perioperative care of the craniosynostosis patient. *AORN Journal* **44** (4): 554–62.

Kirby PJ, Beverley DW, Batchelor AG (1993) Frequency of craniosynostosis in Yorkshire, UK. *The Lancet* **341**: 1412–3.

Lee S, Seto M, Sie K, Cunningham M (2002) A child with Saethre-Chotzen syndrome, sensorineural hearing loss, and a TWIST mutation. *Cleft Palate–Craniofacial Journal* **39** (1): 110–14.

MacKenzie N (1990) Cranio-facial surgery. *Paediatric Nursing* **2** (6): 24–5.

May L (2001) *Craniosynostosis*. In May L (ed.) *Paediatric Neurosurgery: A Handbook for the Multidisciplinary Team*. Whurr Publishers, London.

May L (1992) Craniosynostosis – corrective surgery for a cosmetic defect. *Professional Nurse* **8** (3): 176–8.

Moos K, Hide R (1993) Craniofacial surgery – surgical correction of congenital deformities. *Surgery* **11** (8): 457–65.

Mouradian WE (1998) Controversies in the diagnosis and management of craniosynostosis: a panel discussion. *Cleft Palate–Craniofacial Journal* **35** (3): 190–3.

Mynanthopolous NC (1977) *Malformations in Children from One to Seven Years*. A report from the National Collaborative Perinatal Project. Alan R Liss, New York.

National Craniofacial Association (2003a) *Saethre-Chotzen Syndrome*. Available: www.faces-cranio.org/ Disord/Saethre.htm. Accessed February 2008.

National Craniofacial Association (2003b) *Pfeiffer Syndrome*. Available: www.faces-cranio.org/Disord/ Pfeiffer.htm. Accessed February 2008.

Okkerse JM, Beemer FA, de Jong TH *et al.* (2004) Condition variables in children with craniofacial anomalies: a descriptive study. *Journal of Craniofacial Surgery* **15** (1): 151–6.

Panchal J, Amirsheybani H, Gurwitch R *et al.* (2001) Neurodevelopment in children with single-suture craniosynostosis and plagiocephaly without synostosis. *Plastic and Reconstructive Surgery* **108** (6): 1492–8.

Panchal J, Uttchin V (2003) Management of craniosynostosis. *Plastic and Reconstructive Surgery* **111** (6): 2032–49.

Polley J, Charbel F, Kim D, MaFee MF (1998) Nonsyndromal craniosynostosis: longitudinal outcome following cranio-orbital reconstruction in infancy. *Plastic and Reconstructive Surgery* **102** (3): 619–28.

Sarimski K (2001) Social adjustment of children with a severe craniofacial anomaly (Apert syndrome) *Child: Care, Health and Development* **27** (6): 583–90.

Sarnat HB, Menkes JH (2000) Neuroembryology, genetic programming and malformations of the nervous system. In Menkes JH, Sarnat HB (eds) *Part 2: Malformations of the Central Nervous System*. Lippincott Williams & Wilkins, Philadelphia, PA.

Society of British Neurological Surgeons (2001) *Safe Paediatric Neurosurgery 2001*. SBNS, London.

Speltz ML, Endriga MC, Mouradian WE (1997) Presurgical and postsurgical mental and psychomotor development of infants with sagittal synostosis. *Cleft Palate–Craniofacial Journal* **34** (5): 374–9.

Suttaford T (1993) 'Growing peril'. *The Times* July 8: 15.

Virchow R (1851) Uber dem cretinismus, namentlich in Franken und uber pathologische Schadleformen. *Vehd, Physik Med Gesell Whuzburg* **2**: 230. Cited in Hockley AD (1993) Craniosynostosis. *Lancet* **342**: 189–90.

Warren SM, Greenwald JA, Spector JA *et al.* (2001) New developments in cranial suture research. *Cranial Suture Research* **107** (2): 523–40.

World Craniofacial Foundation (2004) *Carpenter's Syndrome*. Available: www.craniofacial.net/carpenters_syndrome.htm. Accessed February 2008.

7 Brain tumours

Brain tumours are the most common solid tumour and the second most common malignancy in children under 15 years, only leukaemia being more prevalent. Brain tumours are the leading cause of cancer-related death in children under the age of 15 (Hargrave *et al.* 2004). The cause of brain tumours in children remains unknown, although possible contributing factors have been identified. Progress – although slower than in other forms of cancers, notably acute lymphoblastic leukaemia – has been made in the treatment and management of these children and has contributed to the overall reduction in mortality (Stewart and Cohen 1998). Unfortunately, the morbidity of physical and intellectual sequelae in children with brain tumours, from the effects of the tumour itself and aggressive treatments, is significant. Caring for children with brain tumours remains a challenge for healthcare professionals (Strother *et al.* 2002) with a crucial element of care centred around providing adequate and appropriate support to the child and family through diagnosis, treatment and long-term follow up (Freeman *et al.* 2000).

At the end of reading this chapter you will be able to:

Learning outcomes

- Outline the common types of brain tumours in children
- Describe the management options for brain tumours in children
- Understand the long-term care needs of the child and family.

7.1 Incidence, aetiology and classification

Incidence

The precise incidence of childhood brain tumours is difficult to establish due to different data collection methods, but is estimated to be 2–3 children in 100,000 (Leviton 1994). Difficulties in defining true incidence include variations between studies such as differing age ranges included within studies, and the differing inclusion/exclusion of tumour types such as craniopharyngiomas. It has been estimated that 350 children are diagnosed with a brain tumour every year in the UK (CancerBACUP 2005), with evidence to suggest that this figure is increasing (Maria and Menkes 2000). This increase in the number of children diagnosed with a brain tumour may be a result of improvements in diagnostic techniques, a shift in inclusion criteria (Strother *et al.* 2002) and the centralization and development of specialized paediatric neurosurgical services which have contributed to an increase in accurate diagnosis and reporting of brain tumours in children (Hargrave *et al.* 2004). Recent improvements in diagnostic techniques include:

- Increased use of magnetic resonance imaging (MRI)
- Microscopical confirmation of brain stem lesions
- Stereotactic biopsies allowing the histology of previously inaccessible tumours to be identified.

With these improved diagnostic methods, children who would have previously died without a confirmed diagnosis are now being diagnosed. A further factor that could have contributed to the apparent increase in the number of children with brain tumours is a change to the World Health Organization's (WHO) classification of brain tumours. This has resulted in a shift in the classification of tumours, for example some gliomas previously classified as benign are now classified as malignant (Ryan-Murray and Petriccione 2002; Strother *et al.* 2002). The main types of brain tumours that occur in children are presented in Figure 7.1a.

Points to consider

- The incidence of brain tumours is greatest within the first decade of life (Strother *et al.* 2002)
- Under two years of age, brain tumours are most likely to be found in the cerebral hemispheres
- Between two and ten years they are more commonly found in the cerebellum (Strother *et al.* 2002).

Aetiology

A brain tumour occurs as a result of a proliferation of new and abnormal cells which form an expanding intracranial lesion. The lesion occupies space within the intracranial cavity and, along with associated oedema, impinges upon the surrounding structures of the brain. Once the tumour

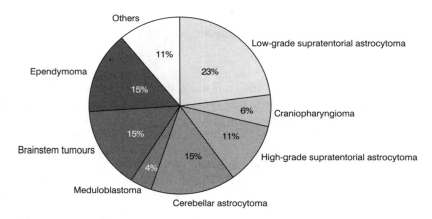

Figure 7.1a The main types of brain tumours in children (Source: Vernon-Levett and Geller 1997)

reaches a size where it invades surrounding structures, the child will become symptomatic. The signs and symptoms are specific to the location of the tumour and the structures damaged. Normally tumours are divided into malignant or benign with the distinction primarily describing the rate of tumour growth and its invasiveness, and therefore its lethalness. However, in the case of the brain it is often the position of the tumour that determines the eventual outcome because damage to vital centres essential for life are fatal and the accessibility of the tumour for surgical treatment will influence management options.

Points to consider

The position of the tumour in the brain is as significant as the type of tumour. A benign tumour which impinges on and damages vital structures within the brain or is inaccessible for surgical treatment can be fatal.

Although the aetiology of brain tumours is unknown possible contributing factors include (Strother *et al.* 2002):

- Exposure to ionizing radiation, for example following radiotherapy, particularly cranial irradiation for acute lymphoblastic leukaemia.
- Association with other cancers or their treatments, for example children with malignant rhabdoid tumours of the kidney.
- Underlying immunosuppression disorders, for example Wiskott-Aldrich syndrome or an acquired immunodeficiency, such as after solid organ transplantation.
- A family history of bone cancer, leukaemia and lymphoma.
- Environmental exposures, for example a possible link with diet, however many environmental links should be treated with caution because of a lack of conclusive evidence.

There is evidence to suggest a genetic component to some types of brain tumours. Brain tumours may be more common in children who have a sibling or parent who has had a brain tumour, and there is familial clustering in children with embryonal tumours and gliomas. There are gender differences in development of brain tumours, for example medulloblastomas are more common in boys than girls, while astrocytomas, affect boys and girls equally. Certain syndromes, such as neurofibromatosis or tuberous sclerosis are associated with the development of brain tumours (Strother *et al.* 2002). Recent advances in molecular biology and cytogenetics have begun to identify possible sites of oncogenesis linked to the development of brain tumours. For example, mutations on chromosome 17 have been associated with the development of medulloblastomas and astrocytomas, and deletions on chromosome 10 have been associated with glioblastoma (Shiminski-Maher and Shields 1995).

Points to consider

Establishing a specific cause for the development of a brain tumour is rarely possible. It is likely that the aetiology of brain tumours is probably multifactoral and there may be links with environmental exposure.

Childhood brain tumours are rare and therefore much of the research into the aetiology is based upon small groups of children or single cases. This can lead to generalizations and reliance on the child's and family's observations of the disease. In attempts to overcome problems relating to studying childhood cancers, they are often considered as a single entity, which includes brain tumours. Whilst this provides larger numbers to study, the cause of children's brain tumours is possibly different from the aetiology of other childhood malignancies, thus larger more general studies may have limited relevance in advancing the care of children with brain tumours.

Classification

Brain tumour classifications can be based on cytogenetics, histology and location of the tumour. The range of classification systems has resulted in confusing terminology and some brain tumours having more than one name. Evolving classifications during the 1990s resulted in the emergence of the term 'primitive neuroectodermal tumour' (PNET), an umbrella category that includes embryonal tumours including medulloblastomas (Strother *et al.* 2002). Tumours with the same histological features arising in the cerebrum or pineal gland are classified as a supratentorial PNET (sPNET) or pineoblastoma respectively.

Although there remains some controversy over the classification of brain tumours, the WHO (2000) classification system is currently accepted (Kleihues and Cavenee 2000). The system includes a grading scale of malignancy: grades I–II representing benign tumours; and grades III–IV malignant tumours (Hargrave *et al.* 2004). Some types of brain tumours are not given a numerical grade, but may be classified as being high grade or low grade (CancerBACUP 2005). The main types of brain tumours occurring in children are depicted in Figure 7.1b. The classification system for the common paediatric brain tumours are shown in Table 7.1a.

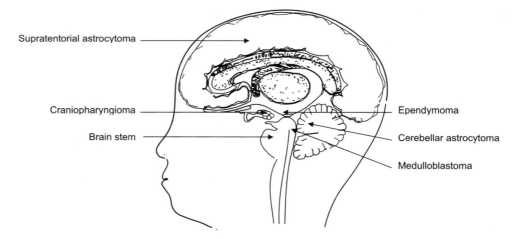

Figure 7.1b Location of common brain tumours in children

Table 7.1a Common paediatric brain tumours

Astrocytic tumours	Grade I: Pilocytic astrocytoma Grade II: Low-grade fibrillary astrocytoma Grade III: Anaplastic or high-grade astrocytoma Grade IV: Glioblastoma multiforme
Ependymal tumours	Grade I: Myxopapillary ependymoma and subependymoma Grade II: Ependymoma Grade III: Anaplastic ependymoma
Embryonal tumours	Grade IV: Medulloblastoma Grade IV: Supratentorial primitive neuroectodermal tumours
Neuroepithelial tumours	Grade IV: Pineoblastoma
Other tumours	Craniopharyngioma

Source: Kleihues and Cavenee (2000)

7.2 Pathophysiology

Astrocytoma

Astrocytomas occur in adults and children. Childhood astrocytomas are found throughout the brain and are relatively slow growing compared to those found in adults, which are predominantly located within the cerebral hemispheres and usually grow rapidly. The peak incidence of astrocytomas in children is five to nine years, affecting both sexes equally (Fenichel 1997), with the exception of cerebellar astrocytomas which have a higher incidence in boys compared to girls (Strother *et al.* 2002). Astrocytomas arise from glial astrocyte cells (Ryan-Murray and Petriccione 2002). The appearance of the astrocytoma can vary and in children, it has a tendency to form cysts that may become much larger than the solid portion of the tumour. The cysts contain clear yellow fluid rich in protein. Astrocytomas are graded from I–IV with grade I indicating a benign slow-growing lesion and grade IV being a highly malignant tumour. The majority of astrocytomas in children are pilocytic or low-grade fibrillary astrocytomas regardless of the site of the tumour. Approximately one-tenth of all childhood brain tumours are high-grade astrocytomas or glioblastoma multiforme. Astrocytomas in children mainly occur in the frontal, temporal or parietal lobes of the cerebral hemispheres (Ryan-Murray and Petriccione 2002). Cerebellar astrocytomas of childhood arise in the posterior fossa, in or near the midline of the cerebellum, and occasionally into the brain stem.

Ependymoma

Although the mean age at diagnosis is 15 years (Brett 1997), the peak incidence of ependymomas in children is birth to four years, with both sexes affected equally (Fenichel 1997). Ependymomas originate from the ependymal tissue within the ventricular system (Shiminski-Maher and Shields 1995). Although they can arise from any part of the ventricular system, ependymomas most commonly derive from cells that line the roof and floor of the fourth ventricles (Fenichel 1997; Maria and Menkes 2000). The macroscopic appearance of an ependymoma resembles that of a cauliflower, adjusting in form to its surroundings, such as the constraints of the fourth ventricle (Brett 1997). The histological features vary from a benign tumour composed of uniform glial cells, through to a malignant ependymoma or ependymoblastoma, with similarities to a medulloblastoma and a tendency to metastasize along the cerebral spinal fluid (CSF) pathways (Brett 1997). Ependymomas are graded according to their rate of cell growth as either benign or malignant (Shiminski-Maher and Shields 1995).

Medulloblastoma

The peak age for diagnosis of medulloblastoma is four to eight years, but they can occur throughout childhood. Medulloblastoma is less common in teenagers and adults. Medulloblastoma arises from primitive neuroepithelial cells of the external granular layer of the cerebellum (Worrall 1999). Normally these embryonic cells disappear by 18 months of age; the abnormal persistence of these cells is the basis for the development of this primitive tumour (Worrall 1999). The tumour cells multiply and form a soft tumour mass which usually is without necrosis, cyst formation or calcification. In addition, medulloblastomas do not have a clear line of demarcation from normal tissue (Brett and Harding 1997). There are two opposing views regarding the exact site of origin of medulloblastomas:

1   The roof of the fourth ventricle, growing into the lumen of the fourth ventricle and extending towards the dorsum of the cerebellar vermis (Brett and Harding 1997)
2   The midline of the cerebellar vermis, spreading through the cerebellum and into the floor of the fourth ventricle where it grows and frequently fills the fourth ventricle, until it infiltrates the ventricle walls and floor (Friedman *et al.* 1991; Halperin *et al.* 1994).

Although there remains controversy regarding the exact origin of medulloblastoma tumours (Heideman *et al.* 1997), it is generally accepted that the tumour develops within the fourth ventricle, then permeates along the CSF pathways, ascends into the cerebral aqueduct, then descends inferiorly to the cisterna magna and extends laterally via the foramina of Luschka into the cerebellopontine angle. By this stage CSF circulation has generally been blocked resulting in obstructive hydrocephalus (Louis and Cavenee 1997). Hydrocephalus is outlined in detail in *Chapter 4*.

Craniopharyngioma

Craniopharyngiomas are not common and account for 6–8 per cent of all children presenting with primary cerebral lesions (Greenwood 1992, Vernon-Levett and Geller 1997). Craniopharyngiomas are benign, slow-growing tumours, rarely producing symptoms before the age of four years, although the tumour itself is probably present from birth or prenatally. Occasionally symptoms occur in the newborn period (Brett 1997). Craniopharyngioma is a deep-seated midline tumour usually found around the pituitary gland. It is composed of a solid mass of epithelial tissue and cysts. The multiplication of tumour cells results in compression of neighbouring structures, such as the optic nerves, the internal carotid arteries, pituitary gland and the hypothalamus, and impairs their function (Greenwood 1992). Despite the clinically benign features, many of these tumours possess characteristics that result in significant morbidity and mortality (Strother *et al.* 2002). Craniopharyngiomas are usually difficult to treat due to their anatomical location and because the abnormal connective tissue adheres to surrounding tissues preventing normal function. Involvement of the pituitary gland has an impact on endocrine function. Obstruction of the third ventricle or one or both foramina of Monro results in the development of hydrocephalus, outlined in detail in Chapter 4.

Brain stem tumours

The peak incidence of brain stem tumours is between five and eight years of age (Brett 1997). The majority of these tumours are fast growing, diffuse and highly malignant with extensive branching that respond poorly to treatment (Ryan-Murray and Petriccione 2002). Advances in MRI techniques have allowed better visualization of the interior of the brainstem; however a definitive diagnosis may not be possible because the position of the tumour may not allow for a biopsy to be undertaken safely (Brett 1997). Nearly all brain stem tumours are thought to be high-grade astrocytomas (Brett 1997).

The types of childhood tumours according to age, location and presenting signs and symptoms are summarized and presented in Table 7.2a.

Table 7.2a Childhood tumours, age and location

Type of tumour	Peak age of child at diagnosis	Most common location of tumour in the brain	Type of cells affected	Presenting signs and symptoms
Supratentorial astrocytoma	5–9 years	Cerebral hemisphere	Glial cells	Headaches, vomiting, seizures, raised intracranial pressure
Cerebellar astrocytoma	5–9 years	Cerebellum	Glial cells	Headaches, clumsiness, awkward gait, ataxia, vomiting. Symptoms usually occur gradually
Ependymoma	Birth–4 years	Fourth ventricle	Ependymal tissue	Raised intracranial pressure, hydrocephalus, ataxia, awkward gait, vomiting, headaches, stiff neck and shoulders, weakness of face, pharynx and tongue. Symptoms usually occur gradually
Medulloblastoma	4–8 years	Cerebellum extending into the fourth ventricle	Primitive neuroepithelial cells	Ataxia, clumsiness, awkward gait, vomiting. Symptoms usually occur rapidly
Craniopharyngioma	4 years, but probably present at birth	Midline, usually around the pituitary gland	Epithelial tissue	Raised intracranial pressure, hydrocephalus, visual disturbances, delayed skeletal growth, delayed sexual maturation, drowsiness, obesity, diabetes insipidus
Brain stem tumours	5–8 years	Brain Stem	Glial cells	Cranial nerve palsies, hemiparesis

7.3 Presentation, diagnosis and management options

Presentation

The presenting signs and symptoms vary depending on the site, growth rate of the tumour, age and developmental stage of the child (Table 7.2a).

Specific or focal symptoms associated with a brain tumour usually correlate with the functional area of the brain that is affected. Figure 7.3a and Table 7.2a outline the links between altered function, tumour location and signs and symptoms of specific tumours.

> **Points to consider**
>
> Symptoms occurring within a short duration of time usually indicate a rapidly growing or aggressive tumour with more gradual symptoms more likely to be caused by a low grade or benign tumour (Stewart and Cohen 1998).

> **Points to consider**
>
> The general symptoms of a brain tumour include:
>
> - Vomiting, often projectile and without nausea; this is common in children with posterior fossa tumours (Gibson 1995; Chadwick *et al.* 1989)
> - Headaches are experienced by the majority of children with a brain tumour and are the result of traction, distortion or irritation of structures within the brain (Kaye and Laws 1995); most often occur upon waking in the morning and often relieved once the child adopts an erect posture (Gibson 1995)
> - Headaches are made worse by activities such as coughing, sneezing, straining and bending because these activities cause a transient rise in intracranial pressure (Allan 1986)
> - In young children cerebral dysfunction may initially present as irritability and lethargy (Chadwick *et al.* 1989)
> - Changes in mental function such as forgetfulness and memory loss in older children (Chadwick *et al.* 1989)
> - Pappilloedema causes blurred vision, and there may be momentary loss of vision whilst moving
> - Seizures occur in approximately one-third of children with a brain tumour (Chadwick *et al.* 1989). They are probably a result of irritative effects of the tumour but can also occur when intracranial pressure rises (Wong 1995)
> - Alteration in consciousness in children with brain tumours is caused by: raised intracranial pressure, the alteration in function of the structures that maintain arousal, or as a result of brain stem compression and herniation (Kaye and Laws 1995; Gibson 1995).

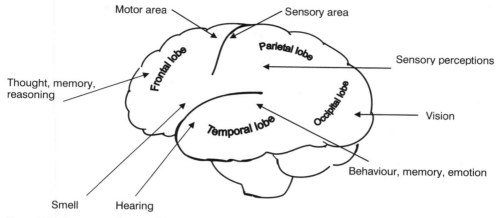

Motor area

Sensory area

Parietal lobe

Sensory perceptions

Frontal lobe

Thought, memory,
reasoning

Occipital lobe

Vision

Temporal lobe

Behaviour, memory, emotion

Smell   Hearing

Figure 7.3a Summary of areas of the brain relating to function

Most childhood brain tumours are associated with an increase in intracranial pressure. As the tumour expands it will fill any available space within the brain, for example in the case of a medulloblastoma the lesion usually grows until it fills the fourth ventricle (Halperin *et al.* 1994). Once the tumour has filled any available space it will continue to expand, compressing surrounding structures and causing an increase in intracranial pressure, or it will grow along the CSF pathways and block CSF circulation causing obstructive hydrocephalus, which is outlined in detail in Chapter 4 (Louis and Cavenee 1997). The management of raised intracranial pressure is outlined in Chapter 5, Section 3. The signs of raised intracranial pressure include:

- Progressively sluggish pupil reactions to light.
- The pupils may eventually become fixed and dilated.
- Cushing's response, where the child has an increase in blood pressure, decrease in pulse and a decrease in respirations, this is probably due to brain shifts and brain stem compression (Kaye and Laws 1995; Hudak *et al.* 1998, Hickey 2003). This is a late response and irreversible damage may have already occurred (Hickey and Armstrong 1997; Shiminski-Maher and Shields 1995).

Supratentorial lesions may cause hemiparesis, hemisensory loss, hemivisual defects and seizures (Stewart and Cohen 1998). Astrocytomas originating near the motor cortex typically present with hemiparesis and focal seizures. Seizure patterns may help to locate the tumour location, for example complex seizures are associated with temporal lobe tumours and focal motor seizures typically occur with frontoparietal tumours. Occipital lobe tumours result in visual field abnormalities. Hemispheric gliomas often present with subtle symptoms such as sensory loss, personality changes and a decline in academic performance. Deep-seated tumours, such as hypothalamic and optic pathway tumours present with visual deficits, memory and cognitive dysfunction and endocrinopathies (Shiminski-Maher and Shields 1995). If the tumour is in the temporal lobe, the child may loose the ability to recognize sounds and speech (Ryan-Murray and Petriccione 2002).

Many childhood brain tumours occur in the posterior fossa, for example medulloblastomas and cerebellar astrocytomas, and affect the function of the cerebellum (Halperin *et al.* 1994). Damage or compression to any of the structures within the cerebellum results in lack of coordinated muscular movements, a staggering wide-based gait and inability to carry out fine movements in a steady and precise action (Ross and Wilson 1985). When walking, the child will tend to deviate towards the side of the injury because information is not transferred between cerebellar hemispheres (Hinchliff and Montague 1992). If only one of the cerebellar hemispheres is affected, head tilt, asymmetrical ataxia and nystagmus are likely to be presenting features (Brett 1997). Occasionally acute raised intracranial pressure can be the first indication of a cerebellar astrocytoma but generally, unlike children with medulloblastoma, the symptoms occur gradually (Brett 1997). Consequently, the history with cerebellar astrocytoma is much longer and the child may appear less unwell at initial diagnosis.

The child with a brain stem tumour often presents with a short history and hemiparesis (Ryan-Murray and Petriccione 2002). Brain stem tumours can cause cranial nerve palsies, in particular the sixth cranial nerve, which manifests as loss of lateral gaze (Stewart and Cohen 1998). Signs and symptoms of raised intracranial pressure in the child at diagnosis are usually indicative of a tumour that has advanced significantly (Brett 1997).

The clinical features of ependymomas evolve slowly and therefore it is often several months before medical consultation is sought and a diagnosis made (Fenichel 1997). As the tumour tends to invade the fourth ventricle and obstructs CSF flow it is likely to cause raised intracranial pressure and hydrocephalus. Cerebellar signs are common, such as ataxia, coordination and gait disturbances, vomiting and headaches. The child may complain of stiffness of the neck and shoulders because of a downward extension of the tumour into the cervical spinal cord. There may be cranial nerve involvement and associated weakness of the face, pharynx and tongue (Brett 1997).

Symptoms of craniopharyngiomas are insidious because the tumour growth is slow and may not become apparent until later in life. Diagnosis can be time consuming and often delayed because vague signs are not always linked to the possibility that they are the result of a brain tumour (Greenwood 1992). The child may feel lethargic and present with a low blood pressure. Compression of the optic nerves leads to visual field defects and hypothalamic disturbances and may cause drowsiness, obesity and diabetes insipidus (Brett 1997). Pituitary function may be disturbed with delayed skeletal growth and sexual maturation.

Points to consider

Many of the signs and symptoms of brain tumours are insidious, non-specific and develop gradually. There is often a time delay between the onset of symptoms and obtaining a diagnosis.

Diagnosis

Cancers in children are uncommon. The diagnosis of a brain tumour in a child is often difficult because the presenting symptoms can be vague and non-specific or similar to the symptoms of other more common childhood illnesses (Stewart and Cohen 1998). Many general practitioners will rarely, if ever, be presented with a child with cancer, and even fewer will be presented with a child with a brain tumour (National Institute for Health and Clinical Excellence (NICE) 2005a). Guidelines are available to assist primary healthcare professionals in making prompt and appropriate referrals when a child presents with vague signs and symptoms and a brain tumour is a possible diagnosis (NICE 2005b). Primary healthcare professionals must be willing to reassess the child or to seek a second opinion from a colleague if a child fails to recover as expected from an alternative diagnosis.

Essential care

Primary healthcare professionals should recognize that parents are usually the best observers of their child, and therefore must listen carefully to their concerns (NICE 2005a).

Best practice recommendations

Recommendations for primary healthcare professionals referring a child with a suspected brain tumour to a specialist centre are (NICE 2005b):

1   Children aged two years and over:
    - Persistent headache
    - Early morning headaches and vomiting
    - Headaches and vomiting on waking
    - New-onset seizures
    - Cranial nerve abnormalities
    - Visual disturbance
    - Gait abnormalities
    - Motor or sensory signs
    - Unexplained deteriorating school performance or loss of developmental milestones
    - Unexplained behaviour and/or mood changes
    - A reduced level of consciousness

2   Children under two years:
    - New-onset seizures
    - Bulging fontanelle
    - Extensor attacks
    - Persistent vomiting
    - Abnormal increase in head size
    - Arrest or regression of motor development
    - Altered behaviour
    - Abnormal eye movements
    - Lack of visual following
    - Poor feeding/failure to thrive
    - Squint.

Essential care

A child who presents with a reduced level of consciousness requires emergency admission to hospital.

Unfortunately delays in referring the child to a specialist centre are a key concern and source of frustration for many families and their concerns need to be handled sensitively (NICE 2005a). Once referred to the specialist centre, a detailed history and clinical examination will be undertaken by a paediatric neurologist or a neurosurgeon. If a brain tumour is suspected an MRI or CT scan of the head and spine will be requested. MRI is the investigation of choice because the image of the brain is in three different planes and can assist the neurosurgeon when planning future tumour resection or biopsy (Stewart and Cohen 1998). However, in certain situations CT scans have advantages, particularly in demonstrating calcium deposits in tumours such as a craniopharyngioma and in assisting assessment of sudden changes in neurological status, such as the presence of haemorrhage or hydrocephalus. Children with medulloblastoma will require a lumbar puncture because this malignant tumour can spread outside the central nervous system and these investigations help to determine the extent of metastases.

Essential care

Lumbar puncture is usually performed when the child has recovered from the initial surgical procedure. Caution is essential when undertaking a lumbar puncture in children with raised intracranial pressure and the procedure can only be performed if the child does not have any acute signs or symptoms of raised intracranial pressure.

Management options

Many children diagnosed with a brain tumour will require multimodal therapy: surgery, radiotherapy, chemotherapy and symptom management (Walker *et al.* 1999). The order in which treatment is given varies for different diseases. The goal of treatment is to maximize the benefits of each type of therapy whilst minimizing the potential side effects. In most cases, the ultimate aim of treatment is to cure with the least possible morbidity.

Points to consider

Following initial diagnosis a short course of corticosteroids, primarily dexamethasone, are usually prescribed to reduce cerebral swelling and provide temporary relief from presenting symptoms (Walker *et al.* 1999).

Surgery

Surgery is usually the definitive treatment for children with a brain tumour with the exact surgical procedure dependant on the site of the tumour (Brett 1997). Complete removal of the tumour is the most effective treatment for brain tumours and improves survival (Shiminski-Maher and Shields 1995). Unfortunately, complete removal of a brain tumour is not always possible, part – or in some cases all – of the tumour may be deep within the brain or attached to vital structures making the tumour inaccessible to the surgeon. In addition, tumours that have metastasized will be unable to be removed in entirety. In these situations the surgeon will remove as much of the tumour as possible. Tumour resection may relieve obstruction and re-establish patent pathways for CSF circulation in children who have developed obstructive hydrocephalus as a direct result of compression of CSF pathways. In some children hydrocephalus may be permanent requiring a ventricular shunt. The management of ventricular shunts is outlined in detail in Chapter 4, Section 4.

The main objectives of surgery are to (Turini and Redaelli 2001):

- Remove the tumour and provide a cure whenever possible
- Remove as much tumour as possible
- Obtain a biopsy of the tumour so that a definitive diagnosis can be made
- Manage raised intracranial pressure
- Provide access for other treatments, e.g. chemotherapy.

Best practice recommendations

Children's Surgical Forum of the Royal College of Surgeons guidelines (2000) relating to neurosurgery in children recommend:

- Only dedicated paediatric neurosurgeons should undertake neurosurgery on children and at least 50 per cent of their practice must be with children
- Occasional paediatric practice is not recommended.

Neurosurgical procedures should only be performed in centres that can support the needs of the child and family. This requires the centre to have appropriate equipment and staff with the appropriate skills and experience in caring for children following neurosurgery in all areas, including the theatre environment, children's wards and children's intensive care facilities (Chumas *et al.* 2002; Department of Health (DH) 2002). Healthcare professionals must be able to develop and build expertise in caring for these children if their needs are to be met (Stewart and Cohen 1998). The principles of care for the child undergoing neurosurgery are outlined in Chapter 3 and apply to children undergoing surgical procedures for brain tumour resection or removal.

Radiotherapy

The use of radiotherapy for the treatment of brain tumours has been established since the 1890s (Moore 1995). Radiotherapy inhibits the ability of cells to divide by targeting and disrupting the action of DNA (deoxyribonucleic acid) (Shiminski-Maher and Shields 1995). Genes are composed of DNA, which directs the synthesis of cellular proteins and therefore cellular actions. DNA replication is essential for cell division. Radiation primarily affects cells during the division phase, therefore rapidly growing tumour cells are especially sensitive to exposure to radiation (Vernon-Levett and Geller 1997). However, radiation also affects normal healthy cells. Therefore, the goal of radiotherapy is to deliver therapeutic doses of radiation which prevent cell division and cause cellular destruction of the tumour cells, whilst minimizing the toxic effects to the surrounding healthy tissue. Technological evolution of more sophisticated equipment including linear accelerators and computer-assisted equipment has made radiotherapy more precise by ensuring accurate delivery to the tumour site.

Points to consider

Radiotherapy is used for children with brain tumours:

- As a substitute for surgery if the brain tumour is inoperable
- To treat benign or malignant tumours that are incompletely removed during surgery
- After surgery to destroy any remaining seeds of tumour cells
- To relieve symptoms of rapidly growing tumours by shrinking tumour size
- To minimize secondary metastasis within the brain

(Turini and Redaelli 2001)

Essential care

Radiotherapy is not usually appropriate for children under three years because of the high susceptibility of the immature developing brain to radiation damage and long-term complications (Chapter 7, Section 5).

Depending on the reasons radiotherapy is required it is usually administered five times a week for approximately six weeks, two to three weeks following surgery or diagnosis (Walker *et al.* 1999). Some brain tumour management protocols suggest the use of hyperfractionated irradiation, where smaller doses of irradiation are given twice a day (6–8 hours apart). This achieves a higher total daily dose of radiation with reduced effects to surrounding brain tissue (Shiminski-Maher and Shields 1995). Treatment planning is vital because during radiotherapy the child requires immobilizing within an individually constructed mould. This is essential for ensuring precise and consistent positioning of the treatment area during every radiotherapy session (Lew and LaVally 1995).

Chemotherapy

Chemotherapy rarely provides a cure for children with brain tumours but offers an opportunity to limit tumour expansion in the young child until radiotherapy can be delivered (Duffner *et al.* 1993). The use of chemotherapy as a treatment modality has increased the long-term survival rates of children with brain tumours (Shiminski-Maher and Shields 1995). Chemotherapy is used increasingly as an adjunctive therapy with surgery and radiotherapy. The main complication with using chemotherapy as a primary treatment for brain tumours is poor drug penetration across the blood–brain barrier due to the tight junctions between endothelial cells in the brain capillaries. This impermeability prevents most of the chemotherapeutic agents, at conventional dosage, from gaining access to the brain parenchyma (Mastrangelo *et al.* 1999).

Points to consider

The three main techniques for overcoming the blood–brain barrier when administering chemotherapeutic agents are:

1   *Blood–brain barrier disruption*
    Disruption of the junctions between brain capillaries or endothelial cells by the administration of drugs such as mannitol, which facilitate chemotherapeutic agents to enter normal brain tissue. However, these techniques may cause transient exacerbation of symptoms or seizures

2   *Combination chemotherapy*
    Multi-drug combinations may be useful if there is more than one tumour cell type and can be more effective and better tolerated than a single agent chemotherapy regimen.

3   *High-dose chemotherapy*
    Administrations of high doses of chemotherapeutic agents such as methotrexate, which is followed by the administration of an antidote, such as folinic acid rescue therapy, which reverses the excess drug.

(Turini and Redaelli 2001)

It is likely that future success in treating brain tumours in children will concentrate on new and better chemotherapy agents and regimens, particularly as aggressive surgery and radiotherapy can have detrimental effects for the child (Stewart and Cohen 1998). Research relating to improving treatment includes the administration of high-dose chemotherapeutic agents with stem cell rescue or autologous bone marrow rescue. This could be used to treat a number of high-grade tumours including high-risk or recurrent medulloblastoma, high-grade glioma and pineoblastoma (Stewart and Cohen 1998). As a consequence of such advances, the treatment and care of children with brain tumours is likely to become more complex.

All children with a brain tumour undergoing chemotherapy and/or radiotherapy, should be cared for in one of the 17 UK Children Cancer Study Group (UKCCSG) accredited centres (NICE 2005a). Some children may receive care in a shared-care centre; however the major elements of treatment and all management planning should take place at a UKCCSG centre (NICE 2005a). At each of the UKCCSG centres, treatment protocols are adapted to incorporate the current evidence, and outcomes are monitored, with the potential to influence future developments (Lashford and Walker 1997).

7.4 Principles of nursing care for a child with a brain tumour

The diagnosis of a brain tumour is devastating for the child and family and both will require extensive psychological support from the multidisciplinary team. The family will have many questions about the cause of the tumour and will be frustrated that answers will not be available until after the initial investigations and histology results. Anxiety and stress may cause the family to perceive investigations as taking an excessively long time. The family may be angry that vague signs and symptoms have gone unnoticed and there will be fears about the planned treatment and prognosis. These emotions will affect the family's ability to comprehend information given to them. It is essential that the family is provided with opportunities to ask questions, and provided with clear, accurate and honest responses (Jackson *et al.* 2007). It will be necessary to repeat information regularly especially during the stressful period around diagnosis and throughout treatment as care needs change (Jackson *et al.* 2007). The child and family need input and support from different healthcare professionals at various stages of treatment. The support required will vary, depending upon the unique needs of the child and family, the stage of treatment and the child's response to treatments (Freeman *et al.* 2000). Meeting the emotional and psychological needs of the child and family is outlined in Chapter 2, Section 7.

Points to consider

It is important to include the child in discussions about their diagnosis and the subsequent care they will require at a level appropriate to their age and stage of development. It is essential that information shared with the child and family is communicated effectively between multidisciplinary team members to prevent confusion and to ensure a consistent approach to care. This can be achieved through shared goals and regular multidisciplinary team meetings

Principles of care relating to the surgical procedure

Preoperative care

The general principles that apply to a child (and family) undergoing surgery for any procedure equally apply to the child undergoing a brain tumour resection. The principles of caring for the child undergoing surgery are described in detail in Chapter 3. Only specific aspects of care relating to brain tumour resection will be discussed. The overall aims of care are to safely prepare the child for theatre, detect acute neurological sequelae in the peri-operative period by accurate and timely neurological assessments, and support the child and family.

Preoperatively the child will require a full neurological assessment, a detailed ophthalmic assessment, endocrine assessment (depending on the location of the tumour) and monitoring for signs and symptoms of raised intracranial pressure (Chapter 2, Sections 2 and 3). Corticosteriods, primarily dexamethasone, are usually prescribed preoperatively. There will be a need to administer additional corticosteroids on induction of the anaesthetic. Obstructive hydrocephalus may require treating before tumour resection if there is a sudden acute rise in intracranial pressure caused by compression of CSF pathways (Vernon-Levett and Geller 1997). This is usually achieved by surgically inserting an external ventricular drain (EVD). The management of EVDs are outlined in Chapter 4, Section 4.

Postoperative care

The general principles of caring for a child following neurosurgery described in Chapter 3 will apply to the child who has had resection of a brain tumour. Postoperatively, it is vital that the child is cared for in an environment that can offer maximum observations by staff skilled in the care of the child with a neurological problem (NICE 2005a).

Points to consider

Immediate postoperative complications include:

- Cerebral oedema, due to a generalized inflammatory response caused by the manipulation of delicate tissue during the surgical resection
- Haemorrhage, damage to small capillaries will result in a slow oozing of blood and will contribute to any rises in intracranial pressure. Damage and failure to effectively cauterize large vessels during theatre will result in the rapid development of a haematoma and sudden rise in intracranial pressure
- Development or progression of an existing hydrocephalus.

The management of children following removal or resection of a brain tumour requires effective teamwork and the support of facilities, such as rapid access to CT scanning and an emergency operating theatre suite. The child who has had surgery to remove a tumour situated within the posterior fossa, which contains vital control centres, is at particular risk of respiratory or cardiovascular instability (May 2001). These children will require ventilatory support and invasive monitoring of blood pressure and therefore will require intensive care facilities post-surgery. Nursing care will be directed towards detecting, treating and minimizing the consequences of increased intracranial pressure (Chapter 5, Section 3). An MRI scan is usually performed 24–48 hours postoperatively to assess the extent of tissue resected and the extent of residual tumour. For tumours of the posterior fossa the MRI will include imaging the spine because these tumours have a tendency to metastasize along the CSF.

Posterior fossa syndrome is a collection of symptoms that occur in a small group of patients following posterior fossa surgery. Initially the child will appear to be making a satisfactory postoperative recovery, but within 18–72 hours facial weakness, drooling and nystagmus followed by mutism, inability to follow commands, difficulty verbalizing, emotional lability and upper and lower extremity weakness develop (Dailey *et al.* 1995). The cause of posterior fossa syndrome is unknown. The symptoms are disturbing and debilitating and can prolong recovery (Vernon-Levett and Geller 1997). Patients and families often view posterior fossa syndrome as an added burden to an already frightening diagnosis with an uncertain neurological outcome. Outlining posterior fossa syndrome as a potential complication to the child and family should form part of preoperative discussions. Children with posterior fossa syndrome will require speech and language therapy, physiotherapy, occupational therapy and psychological support (Vernon-Levett and Geller 1997). Early recognition of symptoms and careful assessment of cranial nerve function and nutritional status are important aspects of care. Failure to tolerate oral feeding because of the loss of swallow and gag reflexes or psychological factors may require enteral or parenteral nutrition. Communication devices may lessen frustration. Safety measures such as padded side rails can prevent physical injury.

Principles of care relating to radiotherapy

Planning for radiotherapy involves precise mapping of the treatment area using radiological imaging. The first stage of the process requires fitting the child with a mould or cast, which is used to immobilize the child and ensure consistent positioning during every treatment session. Children with posterior fossa tumours will be required to lie face down and be immobilized in a prone position to allow the radiation to be directed to the posterior base of the skull. Lying in a face down prone position can be distressing for the child (Shiminski-Maher and Shields 1995). An important aspect of care, particularly for young children, is preparation for radiotherapy treatment, which must include allowing the child opportunity to adjust to the procedure. Play therapists are valuable in preparing and supporting the child during radiotherapy. This preparation usually includes encouraging the young child to make and paint masks before they have their own mould made. Many centres allow the child to keep their mould after treatment has been completed. Where time allows, families are invited to visit the radiotherapy unit before treatment begins to meet staff and become familiar with the equipment used. A 'dry run' in the final stages of planning, during which the child experiences all aspects of the treatment is a valuable opportunity to identify any potential problems before treatment begins (Vernon-Levett and Geller 1997).

The psychological needs of the child are important and for the young child sedation or even general anaesthesia may be the only option. However, where possible, sedation and anaesthesia are avoided because both have potential risks. Many children can take a considerable length of time to recover from sedation with a potential for dehydration. When considering treatment is usually five days a week for six weeks, the use of sedation or anaesthesia on a daily basis has the potential to affect the child's ability to undertake other activities and compounds the effects of the treatment.

Acute toxicity may occur during or immediately following radiotherapy. Initially radiotherapy can cause oedema of the tumour and surrounding area, resulting in pressure on adjacent brain structures (Vernon-Levett and Geller 1997). The child must be monitored for signs of increasing intracranial pressure, including depressed conscious levels and respiratory effort. Increased pressure within the brain stem can result in cranial nerve dysfunction, with loss of protective mechanisms such as gag and swallowing reflexes. Corticosteroids, usually dexamethasone, are used to reduce radiotherapy-induced oedema. Other immediate side effects of radiotherapy include nausea, vomiting, headaches, loss of appetite, fluid and electrolyte disturbances and localized skin irritation (Vernon-Levett and Geller 1997).

Children receiving radiotherapy are also at risk of developing a condition known as radiotherapy somnolence, characterized by excessive drowsiness (up to 20 hours a day), lethargy and malaise. Additional symptoms can include fever, headaches, nausea, dysphasia, ataxia and pappilloedema. Radiotherapy somnolence typically develops several weeks to three months after completion of radiotherapy treatment. The cause is unclear, but it could relate to damage to supportive oligodendroglia cells, inhibition of myelin formation and transient myelin degeneration (Moore 1995). Treatment consists of low-dose corticosteroids such as dexamethasone. The condition is self-limiting and does not appear to have any long-term detrimental effects (Vernon- Levett and Geller 1997).

Principles of care relating to chemotherapy

Over the past decade, chemotherapy has emerged as an important adjunctive therapy in the treatment of children with many types of brain tumours (Vernon-Levett and Geller 1997). This has resulted in an increase in the number of children with brain tumours requiring admission to children's oncology wards both for chemotherapy and to treat the complications of chemotherapy (Shiminski-Maher and Shields 1995). This has required nurses to be responsive to change and to develop their knowledge and clinical skills in caring for the child with a neuro-oncology problem (Smith 1999). Children with brain tumours and their families are referred to the oncology ward at a different time in the illness trajectory compared to most other children treated for other types of malignancies. Most other children attending the children's oncology ward will be doing so as newly diagnosed patients; children with brain tumours and their parents have usually been diagnosed and undergone initial treatment on a specialized children's neurological ward. The child may have already had a lengthy inpatient stay, had a period in intensive care, had surgery and/or radiotherapy and has probably been seen in a children's oncology outpatient clinic prior to admission to the ward for chemotherapy. The child and family will have already experienced a range of healthcare professionals and different specialist teams. In many trusts, these specialist areas are on different hospital sites, therefore it is vital the multidisciplinary team have established channels of communication to ensure consistent information is given to the child and family and to prevent unnecessary repetition of information. The introduction of specific key workers, such as neuro-oncology liaison nurses, and joint clinics can help to bridge the potential divisions between different departments and staff caring for the child with a brain tumour.

The nurse on the children's oncology ward needs to use a variety of communication skills to ensure families and children feel welcome and receive the required amount of psychological support. Nurses need to understand the frustrations experienced by the child and family, who are meeting and dealing with a new set of staff and a different environment. This may also be the time at which the child and family are beginning to understand the reality that their child has a brain tumour. The nurse caring for the child with a brain tumour undergoing chemotherapy needs to have knowledge of the surgical procedures and potential complications, including recognition of the signs and symptoms of increasing intracranial pressure, especially as many of the signs, such as vomiting, irritability and lethargy, are similar to the side effects of chemotherapy.

It is likely that around the time of the admission to the oncology ward, the child will need a central line inserted so that intravenous chemotherapy can be administered safely (Cancer Backup 2007). The nursing and medical team caring for the child will be responsible for ensuring that the child and family are given accurate information about the surgical procedure and the types of central lines available so that the family can give informed consent and make informed choices about the type of central line to be inserted. During this surgical procedure the general principles of preparing a child for theatre outlined in Chapter 3 apply. Following the procedure and before discharge home, the child and parents will need to be given advice regarding central line care, dressings, bathing and flushing the central line as appropriate and in accordance with unit policies.

In addition to the potential neurological problems of the child, during and after chemotherapy the nurse will need to monitor and treat the possible side effects of chemotherapy, such as vomiting, mucositis, pain, bone marrow suppression and infection (Vernon-Levett and Geller 1997). The child will require antiemetics to help prevent and alleviate nausea and vomiting, and education in mouth care to help prevent mucositis. Pain should be recorded using an appropriate pain assessment tool with the aim of providing adequate analgesia to keep the child comfortable. The child must be observed for any signs of infection. A febrile child requires blood to be taken for a full blood count and blood cultures. If the child is febrile and neutropenic antibiotics must be commenced. The child must be observed for signs of anaemia such as lethargy and thrombocytopenia such as bruising, bleeding and petechial rash. Regular blood counts are taken to monitor the child's haemoglobin and platelet counts. A low haemoglobin or platelet count will require the child to undergo a blood transfusion or platelet transfusion. Parents must be educated to observe for side effects of chemotherapy between treatments and to contact the ward or key worker if they have any concerns about their child.

Points to consider

The main side effects of chemotherapy agents are:

- Myelosuppression
  - Anaemia
  - Thrombocytopenia
  - Neutropenia
- Nausea and vomiting
- Hair loss
- Mucositis
- Alterations in taste
- Weight loss
- Lethargy and feeling weak.

(Cancer Backup 2007)

In addition to the general side effects caused by most chemotherapy agents, each chemotherapy agent can cause specific side effects. These specific side effects are outlined in Table 7.4a.

Some children will be prescribed oral chemotherapy. These children and their families will need information and support relating to the safe storage of oral chemotherapy and clear instructions regarding taking the medication.

Essential care

Children prescribed oral chemotherapy and their parents need to be informed about:

- The importance of taking the medicine at the correct time as prescribed

- If the child vomits after taking the medicine parents should be advised to contact the medical team for advice
- If a dose is missed, parents should inform the medical team, continue to take their regular dose and should not take double the dose
- Storing medicines in a dry place away from direct sunlight
- Keeping the medication in a safe place away from children
- Returning any unused medicines to a pharmacy.

(Cancer Backup 2007)

The child and parents will require psychological support from the multidisciplinary team, which must be tailored to meet the individual needs of each child and family. Many children and their families are concerned about the effects chemotherapy and radiotherapy will have on hair loss. The child and family will be offered psychological support and advice on head scarves, hats and wigs, but they should also be informed that following treatment hair may grow back a different colour and change in texture (Cancer BACUP 2005).

Table 7.4a Common chemotherapy drugs used in the treatment of children with brain tumours and their specific side effects

Chemotherapy drug	Method of administration	Specific side effects
Vincristine	Slow intravenous bolus	Peripheral neuropathy, Jaw pain, blurred vision
Carboplatin	Intravenous infusion	Irreversible hearing loss, tinnitus, peripheral neuropathy, temporary kidney damage
Etoposide	Intravenous infusion	Rash which maybe itchy, a temporary excess production of skin pigment causing skin to darken, sleeplessness, headaches, confusion, very rarely a second cancer
Cisplatin	Intravenous infusion	Irreversible hearing loss, tinnitus, kidney damage (intravenous pre and post hyperhydration usually given to maintain kidney function), peripheral neuropathy
Cyclophosfamide	Intravenous infusion	Irritation of the bladder lining (intravenous hydration and mesna given to prevent bladder irritation), temporary liver damage, diarrhoea, temporary skin changes and excess pigment, heart damage, rarely a second cancer
Lomustine (CCNU)	Oral	Changes to lung tissue, temporary liver damage, diarrhoea, very rarely eyesight affected
Temozolomide	Oral capsule – taken on an empty stomach	Constipation, rash which may be itchy, headache, dizziness, breathlessness, pyrexia
Ifosfamide	Intravenous infusion	Irritation of the bladder (hydration fluids and mesna given to prevent bladder irritation), changes to nails (nails become ridged), temporary liver damage, rash which maybe itchy, excess production of skin pigment causing darkened skin, confusion, lethargy, sleeplessness, loss of balance

Source: Cancer Backup (2007)

Supportive therapies, such as enteral feeding and total parenteral nutrition, are increasingly being used. Many children experience weight loss and periods of difficulty in eating or swallowing during chemotherapy and radiotherapy treatment. This is due to the side effects of treatment which can cause nausea and vomiting, mucositis of the mouth and gut, lethargy, fevers and periods of being generally unwell. Nasogastric or gastrostomy feeding are often advocated. Dieticians usually advise on the type and amount of feed to be given and give other nutritional advice tailored to the individual child's requirements. This includes advice on diet, high calorie drinks and milkshakes, and in some cases total parenteral nutrition is prescribed.

Increasingly complementary therapies such as music therapy, art therapy, meditation and yoga are being used, particularly with older children and teenagers as a means to relax and achieve a positive outlook and sense of well-being (Stewart and Cohen 1998).

7.5 Long-term outcomes and ongoing care needs of the child and family

There have been great advances in the treatment of children with brain tumours over the past 10–20 years. The child's prognosis depends on the age of the child at diagnosis, the anatomic location of the tumour and the tumour histology (Stewart and Cohen 1998). Although treatment methods have improved the survival rates for children with brain tumours, the long-term outcomes and complications from treatment are significant.

Points to consider

Infants and young children have the poorest prognosis because:

- Brain tumours in this age group tend to be biologically more aggressive
- There is often a delay in diagnosis because the skull is able to expand to accommodate a rise in intracranial pressure which delays symptoms
- Young children have a poor tolerance to aggressive surgery and the neurotoxic effect of therapies
- Radiotherapy, often the treatment of choice, cannot be administered to the young child.

(Stewart and Cohen 1998)

With an increase in the survival of children with brain tumours there has been an increased emphasis on understanding and managing the long-term sequelae of treatments. The effects of treatments may be evident during or immediately after the treatment, for example posterior fossa syndrome after surgery and radiotherapy somnolence. However, late effects may not fully manifest themselves for several years. Long-term survival is often accompanied by deficits in motor and sensory function, cognitive and learning abilities, vision and hearing, as well as chronic endocrine deficiencies (Lew and LaVally 1995). It has been estimated that 80 per cent of children have delays in neurobehavioral function following surgical resection of a brain tumour, prior to radiotherapy or chemotherapy, and more than half of children treated for medulloblastoma require special educational assistance during their schooling (Lew and LaVally 1995). The child may have learning difficulties in areas such as problem solving, learning new material without repetition and recalling the details or sequences of tasks (Mulhern *et al.* 1998). Fine motor and perceptual difficulties make handwriting, typing and computer-based tasks more difficult (McCabe *et al.* 1995).

The effects of the tumour and aggressive multimodal therapy can result in lifelong disabilities in many children. This is as a result of damage to growing and developing tissues in the brain. Whole brain radiotherapy has been most closely linked to late effects of treatment (Stewart and Cohen 1998). Radiotherapy has been shown to produce alterations in intellectual functioning. Radiotherapy to the whole brain can produce subcortical white matter degeneration, diffuse slowing of electroencephalogram waves, and focal organ damage including hearing and visual deficits (Moore 1995). Following radiotherapy children may have a reduced ability to acquire new skills and information, rather than a loss of previously acquired information and skills, in comparison to healthy peers (Palmer *et al.* 2001).

Endocrine dysfunction may also occur in children treated with cranial radiotherapy to the posterior fossa and may result from pituitary and hypothalamic damage or from suppression of growth hormone-releasing factor in the hypothalamus (Cullen *et al.* 2002). The most common endocrine problem in children following cranial radiotherapy is growth hormone deficiency. Growth hormone replacement is helpful in treating children, with improvements noted in longitudinal growth. Hypothyroidism is the second most common endocrine problem seen in children following radiotherapy for brain tumours and may be a result of either primary injury from irradiation or damage to the hypothalamic pituitary axis. Many children require thyroxine supplements to support thyroid function (Vernon-Levett and Geller 1997). Precocious puberty may occur because radiotherapy can cause premature closure of growth plates (Stewart and Cohen 1998).

Points to consider

Radiotherapy is not usually appropriate for children under three years because of the high susceptibility of the immature developing brain to radiation damage. In children under three years, wherever possible, chemotherapy is used as an initial treatment until the child is older and the developing brain can tolerate radiotherapy (Palmer *et al.* 2001).

Less is known about the long-term effects of chemotherapy and its use in children with brain tumours. This is because it is a relatively recent treatment and it is usually used in combination with surgery and radiotherapy making it difficult to measure the detrimental effects specifically relating to chemotherapy alone. Furthermore, chemotherapeutic agents are constantly changing and being used in new combinations making identification of specific drug side effects difficult to determine. However, chemotherapy has been implicated in causing intellectual deterioration (Vernon-Levett and Geller 1997). Platinum-based chemotherapy agents, such as cisplatin and carboplatin, often used in the treatment of children with brain tumours are known to cause irreversible hearing loss. This hearing loss is even more significant when used in combination with cranial radiotherapy (Huang *et al.* 2002). Systemic chemotherapy has also been associated with hypothyroidism, gonadal dysfunction, nephrotoxicity, peripheral neuropathy and an increased risk of a second malignancy (Freilich *et al.* 1996).

Although advances in the diagnosis and treatment of brain tumours have occurred, and even if the treatment is successful, there is the potential for neurological, cognitive and endocrine morbidity may be significant for the child with a brain tumour (Stewart and Cohen 1998). The child with a brain tumour poses a challenge to the healthcare team because neurodevelopment exists on a continuum throughout life. The healthcare team need in-depth understanding of the exact stage of the child's development before diagnosis to be able to identify subtle changes in the child's condition during the different stages of treatment and to be able to review the child's development over time. Although the initial support required by the child and family will relate to the immediate crisis of diagnosis and treatment, the potential long-term difficulties, and therefore ongoing support, for the child and family cannot be underestimated.

Points to consider

The long-term effects for the child who has a brain tumour include:

- Emotional and behavioural difficulties and lack of interpersonal skills which may impede the development of future relationships
- An inability to live independently and to perform tasks of daily living. The child may require lifelong continual healthcare support

- Reduced future employment options because of lack of ability to concentrate, sequence events, coordinate motor skills, discriminate between left and right, use non-verbal memory and perceptual motor reasoning. The ability to undertake skills such as learning to drive a car may be unachievable.
- Lower levels of achievement in reading, spelling and arithmetic, which has implications for daily communications and management of personal finances.

(McCabe *et al.* 1995)

The child's performance at school is compromised because of learning problems as a consequence of treatments, prolonged absences from school and psychosocial problems (Upton and Eiser 2006). It has been estimated that approximately half of children who have been treated for a brain tumour have significant ongoing neurological problems and will require special help with schooling (Upton and Eiser 2006).

Healthcare professionals will need to perform regular assessments for the child's neurological, physical, psychological, educational, vocational and social needs to effectively plan for the child's long-term care needs. This requires a multi-professional team approach to care with input from many healthcare professionals including: paediatric neurologists, neurosurgeons, neuro-oncologists, radiotherapists, endocrinologists, neuropathologists, ophthalmologists, neuropsychologists, rehabilitation nurses, teachers and social workers. The approach to care needs to be family centred, and the importance of the role of the family as an integral part of the healthcare team must be recognized. The nurse plays a vital role in this team in aiding communication and coordination of care (Challinor *et al.* 2000). The follow-up care for children following treatment for brain tumours is a lifelong process so that potential late complications can be identified and ongoing support can be given to the child and family.

Key messages from this chapter

- Brain tumours are the leading cause of cancer-related death in children under the age of 15
- The position of the tumour within the brain is as significant as the type of tumour. A benign tumour which damages vital structures within the brain essential for life or a tumour which is inaccessible to the surgeon can still be devastating
- Establishing a specific cause for the development of a brain tumour is rarely possible
- Symptoms occurring within a short duration of time usually indicate a rapidly growing or aggressive tumour, with gradual symptoms more likely to be caused by a low-grade or benign tumour
- Many of the signs and symptoms of brain tumours are insidious, non-specific and develop gradually
- Many children diagnosed with a brain tumour will require multimodal therapy: surgery, radiotherapy, chemotherapy and symptom management

- Radiotherapy is not usually appropriate for children under three years because of the high susceptibility of the immature developing brain to radiation damage
- Long-term survival is often accompanied by deficits including motor and sensory dysfunction, cognitive and learning disabilities, visual and hearing deficits and chronic endocrine deficiencies.

Web resources

Candelighters
provides support and acts as an advocate for families of children with cancer, survivors of childhood cancer, healthcare professionals and educators.
www.candlelighters.org
CancerBACUP
provides information and support for individuals with cancer, families and healthcare professionals, and includes access to online booklets and other resources.
www.cancerbacup.org.uk

References

Allan D (1986) Raised intracranial pressure. *Professional Nurse* **2** (3): 78–80.
Brett EM (1997) Ataxia. In Brett EM (Ed) *Paediatric Neurology,* 3rd edn. Churchill Livingstone, London
Brett EM, Harding BN (1997) Intracranial and spinal cord tumours. In Brett EM (Ed) *Paediatric Neurology,* 3rd edn. Churchill Livingstone, London.
Cancer Backup (2007) Individual chemotherapy drugs. Available: www.cancerbacup.org.uk/Treatments/Chemotherapy/Individualdrugs. Accessed February 2008.
CancerBACUP (2005) *Children's Cancers – Brain Tumours in Children.* CancerBACUP, London.
Chadwick D, Caetlidge N, Bates D (1989) Raised intracranial pressure and cerebral tumours. In Chadwick D (Ed) *Medical Neurology.* Churchill Livingston, Edinburgh.
Challinor J, Miaskowski C, Moore I, Slaughter R, Franck L (2000) Review of research studies that evaluated the impact of treatment for childhood cancers on neurocognition and behavioral and social competence: nursing implications. *Journal of the Society of Pediatric Nurses* **5** (2): 57–74.
Children's Surgical Forum of the Royal College of Surgeons (2000) *Children's Surgery: A First Class Service.* Royal College of Surgeons, London.
Chumas P, Hardy D, Hockley A *et al.* (2002) Safe paediatric neurosurgery 2001. *British Journal of Neurosurgery* **16** (3): 208–10.
Cullen PM, Derrickson JD, Potter JA (2002) Radiation therapy. In Baggott CR, Kelly KP, Fochtman D, Foley GV (eds) *Association of Pediatric Oncology Nurses. Nursing Care of Children and Adolescents with Cancer,* 3rd edn. W.B. Saunders, Philadelphia, PA.
Dailey AT, McKhann GM, Berger MS (1995) The pathophysiology of oral pharyngeal apraxia and mutism following posterior fossa tumor resection in children. *Journal of Neurosurgery* **83** (3): 467–75.
Department of Health (2002) *Specialised Services for Children – Definition No.23.* Available: www.dh.gov.uk/en/Managingyourorganisation/Commissioning/Commissioningspecialisedservices/Specialisedservicesdefinition/DH_4001699. Accessed February 2008.
Duffner PK, Horowitz ME, Krischer JP *et al.* (1993) Postoperative chemotherapy and delayed radiation in children less than three years of age with malignant brain tumors. *New England Journal of Medicine* **328** (24): 1725–31.

Fenichel GM (1997) Disorders of cranial volume and shape. In Fenichel GM (Ed) *Clinical Pediatric Neurology. A Signs and Symptoms Approach*, 3rd edn. W.B. Saunders, Philadelphia, PA.

Freeman K, O'dell C, Meola C (2000) Issues in families of children with brain tumors. *Oncology Nursing Forum* **27** (5): 843–8.

Freilich RJ, Kraus DH, Budnick AS, Bayer LA, Finlay JL (1996) Hearing loss in children with brain tumors treated with cisplatin and carboplatin-based high-dose chemotherapy with autologous bone marrow rescue. *Medical and Pediatric Oncology* **26** (2): 95–100.

Friedman HS, Oakes WJ, Bigner SH, Wikstrand CJ, Bigner DD (1991) Medulloblastoma: tumor biological and clinical perspectives. *Journal of Neuro-Oncology* **11** (1): 1–15.

Gibson I (1995) Making sense of external ventricular drainage. *Nursing Times* **91** (23): 34–5.

Greenwood I (1992) A benign tumour with lifelong effects. Treatment and management of craniopharyngioma. *Professional Nurse* **7** (6): 358–61.

Halperin EC, Constine lS, Tarbell NJ *et al.* (1994) Tumors of the posterior fossa of the brain and the spinal canal. In Halperin EC, Constine lS, Tarbell NJ *et al.* (eds) *Pediatric Radiation Oncology*, 2nd edn. Raven Press, New York.

Hargrave DR, Messahel B, Plowman PN (2004) Tumours of the central nervous system. In Pinkerton R, Plowman PN, Pieters R (Eds) *Paediatric Oncology*, 3rd edn. Arnold, London.

Heideman RL, Packer RJ, Albright LA *et al.* (1997) Tumours of the central nervous system. In Pizzo PA, Poplack DG (Eds) *Principles and Practice of Pediatric Oncology*, 3rd edn. Lippincott-Raven, Philadelphia, PA.

Hickey JV (2003) Neurological assessment. In Hickey JV (Ed) *The Clinical Practice of Neurological and Neurosurgical Nursing*, 5th edn. Lippincott Williams & Wilkins, Philadelphia, PA.

Hickey JV, Armstrong, T (1997) Brain tumors. In Hickey JV (Ed) *The Clinical Practice of Neurological and Neurosurgical Nursing*, 5th edn. Lippincott Williams & Wilkins, Philadelphia, PA.

Hinchliff S, Montague S (1992) *Physiology for Nursing Practice*, 4th edn. Baillière Tindall, London.

Huang E, Teh BS, Strother DR *et al.* (2002) Intensity-modulated radiation therapy for pediatric medulloblastoma: early report on the reduction of ototoxicity. *International Journal of Radiation Oncology, Biology and Physics* **52** (3): 599–605.

Hudak C, Gallo BM, Morton PG (1998) *Critical Care Nursing: A Holistic Approach*, 7th edn. Lippincott-Raven, Philadelphia, PA.

Jackson AC, Stewart H, O'Toole M *et al.* (2007) Pediatric brain tumor patients: their parents' perceptions of the hospital experiences. *Journal of Pediatric Oncology Nursing* **24** (2): 95–105.

Kaye AH, Laws ER (1995) *Brain Tumours. An Encyclopaedic Approach*. Churchill Livingston, Edinburgh.

Kleihues P, Cavenee WK (2000) *Pathology and Genetics of Tumours of the Nervous System*. World Health Organization Classification of Tumours series. WHO/IARC, Lyon, France.

Lashford LS, Walker DA (1997) Improving care for central nervous system tumours: a mood for change. *Archives of Disease in Childhood* **76** (2): 88–90.

Lew CM, LaVally B (1995) The role of stereotactic radiation therapy in management of children with brain tumors. *Journal of Pediatric Oncology Nursing* **12** (4): 212–22.

Leviton A (1994) Principles of epidemiology. In Cohen ME, Duffner P (Eds) *Brain Tumours in Children: Principles of Diagnosis and Treatment*, 2nd edn. Raven Press, New York.

Louis D, Cavenee WK (1997) Neoplasms of the central nervous system. In Devita VT, Hellman S, Rosenberg SA (eds) *Cancer: Principles and Practice of Oncology*, 4th edn. Lippincott-Raven, Philadelphia, PA.

May L (2001) Brain tumours. in May L (ed.) *Pediatric Neurosurgery: A Handbook for the Multidisciplinary Team*. Whurr Publishers, London.

McCabe MA, Getson P, Brasseux C *et al.* (1995) Survivors of medulloblastoma: implications for program planning. *Cancer Practice* **3** (1): 47–53.

Maria BL, Menkes JH (2000) Tumors of the nervous system. In Menkes JH, Sarnat, HB (Eds) *Child Neurology*. Lippincott Williams & Wilkins, Philadelphia, PA.

Mastrangelo S, Tornesello A, Mastrangelo R (1999) Perspectives: chemotherapy of medulloblastoma. *Medical and Pediatric Oncology* **33** (2): 116–19.

Moore IM (1995) Central nervous system toxicity of cancer therapy in children. *Journal of Pediatric Oncology Nursing* **12** (4): 203–10.

Mulhern RK, Kepner JL, Thomas PR *et al.* (1998) Neuropsychologic functioning of survivors of childhood medulloblastoma randomized to receive conventional or reduced-dose craniospinal irradiation: a Pediatric Oncology Group study. *Journal of Clinical Oncology* **16** (5): 1723–8.

National Institute for Health and Clinical Excellence (2005a) *Guidance on Cancer Services. Improving Outcomes in Children and Young People with Cancer.* NICE, London.

National Institute for Health and Clinical Excellence (2005b) *Referral Guidelines for Suspected Cancer.* Clinical Guideline 27. NICE, London.

Palmer SL, Goloubeva O, Reddick WE *et al.* (2001) Patterns of intellectual development among survivors of pediatric medulloblastoma: a longitudinal analysis. *Journal of Clinical Oncology* **19** (8): 2302–8.

Ross JS, Wilson KJW (1985) *Foundations of Anatomy and Physiology*, 5th edn. Churchill Livingstone, Oxford.

Ryan-Murray J, Petriccione MM (2002) Central nervous system tumors. In Baggott CR, Kelly KP, Fochtman D, Foley GV (Eds) *Association of Pediatric Oncology Nurses. Nursing Care of Children and Adolescents with Cancer,* 3rd edn. W.B. Saunders, Philadelphia, PA.

Shiminski-Maher T, Shields M (1995) Pediatric brain tumors: diagnosis and management. *Journal of Pediatric Oncology Nursing* **12** (4): 188–98.

Smith J (1999) Specialist courses: education for the future. *Paediatric Nursing* **11** (4): 19–21.

Stewart ES, Cohen DG (1998) Central nervous system tumors in children. *Seminars in Oncology Nursing* **14** (1): 34–42.

Strother DR, Pollack IF, Fisher PG *et al.* (2002) Tumors of the central nervous system. In Pizzo PA, Poplack DG (Eds) *Principles and Practice of Pediatric Oncology,* 4th edn. Lippincott Williams & Wilkins, Philadelphia, PA.

Turini M, Redaelli A (2001) Primary brain tumours: a review of research and management. *International Journal of Clinical Practice* **55** (7): 471–5.

Upton P, Eiser C (2006) School experiences after treatment for a brain tumour. *Child: Care, Health and Development* **32** (1): 9–17.

Vernon-Levett P, Geller M (1997) Posterior fossa tumors in children: a case study. *AACN Clinical Issues* **8** (2): 214–26.

Walker DA, Punt JAG, Sokal M (1999) Clinical management of brain stem glioma. *Archives of Disease in Childhood* **80** (6): 558–64.

Wong DL (1995) *The child with cerebral dysfunction.* In Wong DL (ed.) *Whaley and Wong's Nursing Care of Infants and Young Children,* 5th edn. Mosby, New York.

Worrall L (1999) Medulloblastoma. In Miaskowski C, Buchel P (eds) *Oncology Nursing – Assessment and Clinical Care.* Mosby, St Louis, MO.

8 Surgical management of epilepsy in children

Epilepsy is one of the most common neurological conditions in adults and children. Although there is no uniform definition, epilepsy can be thought of as a condition that is characterized by recurrent, unprovoked seizures (Panayiotopoulos 2005). An epileptic seizure is an episode of excessive neuronal activity that interrupts cerebral function. The management of acute seizures and status epilepticus in children are outlined in Chapter 2, Section 5. This chapter will provide a brief overview of the epidemiology, classification and general management of epilepsy in children. The main focus of the chapter will relate to the principles of caring for the child and family, where the child requires surgery for epilepsy.

At the end of reading this chapter you will be able to:

Learning outcomes

- Describe the International League Against Epilepsy's system for classifying epilepsy (Engel 2001)
- Outline the management of epilepsy in children
- Describe the principles of care for the child and family, where the child requires surgery to treat epilepsy
- Discuss the long-term care needs of the child and family.

8.1 Incidence, classification and aetiology

Incidence

Approximately 1 person in 2,000 is diagnosed with epilepsy each year (Heaney *et al.* 2002). The risk of developing epilepsy increases to 1 in 500 in children less than 1 year of age, and the estimated prevalence rate in children is 1 in 200 (Royal College of Paediatrics and Child Health 2000; Heaney *et al.* 2002). The incidence of epilepsy related to age is presented in Figure 8.1a.

Classification

Epilepsy can manifest in a range of seizure presentations that respond differently to the treatments available and have differing prognoses. It is essential to establish a correct diagnosis because identifying the type of epilepsy ensures an appropriate treatment plan is initiated (Panayiotopoulos 2005). The current classification of epilepsy is based on the 2001 International

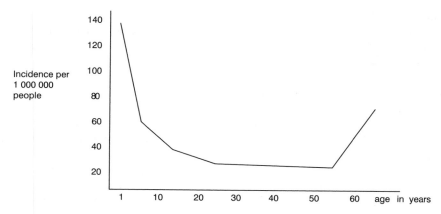

Figure 8.1a Incidence of epilepsy related to age (Source: Appleton 1995)

League Against Epilepsy (ILAE) system (Panayiotopoulos 2005). The types of epileptic seizures, according to the ILAE classification, are presented in Table 8.1a. Generalized seizures are those where the seizure activity is generated in both cerebral hemispheres (Panayiotopoulos 2005). Focal seizures are those where the seizure activity is generated within a localized area of the brain (Panayiotopoulos 2005).

Table 8.1a Types of epileptic seizures

Focal (or local) seizures	Focal sensory seizures
	Focal motor seizures
	Gelastic seizures
	Hemiclonic seizures
	Secondary generalized seizures
	Reflex seizures in focal epilepsy syndromes
Generalised seizures	Tonic–clonic seizures
	Clonic seizures
	Typical absence seizures
	Atypical absence seizures
	Mycological absence seizures
	Tonic seizures
	Spasms
	Myoclonic seizures
	Eyelid myoclonia
	Myoclonic atonic seizures
	Negative myoclonus
	Atonic seizures
	Reflex seizures in generalised epilepsy syndromes
Unclassified epileptic seizures	Neonatal seizures such as rhythmic eye movements, chewing, swimming movements
Prolonged seizures	Generalised status epilepticus
	Focal status epilepticus

Source: Engel (2001)

Epileptic syndromes

An epileptic syndrome is an epileptic disorder that is characterized by a cluster of signs and symptoms usually occurring together (Commission on Classification and Terminology of the International League against Epilepsy 1989). The three most common epilepsy syndromes in childhood are (Panayiotopoulos 2005):

• Benign childhood focal seizures: the most common type of epilepsy in children and usually develops during early childhood. Seizures start with an aura (abnormal sensations), followed by hemifacial motor seizures and a tendency to evolve into a generalized tonic-clonic seizure. The seizures usually remit after a few years. The child may or may not require antiepileptic drugs
• Juvenile myoclonic epilepsy: a fairly common type of epilepsy and usually develops during adolescence; seizure types include tonic-clonic seizures, myoclonic jerks and/or absences (being unaware of surroundings). There is a possible genetic link. The seizure activity can usually be managed successfully with antiepileptic drugs
• Hippocampal epilepsy: a fairly common type of epilepsy usually developing in adolescence. Seizure types are commonly focal seizures and start with an aura, which progress to complex seizures. Seizures may be well controlled with carbamazepine but for a number of individuals the seizures may be difficult to control

Two examples of rare epilepsy syndromes in childhood are:

• Infantile spasms or West syndrome: The child presents with repeated clusters of tonic seizures (infantile spasms). The onset is usually between 3–9 months, prognosis is poor, seizure activity is difficult to treat and many infants develop a range of seizure patterns in later life
• Lennox-Gastaut syndrome: This is one of the most severe types of epilepsy. The child presents with multiple seizure types including atonic seizures and atypical absences. The onset is usually between 1–7 years. There is a possible genetic link and there may be identifiable brain abnormalities. The overall prognosis is poor and seizure activity is difficult to treat.

Aetiology

Although a range of causes can potentially result in the development of epilepsy in children, the aetiology of epilepsy can be broadly divided into: genetic and congenital malformations that occur during cerebral development, and irreversible brain damage (Appleton 1995; Sander and Shorvon 1996). Irreversible brain damage provides a focus for seizure activity and can be a result of traumatic brain injury, central nervous system (CNS) infections, perinatal hypoxia, perinatal intraventricular haemorrhage and tumours (Sander and Shorvon 1996). Children with neurodegenerative disorders usually have epilepsy. Epilepsy appears to have a slightly higher incidence in boys and in south Asian populations (Hamdy *et al.* 2007; Sander and Shorvon 1996).

Points to consider

For the majority of children with epilepsy there is no known cause (idiopathic epilepsy) but it is likely that there is a genetic origin and therefore are best termed cryptogenic (Sander and Shorvon 1996).

Points to consider

Although the reasons are not clear, epilepsy is associated with families who are socio-economically disadvantaged (Heaney *et al.* 2002). Poor socioeconomic status is associated with an increased incidence of traumatic births, infections and poor nutrition, which may contribute to the pathophysiological causes of epilepsy in these children. Furthermore, parents who have epilepsy are more likely to have children with epilepsy than those who don't. This may be a confounding factor in attributing to the family's poor socioeconomic state (Heaney *et al.* 2002).

8.2 Clinical presentation, diagnosis and the principles of managing a child with epilepsy

Clinical presentation

Epilepsy can present in a range of seizure types; the common terms used to describe seizure types include:

- Absence: characterized by a sudden and usually brief loss of awareness of the surroundings and the child may appear to be staring or have rapid eye blinking.
- Atonic: there is a sudden and brief loss of muscle tone resulting in the child falling to the ground, often referred to as a drop attack.
- Aura: a range of abnormal sensations as a result of stimulation of a specific area within the brain, such as visual hallucinations or illusions, auditory, taste or smell hallucinations; may precede other seizure types.
- Automatism: an involuntary repetitive motor activity such as lip smacking.
- Clonic: there is limb jerking caused by the muscles contracting and relaxing in quick succession.
- Myoclonic: a sudden contraction of the muscles that can affect the trunk or be restricted to one or both arms or legs.
- Tonic: increased muscle tone resulting in stiffness.
- Tonic-clonic: the typical image of a seizure. There is increased muscle tone that results in rigidity followed by the clonic phase were there is rhythmical jerking movements. The jerking movements last for a variable period of time and there may be reflex emptying of the bladder and bowels. The tonic-clonic phase may be preceded by an aura, There may be confusion and lethargy once the seizure activity has ceased.
- Versive movements: clonic or tonic head and eye deviations which are involuntary and result in sustained unnatural positioning of the head and eyes.

Diagnosis

A diagnosis of epilepsy is based on the seizure patterns, electroencephalogram (EEG) findings, neuroimaging findings and neurological examination (Lüders *et al.* 1998). The diagnosis, investigation and classification of epilepsy in children should be made by a paediatrician with training and experience in the care of children with epilepsy in accordance with the National Institute of Health and Clinical Excellence (NICE) guidance relating to the care of children with epilepsy (NICE 2004). An accurate diagnosis is essential and is dependent on taking a good history and detailed description of the seizure activity (Appleton 1995). A diagnosis of epilepsy is usually only made if two or more seizures have occurred. Classifying the type of epilepsy is important because the type of epilepsy will influence treatment decisions and assist in predicting the long-term prognosis for the child. Classification will need to consider, the age of onset of the first seizure, the types of seizure activity, the presence of underlying neurological problems, family history and EEG findings (Appleton 1995).

The principles of managing the child with epilepsy

Best practice recommendations

The treatment and care of the child with epilepsy and their family should consider the principles outlined in the National Institute of Health and Clinical Excellence guidance relating to the care of children with epilepsy (NICE 2004). Decision will need to be made to manage the child conservatively (monitoring and regular review) or to offer treatment. Treatment decisions should be made in partnership with the child and family and must consider the risks and benefits of the treatments, the type of epilepsy, long-term prognosis and lifestyle (NICE 2004).

Antiepileptic drugs

Antiepileptic drugs are the main treatment for epilepsy. The overall aim of drug therapy is to use monotherapy in the lowest possible dose to control the seizures, while minimizing side effects and considering the child's and family's preferences. Monotherapy is successful in the majority of children (Camfield *et al.* 1997) and there is an increasingly wide range of antiepileptic drugs available. The choice of drug will depend on the type of seizures and underlying diagnosis.

Best practice recommendations

Although the NICE guidance relating to the care of children with epilepsy make recommendations relating to drug choice (NICE 2004), there is limited research that directly compares the effectiveness of the different antiepileptic drugs (Marson *et al.* 2003).

Traditionally sodium valproate has been the first choice for generalized seizures and carbamazepine for partial seizures (Marson *et al.* 2003, 2007a). However, newer antiepileptic drugs such as vigabatrin and lamotrigine are becoming more established (Marson *et al.* 2007b). A combination of drugs should be considered if monotherapy is not successful. Combined drug therapy should be undertaken at specialist services and follow recommended guidance (NICE 2004). Children who do not respond to monotherapy are more likely to have complex neurological problems and a range of seizure patterns.

Essential care

The care of the child and family, where the child is prescribed antiepileptic drugs must include providing adequate details relating to the action of the drugs, drug dosages, side effects, drug toxicity monitoring and possible drug interactions including over the counter drugs.

There has been an increased focus relating to tapering and discontinuing antiepileptic drugs in a child who has been seizure-free for two years (Tennison *et al.* 1994). The withdrawal of drugs should be undertaken by specialist services and follow recommended guidance (Lhatoo *et al.* 2001; NICE 2004). The usual practice is to taper off the drugs over a six-week period (Tennison *et al.* 1994). This will be an extremely anxious time for the child and family and support from an epilepsy nurse specialist will be invaluable. Only about 30 per cent of these children will remain seizure-free without future medication (Bouma *et al.* 2002).

Intractable epilepsy only occurs in about 4 per cent of children with epilepsy (Camfield *et al.* 1997). Intractable epilepsy had been defined as persistent seizures after two years of treatment and failure to respond to at least two treatment trials (Dlugos 2001; Cross 2002). This definition may not be appropriate for children because of pressures to suppress seizure activity early to reduce developmental morbidity (Cross 2002). Consequently, a greater number of drugs and drug combinations may have been tried over a shorter period. Unfortunately intractable epilepsy is difficult to manage even with multiple drug therapy. Additional treatment options, which may offer opportunity to reduce seizure activities in these children, include the ketogenic diet, vagal nerve stimulation and surgery.

Ketogenic diet

Observations of people with epilepsy who required surgery suggested that during periods of fasting seizure activity is reduced. The ketogenic diet, a diet high in fat but low in carbohydrate, is thought to have similar fasting effects on the body, where fat is the main energy source, rather than glucose. The metabolism of fats results in the production of ketones, which are thought to have antiepileptic properties (Levy and Cooper 2003). Although, there is no reliable evidence to support the use of a ketogenic diet in the management of epilepsy, it appears to be effective for some children (Levy and Cooper 2003).

There are a range of complications associated with the ketogenic diet (Hassan *et al.* 1999), including:

- The development of renal stones
- Low levels of vitamins, minerals and proteins resulting in restricted growth and development
- Thiamine deficiency resulting in optic nerve neuropathy

- Increased risk of infections because of impaired neutrophil functioning and malnutrition
- Nausea and vomiting due to an inability to tolerate the diet.

Essential care

The length of time a child can be maintained on a ketogenic diet will depend on the child's clinical response and the impact on the child's growth and development, with the average length being 6–8 months (Hassan *et al.* 1999). However, the diet is extremely unpalatable and non-compliance is a particular problem in older children. Children who do manage to remain on the diet require close monitoring and regular biochemical screening.

Vagal nerve stimulation

Vagal nerve stimulation is a recent adjunct to the treatment of seizures in children who have a poor response to antiepileptic drug therapy (Murphy 1999). The vagal nerve stimulator is an electronic device that is placed under the skin in the left upper chest and is connected to the left vagal nerve by electrodes (Figure 8.2a). The stimulator can then be programmed to deliver periodic electrical stimuli. Although the vagus nerve connects to various areas within the brain, the exact mechanisms of reducing seizure activity by stimulating the nerve are unknown (Kirse *et al.* 2002). It has been estimated that approximately 40 per cent of children who undergo vagal nerve stimulation treatment, in conjunction with antiepileptic drug therapy, achieve a reduction in seizure frequency (Murphy 1999).

The stimulator is activated and adjusted magnetically, usually when the child and family attend the first outpatient clinic review after insertion of the device. The stimulator can deliver electric currents between 0.5–1.25mA, which along with the frequency of the stimulations, can be altered at subsequent outpatient visits depending upon clinical need and the presence of side effects. The side effects of inserting a vagal nerve stimulator include wound infections, mechanical failure, degeneration of the electrode cables, hoarse voice and the development of a cough when the stimulator is active, as well as communication and swallowing difficulties (Murphy 1999; Kirse *et al.* 2002). However, side effects are usually not severe enough to require removal of the stimulator (Murphy 1999).

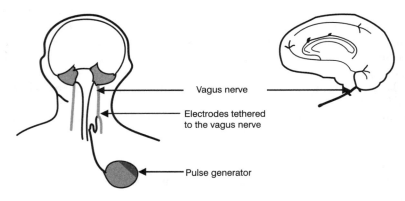

Vagus nerve

Electrodes tethered
to the vagus nerve

Pulse generator

Figure 8.2a Position of the vagus nerve and vagal nerve stimulator

In general there are few specific peri-operative requirements for the child requiring insertion of a vagal nerve stimulator, with the majority of children being able to undergo the procedure as a day case (Kirse *et al.* 2002). Chapter 3 outlines the general principles of a child requiring surgery. Prophylactic antibiotics may be prescribed to reduce the risk of postoperative wound infections (Kirse *et al.* 2002). Nursing care should include discussing with the child and family issues relating to altered body image, which may cause concern as a result of the stimulator protruding under the skin incision and the presence of surgical scars.

Surgery

Surgery for epilepsy can successfully reduce seizure activity in some children with drug resistant epilepsy (Lendt *et al.* 2000; Loddenkemper *et al.* 2007). Surgical procedures can be broadly divided into resective or functional surgery (Cross 2002). Resective surgery aims to remove the site of seizure generation and includes focal cerebral resections and hemispherectomy. Functional surgery aims to moderate brain functioning, for example performing a callosotomy where the corpus callosum is divided preventing seizure activity generated in one hemisphere spreading to the other. Complex neurosurgery, including surgery for children with epilepsy, has been identified as a subspecialty of neurosurgery and therefore should only be undertaken in designated centres where there are appropriate facilities, expertise and a multidisciplinary approach to care (Chumas *et al.* 2002). The principles of caring for a child requiring surgical management of epilepsy are described in Section 3 of this chapter.

General principles of caring for a child with epilepsy and their family

Healthcare professionals working with the child and family, where the child has epilepsy must be able to provide appropriate up-to-date information to enable them to contribute to the decisions about treatment options (NICE 2004). Although information should be tailored to meet specific needs, it must include general information about epilepsy, seizure types and control, treatment options, lifestyle issues and maintaining the child's safety. There remains a social stigma attached to epilepsy. The responsibility for educating school staff, social care staff and healthcare professionals is an important role for professionals caring for the child with epilepsy (NICE 2004). However, the organization of structured training packages is usually the role of the epilepsy nurse specialist.

Best practice recommendations

The treatment and care of the child with epilepsy and their family should consider the principles in the NICE guidance relating to the care of children with epilepsy (NICE 2004). These principles include:

* Empowering the child, with support from specialist epilepsy services, to actively participate in the management of their condition
* Referring children with recent onset seizures to specialist services
* Referring children with seizures which are difficult to control to tertiary services
* Specialist services should include an epilepsy nurse specialist who can act as a key worker and be available to support the child and family by providing training and information to the child, family and main carers.

The nursing care of the child with epilepsy involves supporting the child and family during diagnosis, seizure management and understanding treatment modalities. Ideally, care should be directed by a children's epilepsy nurse specialist. The nurse must work in partnership with the child and family to ensure care plans meet individual needs (Shuttleworth 2004). The care plan should include comprehensive details relating to managing drug therapy and potential side effects. The cognitive and behavioural side effects associated with antiepileptic drugs (Tennison *et al.* 1994) may be particularly distressing and parents will require advice in managing difficult behaviours and ensuring their child can reach their full potential.

Children with intractable and complex epilepsy may require additional support to complete activities of daily living and to promote social, motor and cognitive functioning. The child is particularly at risk of under-nourishment because of an increased metabolic rate during seizures and disruption to normal eating patterns. Children with epilepsy are at risk of injury as a direct result of seizure activity and as a potential consequence of altered cognitive functioning that may affect the danger perception. The child's safety is paramount; the family, carers and school teachers will require the knowledge and skills necessary to maintain the child's safety during a seizure and ensure a safe environment without putting undue restrictions upon the child. The family will require support and advice relating to maintaining childhood activities. Healthcare advice will need to be tailored to the individual child, taking into consideration the child's diagnosis and the family's lifestyle. For example, childhood immunization programmes will need to be individually designed in conjunction with appropriate government guidelines.

Transition from child to adult services needs to be carefully planned (NICE 2004) and is an opportunity to review the young person's treatments and changing needs. The normal challenges of adolescence will be increased for the young person with epilepsy. The young person will need support and advice about lifestyle choices such as independent living, career opportunities, learning to drive, insurance issues, the need to continue medication, contraception and planning a family (NICE 2004).

Points to consider

There is an increased neonatal and childhood morbidity rate for children exposed to antiepileptic drugs *in utero* (Dean *et al.* 2002).
Conditions associated with antiepileptic drug exposure *in utero* include: neonatal drug withdrawal, developmental delay, congenital malformations such as neural tube defects, inguinal hernia, congenital dislocation of the hips and talipes, and behavioural disorders (Dean *et al.* 2002).

Essential care

Maintaining a healthy lifestyle and the risks associated with activities such as alcohol consumption and recreational drug use and the potential impact on seizure activity will need to be discussed. Topics such as sexual activity will need to be handled sensitively. Young people will require advice relating to planning for pregnancy and appropriate review and management of their antiepileptic medication prior to and during pregnancy.

8.3 Principles of caring for a child requiring surgical management of epilepsy

For some children with intractable epilepsy, surgery can result in a reduction of seizure activity and has the potential to improve their overall functioning and improve quality of life (Rydenhag and Silander 2001; Loddenkemper *et al.* 2007). The long-term effects of intractable epilepsy include: brain damage as a result of recurring seizures; antiepileptic drug toxicity; and psychosocial factors, such as excessive dependency and over-protection (Camfield *et al.* 1997). Reducing seizure activity can potentially minimize the risk of injury and sudden unexplained death associated with seizure activity, prevent further cognitive deterioration and improve the psychological consequences of epilepsy (Cross 2002). The child's improvement may be due in part to a reduction in sedating antiepileptic drugs required after surgery (Loddenkemper *et al.* 2007). In some children with intractable epilepsy there are associated behavioural problems such as hyperactivity, attention disorders, social withdrawal and aggression (Lendt *et al.* 2000). For some children, an additional benefit to epilepsy surgery is an improvement in the child's behaviour, which appears to increase as seizure control improves (Lendt *et al.* 2000).

Despite the potential benefits of epilepsy surgery in children, there is often a delay in recommending surgery because of the possibility of causing additional neurological deficits, difficulties in identifying the children who will benefit and the potential for epilepsy in childhood to remit with time (Cross 2002). Epilepsy surgery is a highly invasive procedure with the potential to cause long-term neurological deficits such as cranial nerve palsy, hemiparesis, hemianopia and dysphasia (Behrens *et al.* 1997; Rydenhag and Silander 2001).

Points to consider

Deciding if surgery is appropriate for the child and family is a balance between ensuring the time for potential remission has been sufficient but that the long-term effects of intractable epilepsy which may increase with time are minimized (Dlugos 2001; Cross 2002).

It is thought that clinical prediction models could assist in calculating the outcome of epilepsy surgery (Dlugos 2001). These models can aid in the decision-making processes relating to the child's suitability for epilepsy surgery. The models take into account factors such as the age of the child at the onset of epilepsy, family history of epilepsy, response to antiepileptic drug treatments, number and type of seizures, presence of developmental delay and cognitive deficits, as well as MRI results and EEG findings (Dlugos 2001). Children suitable for epilepsy surgery include those children with intractable epilepsy who have not responded to antiepileptic drug therapy or those children who have a clearly identified structural lesion.

Clinical assessment of the child prior to epilepsy surgery

The main aim of the pre-surgical assessment of children who are likely to undergo epilepsy surgery is to determine if there is a specific area of the brain that is the focus of seizure activity and to ensure the removal of this area of the brain will not compromise the child's ability to function (May 2001; Cross 2002).

Points to consider

It is important that the child who may potentially benefit from epilepsy surgery undergoes a full assessment including: neuropsychological function, structural neuro-imaging such as MRI, and functional neuro-imaging such as positron emission tomography (PET), SPECT and EEG video telemetry.

Non-invasive approaches to investigations are preferable in children and as techniques become more sophisticated they may negate the need for the invasive approaches (Kilpatrick *et al.* 1997; Cross 2002). Chapter 2, Section 1 provides an overview of neurological diagnostic procedures. In addition to the non-invasive neurological investigations, invasive EEG monitoring may be necessary because routine recordings, obtained by electrodes placed on the scalp surface, may not precisely locate the site where initiation of the seizure activity occurs. Other functional areas of the brain including those responsible for speech, language, sensory and motor functions can also be identified (May 2001). Invasive EEG monitoring involves placing electrodes either on the surface of the brain, subdurally or deep within the cortex. These procedures require the child to undergo a craniotomy to enable the electrode grids to be positioned. The external cable of the electrode grids enable the child to be connected to the EEG. Following insertion of the electrodes, the child is monitored for a period of one to two weeks using video telemetry techniques to gain detailed information about the child's brain function. The results will assist in planning the extent of the surgery and the exact area of the brain that will be resected. During the procedure the child's antiepileptic drugs may be withheld to enable the range of seizures experienced by the child to be recorded (May 2001).

Essential care

The priorities for nursing care during invasive EEG monitoring include: maintaining the position of the electrodes, maintaining safety during periods of seizure activity and managing seizures in accordance with unit protocols. It is essential that the nursing staff work in partnership with the child and family to minimize distress that may occur as a result of constant surveillance, repeated seizure activity and a restricted environment.

A full neuropsychological assessment is essential to provide and record the child's baseline level of cognitive functioning, to identify current impairments and possible relocation of functional areas as a result of cerebral adaptation and identify cerebral dominance (Cross 2002). Neuropsychological assessments need to be performed by a neuropsychologist, who will be able to apply standard psychological and development tests, while taking into account any specific behavioural or cognitive difficulties. The range of tests include: cognitive functions, such as intelligence quotient scoring, long- and short-term memory tests, receptive and expressive language tests, visuospatial function, information processing and educational achievements (May 2001). In addition to evaluating the child's cognitive abilities prior to surgery, postoperative neuropsychological assessment is an essential part of assessing the quality and outcomes related to epilepsy surgery (Helmstaedter 2004).

Preoperative care

The general principles of caring for a child undergoing a craniotomy described in Chapter 3 will apply to the child undergoing surgery for epilepsy. The preoperative evaluation of a child has already been described. The investigations are complex and can be invasive. Therefore, it is essential that the child and family have access to an epilepsy nurse specialist who can provide support and advice during the long process of assessment through to actual surgery (May 2001). The epilepsy nurse specialist will have a key role in managing parents' expectations, so the nurse must be able to discuss the implications of the surgery. The potential benefits and complications, both of the invasive investigations and the therapeutic surgical procedure, must be outlined to the child and family to enable them to contribute to the decision-making process.

In general there is no specific preoperative preparation for a child undergoing surgery for epilepsy. Blood profiling should include clotting studies which may become altered as a result of anticonvulsant medication. In addition there should be adequate amounts of blood available as large blood losses will require rapid transfusions during the procedure.

Postoperative care

The management of children following surgery for epilepsy requires effective teamwork. The support of facilities such as rapid access to CT scanning and an emergency operating theatre suite are essential to treat and manage complications promptly. The length of the procedure may mean the child requires ventilatory support and invasive blood pressure monitoring and will require the child to be nursed in intensive care for the first 24–48 hours. The specific details of care relating to the postoperative management of the child following craniotomy, covered in Chapter 3, will also apply to the child who has undergone surgery for epilepsy.

Points to consider

Immediate postoperative complications include:

- Cerebral oedema due to generalized inflammatory response caused by tissue damage during the surgical resection
- Although haemorrhage does not appear to be a common complication its affects can be catastrophic (Behrens *et al.* 1997; Rydenhag and Silander 2001), and appears to be a more significant problem following hemispherectomy (Devlin *et al.* 2003). Haemorrhage is a result of damage to small capillaries that will cause slow oozing of blood which will contribute to intracranial pressure over time. Damage and failure to effectively cauterize large vessels intra-operatively will result in the rapid development of a haematoma and sudden rise in intracranial pressure.
- Postoperative fever
- Seizures.

Nursing care will be directed towards the detection, minimizing the development of and treating increased intracranial pressure, managing blood loses and managing seizures effectively, discussed in detail in Chapter 2, Section 3 and Chapter 5, Section 3. Maintaining fluid and electrolytes is a balance between ensuring adequate circulatory blood volume to maintain good cerebral perfusion and preventing over-hydration, which will add to cerebral oedema and blood loss at the capillary beds. The amount of blood loss and circulating fluid volumes must be regularly assessed and the child will require repeated blood sampling to monitor full blood count, urea and electrolytes, clotting factors and serum osmolality. Clinical assessment is necessary, including the monitoring of drainage from surgical drains and circulatory assessment (May 2001). Initially the child will require continual cardiac, arterial and central venous pressure monitoring. Management of fluids will be specific to each child's needs, as will haemoglobin levels and urea and electrolyte profiles. Colloids will be required to treat hypovolaemia and blood transfusion(s) will be indicated if the haemoglobin levels fall, usually when less than 9g/dL. The child's fluid balance must be recorded and monitored. Oral feeds may be introduced to non-ventilated children as soon as the cough and gag reflexes have returned, and once fully recovered from the anaesthetic.

The child's temperature must be monitored, as an elevated temperature could be an indication of wound infection. However, hyperpyrexia is common after cranial surgery as a result of irritation of cerebral tissues by the presence of blood, but this usually subsides after the first 72 hours. Paracetamol, in additional to its analgesic properties, is an antipyretic but may mask the symptoms of infection. Vomiting, lethargy and excessive sleepiness appear to be more persistent following hemispherectomy (May 2001). Vomiting may delay the introduction of oral fluids and the child may require continued support with intravenous fluids; antiemetic therapy will be necessary. Lethargy and excessive sleepiness are best managed by planning care to ensure adequate rest periods.

Complications of surgery: invasive investigations and therapeutic surgical procedures

The potential complications of invasive investigations include hemiparesis, meningitis, subdural haematoma and dislocation of electrode implants (Behrens *et al.* 1997; Rydenhag and Silander 2001). The complications of therapeutic surgical interventions include third nerve palsy, hemianopia (loss of vision in one half of the visual field), dysphasia, hemiparesis, disconnection syndrome, CSF leakage, haematoma, wound infections, meningitis and the development of hydrocephalus (Behrens *et al.* 1997; Rydenhag and Silander 2001, Devlin *et al.* 2003). The majority of these complications are transient, but it is estimated that children who undergo surgery for epilepsy have approximately a 3 per cent risk of long-term complications that affect activities of daily living (Behrens *et al.* 1997; Rydenhag and Silander 2001) which include hemiparesis, hemianopia and disconnection syndrome.

Hemiparesis is a potential complication of all types of epilepsy surgery causing weakness and immobility in the limbs of the affected side of the body. Hemianopia, loss of vision in half of the visual field, is particularly associated with temporal lobectomy. Disconnection syndrome is a potential complication of callosotomy and causes language impairments and disorders of attention, memory and sequencing.

Discharge planning and ongoing needs

If there are no untoward events, the child may be discharged around 5–7 days after surgery. Clips are usually removed after 7–10 days. There must be effective liaison between the hospital and community team to ensure continuing support following discharge. However, an intensive rehabilitation programme will be required for those children who, as a consequence of the surgery, have lost preoperative skills and abilities. The principles of rehabilitation are described in Chapter 2, Section 8.

Discharge planning must involve the multidisciplinary team and consider any additional ongoing needs as a consequence of the surgery. The child's long-term care needs will depend upon the presence of associated neurological deficits such as hemiparesis, hemianopia and disconnection syndrome. The child may require a programme of rehabilitation, ophthalmology evaluation and educational support, discussed in Chapter 2, Section 8. Long-term follow up is essential to evaluate the outcome of the surgery, which should include neuropsychological assessment (Helmstaedter 2004) and seizure monitoring. Many children will be able to have a reduction in the amount of antiepileptic medication (Loddenkemper *et al.* 2007). The reduction of drugs should be undertaken by specialist services and follow recommended guidance (NICE 2004).

8.4 Long-term outcomes and ongoing care needs of a child with epilepsy

Epilepsy is a long-term condition that can affect the child's physical and cognitive functioning and the psychosocial functioning of the child and family (Camfield *et al.* 2001). The effectiveness of antiepileptic drugs achieves protracted remission in 70 per cent of people with epilepsy; the remaining 30 per cent will have an intractable and disabling condition (Hanna *et al.* 2002). Factors that influence everyday life of the child with epilepsy and the family include (Camfield *et al.* 2001):

- Severity of the epilepsy.
- Frequency of seizures.
- Associated neurological problems, behavioural difficulties and developmental problems.
- Complexity of treatments.
- Restrictions to family activities.
- Child and family coping and reaction to the condition.
- Provision of support services.
- Societal myths and misconceptions.

Points to consider

The risk of premature death is 2–3 times higher in people with epilepsy compared to people without epilepsy (Hanna *et al.* 2002). Most of these deaths are sudden, unexpected, and are associated with seizure activity (DH 2003).

The reasons for unexpected deaths in people with epilepsy are unclear but may be a result of apnoea or cardiac arrythmias which occur during a seizure (Langan *et al.* 2000). In general, sudden unexplained deaths are not witnessed. A witness would place the child in the recovery position after a seizure, thereby protecting the airway; that would not occur if the child is alone (Langan *et al.* 2000). This causes a dilemma for parents of children with epilepsy: to ensure the child is safe but still allowed to gain independence. Reducing the risk of sudden unexplained deaths can be best achieved by improving seizure control (Hanna *et al.* 2002).

Many of the children with intractable epilepsy will have complex care needs and will require physical, emotional and social support to maximize their potential. Epilepsy is associated with poor academic achievement, unemployment, low income, poor self-esteem, and social stigma resulting in isolation (Camfield *et al.* 1993; Ellis *et al.* 2000; Heaney *et al.* 2002). The effects of living with a child with epilepsy on the family are far-reaching and place strains on the child and family (Ellis *et al.* 2000). Families of children with epilepsy have high levels of psychological difficulties, and are socially and economically disadvantaged (Ellis *et al.* 2000).

The reported outcomes following epilepsy surgery are variable; studies report a wide range of success in terms of the child becoming seizure free, from 40 to 87 per cent (Cross 2002; Loddenkemper *et al.* 2007). Improved outcomes are associated with a defined focus of seizure activity, identified during neuro-imaging, and the type of seizures (Ferrier *et al.* 1999; Loddenkemper *et al.* 2007). Frontal lobe surgery has a poorer outcome for seizure reduction compared to temporal lobe epilepsy (Ferrier *et al.* 1999). The reasons behind this are unclear and it has been suggested that the area of the brain that is the site of seizure activity is more expansive and difficult to identify in frontal lobe epilepsy (Ferrier *et al.* 1999). Poor outcomes are associated with the presence of autonomic manifestations, eye deviation, contra-lateral head version, and multi-focal sites of epileptogenesis (Ferrier *et al.* 1999). Children with epileptic spasm appear to have a favourable developmental outcome (Loddenkemper *et al.* 2007). Outcomes based on becoming seizure-free do not consider the wider benefits that may be a consequence of epilepsy surgery. These may include a reduction in seizure frequency, a reduction in antiepileptic drug requirements, improvements in future development, and improved behaviour. Unfortunately, it is difficult to qualify if these potential improvements are a direct result of the surgery (Cross 2002).

Key messages from this chapter

- Epilepsy is one of the most common neurological conditions in adults and children
- It is essential to establish a correct diagnosis because identifying the type of epilepsy ensures an appropriate treatment plan is initiated
- For the majority of children with epilepsy there is no known cause
- Antiepileptic drugs are the main treatment for epilepsy, with the choice of drug depending on the type of seizures and underlying diagnosis
- Antiepileptic drugs achieve protracted remission in 70% of people with epilepsy; the remaining 30% have an intractable disabling condition
- For some children with intractable epilepsy, surgery can result in a reduction of seizure activity and has the potential to improve their overall functioning and quality of life
- Epilepsy is a long-term condition that can affect the child's physical and cognitive functioning and the psychosocial functioning of the child and family.

Web resources

The Cochrane Library
holds a range of systematic reviews relating to treatment options for epilepsy. The Cochrane Library can be accessed at the following:
www.cochrane.co.uk
or via the national electronic library for health:
www.nelh.nhs.uk

National Institute for Health and Clinical Excellence
offers evidence-based guidelines relating to the diagnosis and management of epilepsy in children and adults and can be obtained from NICE.
www.nice.org.uk
Epilepsy Action (British Epilepsy Association)
aims to improve the quality of life and promote the interests of people living with epilepsy.
www.epilepsy.org.uk
National Society for Epilepsy
is committed to providing information and support to people with epilepsy.
www.epilepsynse.org.uk

References

Appleton R (1995) Epilepsy in childhood. *Aspects of Epilepsy.* Issue 1.

Behrens E, Schramm J, Zentner J, Konig R (1997) Surgical and neurological complications in a series of 708 epilepsy surgery procedures. *Neurosurgery* **41** (1): 1–10.

Bouma PA, Peters AC, Brouwer OF (2002) Long term course of childhood epilepsy following relapse after antiepileptic drug withdrawal. *Journal of Neurology, Neurosurgery and Psychiatry* **72**: 507–10.

Camfield C, Camfield P, Smith B, Gordon K, Dooley J (1993) Biologic factors as predictors of social outcome of epilepsy in intellectually normal children: a population-based study. *The Journal of Pediatrics* **122** (6): 869–73.

Camfield PR, Camfield CS, Gordon K, Dooley JM (1997) If a first antiepileptic drug fails to control a child's epilepsy, what are the chances of success with the next drug? *The Journal of Pediatrics* **131** (6): 821–4.

Camfield C, Breau L, Camfield P (2001) Impact of pediatric epilepsy on the family: a new scale for clinical and research use. *Epilepsia* **42** (1): 104–12.

Chumas P, Hardy D, Hockley A *et al.* (2002) Safe paediatric neurosurgery 2001. *British Journal of Neurosurgery* **16** (3): 208–10.

Commission on Classification and Terminology of the International League Against Epilepsy (1989) Proposal for revised classification of epilepsies and epileptic syndromes. *Epilepsia* **30** (4): 389–99.

Cross JH (2002) Epilepsy surgery in childhood. *Epilepsia* **43** (Suppl 3): 65–70.

Dean JC, Hailey H, Moore SJ *et al.* (2002) Long term health and neurodevelopment in children exposed to antiepileptic drugs before birth. *Journal of Medical Genetics* **39** (4): 251–9.

Department of Health (2003) *Improving Services for People with Epilepsy.* DH, London.

Devlin AM, Cross JH, Harkness W, *et al.* (2003) Clinical outcomes of hemispherectomy for epilepsy in childhood and adolescence. *Brain* **126** (Pt 3): 556–66.

Dlugos D (2001) The early identification of candidates epilepsy surgery. *Archives of Neurology* **58** (10): 1543–6.

Ellis N, Upton D, Thompson P (2000) Epilepsy and the family: a review of current literature. *Seizure* **9** (1): 22–30.

Engel J (2001) A proposed diagnostic scheme for people with epileptic seizures and with epilepsy: report of the ILAE Task Force on Classification and Terminology. *Epilepsia* **42** (8): 796–803.

Ferrier CH, Engelsman J, Alarcon G, Binnie CD, Polkey CE (1999) Prognostic factors in presurgical assessment of frontal lobe epilepsy. *Journal of Neurology, Neurosurgery, and Psychiatry* **66** (3): 350–6.

Hanna NJ, Black M, Sander JW *et al.* (2002) *National Sentinel Clinical Audit of Epilepsy-Related Death. Epilepsy – Death in the Shadows.* The Stationery Office, London.

Hamdy NA, Ginby D, Feltbower R, Ferrie CD (2007) Ethnic differences in the incidence of seizure disorders in children from Bradford, United Kingdom. *Epilepsia* **48** (5): 913–16.

Hassan AM, Keene DL, Whiting SE *et al.* (1999) Ketogenic diet in the treatment of refractory epilepsy in childhood. *Pediatric Neurology* **21** (2): 548–52.

Heaney DC, MacDonald BK, Everitt A *et al.* (2002) Socioeconomic variation in the incidence of epilepsy: a prospective community based study in south east England. *British Medical Journal* **325**: 1013–16.

Helmstaedter C (2004) Neuropsychological aspects of epilepsy surgery. *Epilepsy & Behavior* **5** (Suppl 1): s45–55.

Kilpatrick C, Cook M, Kaye A, Murphy M, Matkovic Z (1997) Non-invasive investigations successfully select patients for temporal lobe surgery. *Journal of Neurology, Neurosurgery and Psychiatry* **63**: 327–33.

Kirse DJ, Werle AH, Murphy JV *et al.* (2002) Vagus nerve stimulator implantation in children. *Archives Otolaryngology–Head and Neck Surgery* **128** (11): 1263–8

Langan Y, Nashef L, Sander JW (2000) Sudden unexpected death in epilepsy: a series of witnessed death. *Journal of Neurology, Neurosurgery, and Psychiatry* **68** (2): 211–17.

Lendt M, Helmstaedter C, Kuczaty S, Schramm J, Elger CE (2000) Behavioural disorders in children with epilepsy: early improvement after surgery. *Journal of Neurology, Neurosurgery and, Psychiatry* **69** (6): 739–44.

Levy R, Cooper P (2003) Ketogenic diet for epilepsy. (Cochrane Review). *The Cochrane Library*, Issue 4. John Wiley & Sons, Chichester.

Lhatoo SD, Sander JW, Shorvon SD (2001) The dynamics of drug treatment in epilepsy: an observational study in an unselected population based cohort with newly diagnosed epilepsy followed up prospectively over 11–14 years. *Journal of Neurology, Neurosurgery and, Psychiatry* **71** (5): 632–7.

Loddenkemper T, Holland KD, Stanford LD *et al.* (2007) Developmental outcomes after epilepsy surgery in infancy. *Pediatrics* **119** (5): 930–5.

Lüders H, Acharya J, Baumgartner C *et al.* (1998) Semiological seizure classification. *Epilepsia* **39** (9): 1006–13

Marson AG, Williamson PR, Hutton JL, Clough HE, Chadwick DW on behalf of the epilepsy monotherapy trialists (2003) Carbamazepine verus valproate monotherapy for epilepsy (Cochrane Review). *The Cochrane Library*, Issue 4. John Wiley & Sons, Chichester.

Marson AG, Al-Kharusi, Alwaidh M *et al.* (2007a) The SANAD study of effectiveness of valproate, lamotrigine, or topiramate for generalised and unclassifiable epilepsy: an unblinded randomised controlled trial. *Lancet* **369**: 1016–26.

Marson AG, Al-Kharusi, Alwaidh M *et al.* (2007b) The SANAD study of effectiveness of carbamazepine, gabapentin, lamotrigine, oxcarbazepine or topiramate for the treatment of partial epilepsy: an unblinded randomised controlled trial. *Lancet* **369**: 1000–15.

May L (2001) Surgery for epilepsy. In May L (ed.) *Pediatric Neurosurgery: A Handbook for the Multidisciplinary Team*. Whurr Publishers, London.

Murphy JV (1999) Left vagal nerve stimulation in children with medically refractory epilepsy. *The Journal of Pediatrics* **134** (5): 563–6.

National Institute for Health and Clinical Excellence (2004) *The Epilepsies: The Diagnosis and Management of Epilepsy in Children and Adults in Primary and Secondary Care*. NICE, London.

Panayiotopoulos CP (2005) *The Epilepsies: Seizures, Syndromes and Management*. Bladon Medical Publishing, Chipping Norton.

Royal College of Paediatrics and Child Health (2000) *A National Approach to Epilepsy Management in Children and Adults*. RCPCH, London.

Rydenhag B, Silander HC (2001) Complication of epilepsy surgery after 654 procedures in Sweden, September 1990–1995: a multicenter study based on the Swedish National Epilepsy Surgery Register. *Neurosurgery* **49** (1): 51–7.

Sander J, Shorvon S (1996) Epidemiology of the epilepsies. *Journal of Neurology, Neurosurgery and, Psychiatry* **61** (5): 433–43.

Shuttleworth A (2004) Implementing epilepsy guidelines. *Nursing Times* **100** (45): 28–9.

Tennison M, Greenwood R, Lewis D, Thorn M (1994) Discontinuing antiepileptic drugs in children with epilepsy. A comparison of a six-week and a nine-month taper period. *New England Journal of Medicine* **330** (20): 1407–10.

9 Cerebrovascular disorders

Although relatively rare, there are a range of vascular disorders of the nervous system that can affect children. This chapter will provide an overview of the more common cerebrovascular disorders that may present in childhood, namely cerebrovascular malformations, intracranial aneurysms, cerebrovascular accidents, as well as subdural haemorrhage, haematoma and effusions. In addition, the management of a child who has sustained an acute intracranial haemorrhage will be outlined.

At the end of reading this chapter you will be able to:

Learning outcomes

- Describe the common cerebrovascular disorders that may present in childhood
- Outline the management of a child who has sustained an acute intracranial haemorrhage.

9.1 Cerebrovascular malformations

Failure in the development of the embryonic vascular network can result in a range of malformations of the endothelial tissues which can occur within or outside the central nervous system (CNS). Malformations can be divided into two main groups: haemangiomas and vascular malformations (Donnelly *et al.* 2000). Haemangiomas are benign tumours of the endothelial cells which usually develop in a two-stage process (Gampper and Morgan 2002). At birth the lesion may be small, but following birth and over a period of several months, the cells undergo a rapid proliferation, increasing in size. The lesion may have vascular lumens. The second stage is a period of stagnation, when the lesion does not increase in size, which is followed by regression of the lesion. As a consequence of the natural regression of haemangiomas, the majority require no treatment. However, a small proportion of haemangiomas develop life-threatening complications, such as bleeding or compression of vital structures because of the anatomical position of the lesion (Very *et al.* 2002). Cavernous haemangiomas of the brain are composed of sinusoidal blood vessels that are intertwined with brain tissue. Cavernous haemangiomas are usually asymptomatic; however, a large cavernous haemangioma can produce neurological symptoms such as focal neurological deficits and seizures. In these cases removal of the lesion will be necessary.

Vascular malformations are present at birth and enlarge in proportion to the child's growth (Donnelly *et al.* 2000). Depending on the exact histology vascular malformations can be lymphatic, capillary, arteriovenous or mixed in origin. Malformations with an arterial component are considered high flow, and those without an arterial component are considered low flow.

Points to consider

Vascular malformations are associated with a significant morbidity and mortality because vascular damage at the site of the lesion can result in intracranial bleeding (Donnelly *et al.* 2000). Therefore, the child with a vascular disorder is usually referred to a tertiary centre where a range of treatment options can be offered and healthcare specialists are available to support the child and family.

Arteriovenous malformations

Cerebral arteriovenous malformations occur in about 1 in 100, 000 of the population (ApSimon *et al.* 2002). They are the most common cerebrovascular lesions in children. Arteriovenous malformations are congenital lesions which occur as a result of a malfunction in the normal separation of arteries and veins during embryonic development. In arteriovenous malformations the normal capillary bed is replaced by a mass of dilated blood vessels. High pressure arterial blood flows directly into the thin walled venous channels, resulting in an abnormally high blood pressure within the lesion. As a consequence there is abnormal blood flow in the area surrounding the lesion. The high pressure in the lesion places the veins, which are more fragile than arteries, at risk of becoming damaged which may lead to bleeding. Arteriovenous malformations in the CNS are more common above the tentorium, particularly around the middle cerebral artery.

Points to consider

Arteriovenous malformations can be found in many different sites in the body but those located in the brain can have devastating consequences. Arteriovenous malformations are the most common cause of intracranial haemorrhage in children (Levy *et al.* 2000). Following an intracranial bleed many children have resultant functional deficits.

The majority of arteriovenous malformations are asymptomatic. Often these malformations are only discovered incidentally, usually during treatment for an unrelated disorder. Arteriovenous malformations that are symptomatic usually present in young adulthood; the average age of presentation in children is about 10 years of age (Stapf *et al.* 2003). Generalized symptoms include seizures and headaches, additionally, children with an arteriovenous malformation may present with a range of specific focal neurological signs depending on the location of the lesion, such as muscle weakness or hemiplegia, loss of coordination, visual disturbances, abnormal sensations or alterations in cognitive functioning. However, approximately 50 to 80 per cent of arteriovenous malformations present with signs and symptoms of raised intracranial pressure as a result of intracranial haemorrhage (Levy *et al.* 2000; ApSimon *et al.* 2002; Stapf *et al.* 2003). The care of the child who has sustained an intracranial haemorrhage is outlined in Section 4.

Points to consider

There appears to be no real consensus relating to the optimal management of arteriovenous malformations (Levy *et al.* 2000). Management options include medical management, surgery, endovascular embolization and radiotherapy. The decision to treat or not involves balancing the risks of treatment with the likely risk of haemorrhage and must be based on individual assessment. The mortality associated with acute presentation is 16 per cent, and with non-acute presentation is 8 per cent (ApSimon *et al.* 2002). The child and family must be involved in the decision-making processes.

Conservative management is primarily based on periodic radiographic imaging to monitor the size and growth of the aneurysm. Although computerized tomography (CT) scanning should be the first investigative procedure in acute presentations, children who present with generalized signs and symptoms of an arteriovenous malformation will require magnetic resonance imaging (MRI) and angiography to determine the nature and extent of the lesion. Treatment depends on the size and location of the arteriovenous malformation. Surgery involves performing a craniotomy, locating and removing the central portion of the arteriovenous lesion, including the fistula, while attempting to minimize damage to the surrounding neurological structures. Surgery is suitable when the arteriovenous malformation is located superficially in the brain and is relatively small in size. Arteriovenous malformations located deep within the brain generally cannot be approached through a craniotomy because of the increased potential to damage vital structures. Endovascular embolization and radiotherapy are less invasive than surgery and may be a safer option for arteriovenous malformations located deep within the brain.

Treatment options for the child with a cerebrovascular malformation

Endovascular embolization involves inserting embolitic materials directly into the arteriovenous malformation. Embolitic materials are delivered via a catheter inserted into the femoral artery and advanced until it reaches the site of the arteriovenous malformation in the brain. Embolitic materials include biologically inert glues, titanium coils and microscopic balloons. Once the embolitic material is in place, the blood flow within the malformation is altered; it slows through the lesion leading to thrombosis within the malformation. Once thrombosed, the malformation cannot rupture. Radiotherapy involves the administration of focused high-dose radiation aimed directly at the arteriovenous malformation to damages the walls of the blood vessels of the lesion. Over the course of treatment the irradiated vessels gradually degenerate and eventually close, leading to the resolution of the arteriovenous malformation.

Endovascular embolization and radiotherapy may not offer complete or permanent results particularly when an arteriovenous malformation is large. Radiotherapy poses the additional risk of radiation damage to surrounding normal tissues and, even when complete closure of the arteriovenous malformation is possible, the risk of haemorrhage is still present until treatment is complete. However, both techniques offer the possibility of treating previously inaccessible arteriovenous malformations. A combination of treatment approaches may be used, for example embolization therapy before surgical resection will reduce the blood flow through the lesion and has the potential to reduce intra-operative blood losses.

Points to consider

Treatment choices may be influenced by the size of the lesion, anatomical position, structure and age of the child (Levy *et al.* 2000; Mansmann *et al.* 2000). Radiotherapy is not suitable for children under 3 years of age because radiotherapy can significantly affect the growth and development of a young child (Stewart and Cohen 1998; Levy *et al.* 2000).

There is no specific perioperative care for the child requiring surgery to remove an arteriovenous malformation. The principles of perioperative care of the child requiring neurosurgery are outlined in *Chapter 3*. The long-term outcome following surgical removal of an arteriovenous lesion varies from complete absence of neurological deficits to ongoing deficits requiring continual care to maintain activities of daily living (Hartmann *et al.* 2000). Resultant disabilities are estimated to occur in 3 per cent of adults and children following surgical removal of an arteriovenous lesion (Hartmann *et al.* 2000). The child with neurological deficits will require appropriate support and a specific rehabilitation programme, as outlined in Chapter 2, Section 8, to meet the child's and family's ongoing needs.

Venous malformations

Venous malformations are congenital lesions which occur as a result of an uncharacteristic venous system, where there is no recognizable direct arterial input and the veins drain into a dilated venous trunk. They are usually found in the cerebrum, rarely haemorrhage and are usually managed conservatively, which may include endovascular embolization and sclerotherapy. Sclerotherapy involves injecting an irritating solution such as ethanol, sodium tetradecyl sulphate, doxycycline, or OK-432 (a low-virulence strain of group A *Streptococcus pyogenes*), into the lesion to shrink the abnormal veins. For larger lesions sclerotherapy can be combined with surgical excision. Surgical resection may be necessary if there are specific focal deficits. There is no specific perioperative care for the child requiring surgery to excise an arterial venous malformation. The general preoperative care of the child requiring neurosurgery is outlined in *Chapter 3*.

9.2 Intracranial aneurysms

Intracranial aneurysms are sac-like projections occurring in a weakened cerebral blood vessel wall. It is estimated that intracranial aneurysms are found in 2 per cent of the population but the majority are small and insignificant (Rinkel *et al.* 1998). Approximately 8 per cent of individuals with an arteriovenous malformation will have a coexisting aneurysm (Thompson *et al.* 1998). A number of factors appear to contribute to the formation of intracranial aneurysms in adults including: hypertension, smoking, genetic predisposition, and injury or trauma to the blood vessels. However, the exact mechanisms by which intracranial aneurysms develop are unknown (Thompson *et al.* 1998). An aneurysm ruptures when the cerebral blood vessel wall splits. The rupture can be small, in which case only a small amount of blood leaks through the vessels wall, or large, leading to a major haemorrhage.

Points to consider

Rupture of an intracranial aneurysm is the most common cause of non-traumatic subarachnoid haemorrhage in children, but depending on the site of the aneurysm, rupture can result in intracranial haemorrhage or intraventricular haemorrhage (Proust *et al.* 2001; Wanke *et al.* 2002).

The signs and symptoms of an unruptured intracranial aneurysm will partly depend on its size and growth rate. In general, children with a small, unchanging aneurysm are asymptomatic unless the aneurysm ruptures and the child will experience a sudden and severe headache, nausea, vision impairment, vomiting, and loss of consciousness. A large aneurysm that is steadily growing may produce symptoms such as headaches, loss of feeling in the face or visual problems. The child who presents with generalized signs and symptoms of an arteriovenous malformation will require MRI and angiography to determine the nature and extent of the lesion. Diagnostic investigations, their advantages and disadvantages are outlined in Chapter 2, Section 1.

The management of intracranial aneurysms

The management of ruptured and unruptured intracranial aneurysms is challenging. The emergency management of a child who has sustained an intracranial haemorrhage is outlined in *Section 4*. Technological advances in neurosurgery and endovascular techniques have changed the management of unruptured intracranial aneurysms. However, the treatment of intracranial aneurysms must consider the risk of rupture versus the risks associated with treatment (Mansmann *et al.* 2000). Although the natural history of an unruptured aneurysm is unclear (Proust *et al.* 2001), it has been estimated that the risk of an aneurysm rupturing is 2 per cent (Rinkel *et al.* 1998); the mortality rate for a ruptured aneurysm is approximately 20 per cent (Proust *et al.* 2001). The outcome following rupture of an intracranial aneurysm depends on the site and extent of the bleed and appears to have the poorest outcome following a subarachnoid haemorrhage (Proust *et al.* 2001). The morbidity following subarachnoid haemorrhage due to a ruptured aneurysm is 60 per cent, with a high risk of long-term neurological sequelae such as hemiplegia, speech difficulties and learning difficulties (Proust *et al.* 2001).

Treatment options for the child with an intracranial aneurysm

The main treatments for intracranial aneurysms are conservative management, insertion of neurosurgical clips and endovascular techniques, such as insertion of platinum coils within the aneurysm sac. Conservative management is predominantly based on periodic radiographs of the child to monitor the size and growth of the aneurysm. The aim of surgical clips and endovascular coiling is obliteration of the aneurysm. Surgical clipping involves accessing the aneurysm through a craniotomy, dissecting the aneurysm from the surrounding brain tissue and applying a titanium clip either side of the aneurysm, thus occluding the aneurysm from the parent blood vessel.

Endovascular treatment of aneurysms with balloon angioplasty has been replaced by inserting detachable soft wire coils made from platinum into the aneurysm. The coils are inserted via a catheter that is fed into the femoral artery and advanced into the aneurysm. The coils cause the blood flow within the aneurysm to altered; the blood flow slows leading to a thrombosis forming within the aneurysm. A thrombosed aneurysm cannot rupture. The placement of endovascular coils is less invasive than surgical resection of the aneurysm. However, little evidence is available to ascertain if the insertion of coils is a long-term treatment for aneurysms, and not all aneurysms are suitable for the procedure.

Neurosurgical clips and endovascular techniques have a mortality rate of between 4 and 10 per cent, and morbidity rate of 10 per cent (Raaymakers *et al.* 1998; Wanke *et al.* 2002). Complications of neurosurgical clips and endovascular techniques include rupture of the aneurysm at the time of the procedure, causing intracerebral haemorrhage. Although rupture of the aneurysm can have catastrophic consequences during either procedure, surgery probably provides a better opportunity to control the haemorrhage because of direct access to the ruptured aneurysm and the supplying vessels. The long-term effectiveness of treatments is assessed by continued evidence of aneurysm obliteration, absence of reformation of a new blood channel through the blockage and absence of aneurysm regrowth. Coil embolization may have a slightly higher probability of re-rupture compared to surgical clips, but the difference is insignificant (CART Investigators 2006). Children will require ongoing follow-up and regular radiographs to assess the success of treatments.

Aneurysm of the vein of Galen

Aneurysm of the vein of Galen is a rare congenital abnormality that usually presents within the first year of life. The vein of Galen is located within the subarachnoid space, and the presence of an aneurysm interrupts normal cerebrospinal fluid flow. Infants present with increased head circumference and hydrocephalus. Presentation within the neonatal period is complicated by cardiac failure and has traditionally been associated with fatal outcomes. Improved neonatal care facilities and technical advances, including the use of endovascular coil therapy, have improved the outcome for these babies (Mitchell *et al.* 2001).

Arterial intracranial aneurysms

Arterial intracranial aneurysms are very rare in children and are probably a result of a congenital defect in the muscle layer of the arterial wall, a weakness in the wall results in bulging of the blood vessel.

9.3 Intracranial haemorrhage

Rupture of an arteriovenous malformation is the most common cause of intracranial haemorrhage in children (Levy *et al.* 2000). Other causes of intracranial haemorrhage in children include subdural haemorrhage and cerebrovascular accidents.

Subdural haemorrhages, haematomas and effusions

A subdural haemorrhage occurs when the veins, which cross between the cortex of the brain and the dura, shear and bleed into the subdural space. Blood within the subdural space is usually referred to as a subdural haemorrhage in the first three days following the initial bleed (Minns 2005). Normal homeostatic processes operate and the body's clotting system is activated. The first stage of the process is the formation of a blood clot, which aims to prevent further blood loss at the site of injury, followed by fibrinolysis, the process of breaking down and reabsorbing the clot. Fibrinolysis causes expansion of the clot as water and inflammatory mediators are drawn into the clot; the haemorrhage is now termed a subdural haematoma (Minns 2005). If normal cellular responses are prolonged and there is excessive fluid within the lesion a chronic collection may develop, which is termed a subdural effusion (Minns 2005). The process by which a subdural haemorrhage becomes a chronic effusion depends on the initial size of the bleed, repeat bleeding which may hinder normal inflammatory responses, and continued traction on the vessels if the meninges are pulled away from the surface of the brain.

The estimated incidence of subdural haematoma/effusion in infants under 2 years of age is 12.5 per 100,000 infants (Hobbs *et al.* 2005). The causes of subdural haematoma/effusion include non-accidental injury, accidental trauma (commonly road traffic accidents), perinatal trauma, coagulation disorders, vascular malformations and meningitis (Datta *et al.* 2005; Hobbs *et al.* 2005; Feldman *et al.* 2006). Trauma is the most common cause of subdural haematoma/effusion in infants (Hobbs *et al.* 2005).

Points to consider

Recent estimates suggest that approximately 60 per cent of subdural haematoma or effusions in infants are the result of non-accidental injury (Datta *et al.* 2005; Hobbs *et al.* 2005; Feldman *et al.* 2006). Non-accidental head injury can occur as a result of shaking, compressing the brain, or direct force causing impact injuries (Barlow and Minns 2000).

Essential care

Infants presenting with a subdural haemorrhage or subdural haematoma are not only considered a medical emergency but also require a thorough assessment relating to the cause of the injury (Minns 2005).

Over 60 per cent of infants who have sustained a subdural haematoma/effusion will require immediate resuscitation because of the severity of the injury (Hobbs *et al.* 2005). However, presentation can be variable and includes drowsiness or altered consciousness, poor feeding, irritability, seizures, pallor, breathing difficulties, apnoea, decreased muscle tone and increased head size. The diagnostic tool of choice is a CT scan because it is usually readily available, is relatively easy to undertake in the sick child and acute blood loss can be detected (Datta *et al.* 2005). MRI imaging may improve visualization of the haematoma/effusion but may not detect early haemorrhage and is often more difficult to organize (Datta *et al.* 2005). MRI imaging should be performed as a secondary investigation and for ongoing follow up. Other investigations will include full blood count because the child may have a low haemoglobin, and lumbar puncture which may demonstrate blood in the cerebrospinal fluid. In addition, if there are any doubts about the cause of the injury the infant will require ophthalmic assessment to detect the presence of retinal haemorrhages, and a full skeletal survey to identify the presence of additional injuries (Datta *et al.* 2005).

Points to consider

The mortality rate in infants who have sustained a subdural haemorrhage or subdural haematoma is 20 per cent, but there may be significant morbidity due to long-term neurological impairment (Hobbs *et al.* 2005).

Cerebrovascular accidents

A cerebrovascular accident, or stroke, is defined as a clinical syndrome characterized by focal neurological deficits caused by a sudden disruption of the blood supply to the brain, lasting more than 24 hours (World Health Organization 1978). A similar episode with shorter duration and temporary effects is termed a transient ischaemic attack. There are two major types of cerebrovascular accident: ischaemic where there is a blockage in the blood supply to an area of the brain, and haemorrhagic where there is haemorrhage into the brain. Both types result in cellular damage causing altered neurological functions, with the child's specific presentation depending on the area of the brain that is affected. Stroke is much less common in children than in adults. The estimated incidence of stroke in children is approximately 3 in every 100,000 children (Kirkham 1999).

The causes of strokes in children are not the same as in adults (Delsing *et al.* 2001). Strokes in adults are primarily caused by atherosclerotic disease and linked to risk factors such as hypertension, diabetes, excessive alcohol consumption and smoking (Kirkham 1999). Atherosclerotic disease can occur in children but is more likely to be linked to familial hyperlipidaemia. Stroke in children is more likely to occur in the presence of underlying diseases, such as metabolic disorders, haematological disorders (particularly sickle cell anaemia), congenital cardiac disease and moyamoya disease (Kirkham 1999). Moyamoya disease is a syndrome where there is progressive cerebral arterial occlusion as a result of unusual vascular lesions within the artery walls that result in reduced blood flow or obstruction of the major cerebral arteries. However, the cause of the cerebral artery occlusion is not known. The majority of cases of moyamoya disease present before 20 years of age. The disease can result in repeated ischaemic episodes, cerebral infarction, cerebrovascular accidents and seizures.

Points to consider

Approximately 10 to 20 per cent of children who have a stroke have no identifiable cause and are previously well (Delsing *et al.* 2001). However, trigger factors may include infections such as measles and dental infections (Kirkham 1999).

As with adults, the most common presentation of a stroke in children is acute hemiparesis (Kirkham 1999; Delsing *et al.* 2001). In addition, presentation may include facial palsy, seizures, and the child's speech may be affected. Older children may complain of headache at the time of a stroke.

Points to consider

Strokes are more common in children under 6 years of age (De Schryver *et al.* 2000; Delsing *et al.* 2001). This is important because in infants and young children alterations to normal motor functions and speech may be less obvious compared to older children.

Essential care

All children who present with clinical symptoms suggestive of a stroke should have their care managed by a consultant paediatrician and brain imaging performed within 48 hours of presentation (Royal College of Physicians 2004). However, if a child presents with fluctuating levels of consciousness, an urgent CT scan is required

Evidence-based practice

The management and development of services for childhood stroke has, in comparison with research and service developments for adult patients, been a fairly neglected area of healthcare. However, the Royal College of Physicians (2004) has published clinical guidelines for professionals working with a child who has had a stroke regarding diagnosis, management and rehabilitation. Specific medical treatments, depending on the cause of the stroke, in children include: removal of blood clots in the case of haemorrhage, surgery if an aneurysm is evident, exchange transfusion for children with sickle cell disease, and anticoagulation therapy (Kirkham 1999). An overview of the management of stroke in children is outlined in Table 9.3a. There is no evidence to support the effectiveness of thrombolytic agents, such as tissue plasminogen activator, in the treatment of stroke in children (Royal College of Physicians 2004).

Table 9.3a An overview of the management of stoke in children

Underlying cause	Management
Haemorrhagic stroke	Immediate referral to a neurosurgical centre for possible drainage of haematoma/removal of clot
Cerebellar stroke	Immediate referral to a neurosurgical centre for possible brain decompression/treatment of hydrocephalus
Rupture of middle cerebral artery	Immediate referral to a neurosurgical centre for possible brain decompression
Stroke secondary to sickle cell disease	Exchange transfusion
Other causes of stroke	Consider low dose aspirin

Source: Kirkham (1999)

General care of a child who has had a stroke includes maintaining normal temperature, ensuring adequate oxygenation and consideration of aspirin in ischaemic stroke (Royal College of Physicians 2004). In the case of moyamoya disease improvements to cerebral blood flow, as a result of intracranial internal carotid occlusion, can be made by performing vasoreconstructive surgery (Yoshida *et al.* 1999). There are a range of approaches to vasoreconstructive surgery, but the overall aim is to minimize the risk of intracranial haemorrhage by reducing blood flow through the diseased arteries (Yoshida *et al.* 1999; Ishikawa *et al.* 1997). Although bypass surgery appears to improve cerebral circulation and reduce ischaemic episodes, there is as yet insufficient evidence to demonstrate if bypass surgery reduces the incidence of rebleeding and reduces the impact of the long-term cognitive impairments (Ishikawa *et al.* 1997).

The outcome following stroke in children is variable but survival is thought to be better than in adults (Giroud *et al.* 1997). The survival rate following stroke in children has been estimated to be about 85 per cent (Delsing *et al.* 2001). The mortality and morbidity of stroke in childhood appears to be related to the degree of loss of consciousness, presence of seizure at the onset of the stroke and location of the infarct (Delsing *et al.* 2001). Large cortical bleeds appear to have a poor outcome compared to subcortical bleeds. The child's age at time of presentation and underlying disease do not appear to have a significant impact on outcome.

Risk of recurrence of stroke is variable and is estimated to be between 5 and 25 per cent (Delsing *et al.* 2001). However, this figure may be higher, with up to 60 per cent of children with sickle cell disease and 40 per cent of children with moyamoya syndrome likely to have a further stroke (Royal College of Physicians 2004; Dobson *et al.* 2002). Preventative measures aimed at minimizing the risk of recurrence of stroke will depend on the initial cause and include: regular transfusions to ensure haemoglobin S is less than 20 per cent of the total haemoglobin in children with sickle cell disease, vasoreconstructive surgery in children with moyamoya disease, and low-dose aspirin for other conditions (Kirkham 1999).

Although survival following stoke in children is favourable, there is a high incidence of residual deficits (Delsing *et al.* 2001). It has been estimated that complete recovery varies between 25 and 60 per cent, with these children having mild or no motor or cognitive impairments and being able to attend mainstream school (De Schryver *et al.* 2000; Delsing *et al.* 2001). Approximately 30 per cent of children who have sustained a stroke will have severe functional deficits and will require ongoing care and special educational input (De Schryver *et al.* 2000; Delsing *et al.* 2001). Deficits include hemiparesis, poor coordination, poor motor function, problems with continence, swallowing difficulties and learning difficulties (De Schryver *et al.* 2000). In addition, the psychosocial impact on the child and family may affect quality of life, such as additional stress in the family, changes in behaviour, isolation from friends and disruption to usual routines (De Schryver *et al.* 2000).

9.4 Overview of the management of the child who has sustained an intracranial haemorrhage

The child who has sustained an intracranial haemorrhage will require an initial assessment, emergency stabilization and early rehabilitation programmes.

Points to consider

Prompt recognition, early resuscitation and appropriate triage may improve the survival outcome for the child who has sustained an intracranial haemorrhage (Meyer *et al.* 2000).

Once the child is stable and emergency treatment is no longer necessary, the child will require a detailed neurological assessment to establish the nature and extent of the insult. The child will require care from the multidisciplinary team, including a detailed assessment of swallowing, feeding and nutritional needs, communication, pain, moving and handling requirements, positioning requirements and risk of pressure ulcers (Royal College of Physicians 2004). Chapter 2, Section 6 and Chapter 2, Section 8 outline the care of the unconscious child and principles of rehabilitation. There will need to be early liaison and involvement of the community child health services if the child's care is to be managed in the home environment. As with any traumatic event the effects can be far-reaching, and alter the physical, cognitive and affective functions of the child. The child's and family's emotional and psychological needs will need to be considered and incorporated into care, outlined in Chapter 2, Section 7.

Initial stabilization and management

Immediate stabilization of the child will include emergency tracheal intubation to secure the child's airway and ventilation to ensure adequate oxygenation, establishing intravenous access and central venous pressure monitoring (Meyer *et al.* 2000). The child will require frequent neurological assessment as outlined in Chapter 2, Section 2. The child will require stabilization prior to emergency CT scanning, which should be performed within two hours of presentation (Meyer *et al.* 2000). A CT scan should be the first investigative procedure for the child who presents with acute signs and symptoms of intracranial haemorrhage because CT scans are widely available and are able to detect acute blood loss within the cerebral tissues.

Essential care

The child who has sustained an acute intracranial haemorrhage will require a rapid assessment of their airway, breathing, circulation and neurological functions. The child presenting as an emergency with fluctuations in conscious levels and an inability to maintain the airway requires immediate stabilization.

Raised intracranial pressure (RICP) requires appropriate management; the principles of managing a child with RICP are outlined in Chapter 5, Section 3. Emergency surgery may be necessary to decompress the brain by removing the haematoma (Meyer *et al.* 2000). Definitive surgery, for example resection of an arteriovenous malformation, is usually undertaken as a planned procedure (Meyer *et al.* 2000).

The postoperative care of a child who has had a neurosurgical procedure has been outlined in Chapter 3. In addition, the child who has required emergency surgery following an acute intracranial haemorrhage will usually be electively ventilated to ensure oxygen and carbon dioxide levels are maintained within normal limits. Intracranial pressure monitoring usually continues in the immediate postoperative period and the principles of managing a child with RICP will remain applicable (Meyer *et al.* 2000). Postoperative nursing care must include ongoing neurological assessment to detect complications, such as cerebral ischaemia and cerebral oedema, and further intracranial haemorrhage.

Ongoing care needs

The aims of caring for a child who has had an intracranial haemorrhage but does not require emergency resuscitation include minimizing the risk of a further bleed by restricting the child's activities, and detecting changes in the child's neurological functions. This will necessitate the child being nursed in a quiet environment. The child's activities of daily living and psychological needs should be assessed and appropriate care implemented. Care planning should consider the age and the child's stage of development and nursing staff will be required to work in conjunction with the child and family. Stool softeners may be considered to avoid straining. The child will require frequent neurological assessment and residual neurological deficits will necessitate ongoing care and rehabilitation for the child and family. Although the Royal College of Physicians' (2004) clinical guidelines for diagnosis, management and rehabilitation are aimed at professionals working with a child who has had a stroke, many of the issues relating to rehabilitation of children are appropriate for other causes of acquired brain injury. The principles of rehabilitation are outlined in Chapter 2, Section 8.

Key messages from this chapter

- Haemangiomas are benign tumours of the endothelial cells and usually require no treatment
- Vascular lesions, such as arteriovenous and venous malformations, are associated with a significant morbidity and mortality because vascular damage at the site of the lesion can result in intracranial bleeding
- Intracranial aneurysms are sac-like projections occurring in a weakened cerebral blood vessel wall
- Rupture of an arteriovenous malformation is the most common cause of intracranial haemorrhage in children, other causes include subdural haemorrhages and cerebrovascular accidents
- Prompt recognition, early resuscitation and appropriate triage may improve the survival outcome for the child who has sustained an intracranial haemorrhage.

Web resources

The Stroke Association
is a national charity concerned with combating stroke in people of all ages. It funds research into prevention, treatment and better methods of rehabilitation, and helps stroke patients and their families directly through its community services. The association campaigns, educates and informs to increase knowledge of stroke at all levels of society.
www.stroke.org.uk
Brain Help
provides general information for people who have had a brain injury, whatever the cause.
www.brainhelp.co.uk

References

ApSimon HT, Reef H, Phadke RV, Popovic EA (2002) A population-based study of brain arteriovenous malformation: long-term treatment outcomes. *Stroke* **33** (12): 2794–800.

Barlow KM, Minns RA (2000) Annual incidence of shaken impact syndrome in young children. *Lancet* **356**: 1571–2.

CART Investigators (2006) Rates of delayed rebleeding from intracranial aneurysms are low after surgical and endovascular treatment. *Stroke* **37** (6): 1437–42.

Datta S, Stoodley N, Jayawant S, Renowden S, Kemp A (2005) Neuroradiological aspects of subdural haemorrhages. *Archives of Disease in Childhood* **90** (9): 947–51.

Delsing BJ, Catsman-Berrevoets CE, Appel IM (2001) Early prognostic indicators of outcome in ischemic childhood stroke. *Pediatric Neurology* **24** (4): 283–9.

De Schryver EL, Kappelle LJ, Jennekens-Schinkel A *et al.* (2000) Prognosis of ischemic childhood stroke: a long-term follow-up study. *Developmental Medicine and Child Neurology* **42** (5): 313–18.

Dobson SR, Holden KR, Nietert PJ *et al.* (2002) Moyamoya syndrome in childhood sickle cell disease: a predictive factor for recurrent cerebrovascular events. *Blood* **99** (9): 3144–50.

Donnelly LF, Adams DM, Bisset GS (2000) Vascular malformations and hemangiomas: a practical approach in a multidisciplinary clinic. *AJR American Journal of Roentgenology* **174** (3): 597–608.

Gampper TJ, Morgan RF (2002) Vascular anomalies: hemangiomas. *Plastic and Reconstructive Surgery* **110** (2): 572–85.

Giroud M, Lemesle M, Madinier G *et al.* (1997) Stroke in children under 16 years of age. Clinical and etiological difference with adults. *Acta Nerologica Scandinavia* **96** (6): 401–6.

Feldman KW, Bethel R, Shugerman RP *et al.* (2006) The cause of infant and toddler subdural hemorrhage: a prospective study. *Pediatrics* **108** (3): 636–46.

Hartmann A, Stapf C, Hofmeister C *et al.* (2000) Determinants of neurological outcome after surgery for brain arteriovenous malformation *Stroke* **31** (10): 2361–4.

Hobbs C, Childs AM, Wynne J, Livingston J, Seal A (2005) Subdural haematoma and effusion in infancy: an epidemiological study. *Archives of Disease in Childhood* **90** (9): 952–5.

Ishikawa T, Houkin K, Kamiyama H, Abe H (1997) Effects of surgical revascularization on outcome of patients with pediatric moyamoya disease. *Stroke* **28** (6): 1170–3.

Kirkham FJ (1999) Stroke in childhood. *Archives of Disease in Childhood* **81** (1): 85–9.

Levy EI, Niranjan A, Thompson TP *et al.* (2000) Radiosurgery for childhood intracranial arteriovenous malformations. *Neurosurgery* **47** (4): 834–42.

Mansmann U, Meisel J, Brock M *et al.* (2000) Factors associated with intracranial hemorrhage in cases of cerebral arteriovenous malformation. *Neurosurgery* **46** (2): 272–89.

Meyer PG, Orliaguet GA, Zerah M *et al.* (2000) Emergency management of deeply comatose children with acute rupture of cerebral arteriovenous malformations. *Canadian Journal of Anaesthesia* **47** (8): 758–66.

Minns RA (2005) Subdural haemorrhages, haematomas, and effusions in infancy. *Archives of Disease in Childhood* **90** (9): 883–4.

Mitchell PJ, Rosenfeld JV, Dargaville P *et al.* (2001) Endovascular management of vein of Galen aneurysmal malformations presenting in the neonatal period. *AJNR American Journal of Neuroradiology* **22**: 1403–9.

Proust F, Toussaint P, Garniéri J *et al.* (2001) Pediatric cerebral aneurysms. *Journal of Neurosurgery* **94** (5): 733–9.

Raaymakers TW, Rinkel GJ, Limburg M, Algra A (1998) Mortality and morbidity of surgery for unruptured intracranial aneurysms: a meta-analysis. *Stroke* **29** (8): 1531–8.

Rinkel GJ, Djibuti M, Algra A, van Gijn J (1998) Prevalence and risk of rupture of intracranial aneurysms. *Stroke* **29** (1): 251–6.

Royal College of Physicians (2004) *Stroke in Childhood: Clinical Guidelines for Diagnosis Management and Rehabilitation.* RCP, London.

Stapf C, Khaw AV, Sciacca RR *et al.* (2003) Effect of age on clinical and morphological characteristics in patients with brain arteriovenous malformation *Stroke* **34** (11): 2664–70.

Stewart ES, Cohen DG (1998) Central nervous system tumors in children. *Seminars in Oncology Nursing* **14** (1): 34–42.

Thompson RC, Steinberg GK, Levy RP, Marks MP (1998) The management of patients with arteriovenous malformations and associated intracranial aneurysms. *Neurosurgery* **43** (2): 202–11.

Very M, Nagy M, Carr M, Collins S, Brodsky L (2002) Hemangiomas and vascular malformations: analysis of diagnostic accuracy. *Laryngoscope* **112** (4): 612–15.

Wanke I, Doerfler A, Dietrich U *et al.* (2002) Endovascular treatment of unruptured intracranial aneurysms. *AJNR American Journal of Neuroradiology* **23** (5): 756–61.

World Health Organization (1978) *Cerebrovascular Disorders: A Clinical and Research Classification*. WHO, Geneva.

Yoshida Y, Yoshimoto T, Shirane R *et al.* (1999) Clinical course, surgical management, and long-term outcome of moyamoya patients with rebleeding after an episode of intracerebral hemorrhage: an extensive follow-up study. *Stroke* **30** (11): 2272–6.

10 Neural tube defects

Neural tube defects are an important group of congenital malformations that arise early in the gestation period as a result of abnormal embryological development of the neural tube. The embryological development of the neural tube and structure and function of the spinal cord are outlined in Chapter 1, Sections 2 and 8. Neural tube defects include a range of disorders such as anencephaly, encephalocele and spina bifida. Anencephaly occurs when the cephalic end of the neural tube fails to close. The result is an absence of the cranial vault and the presence of an occipital meningocele. Anencephaly is usually incompatible with life and often results in spontaneous abortion. In common with anencephaly, encephalocele occurs when the cephalic end of the neural tube fails to close but the presentation differs; there is a large fluid-filled sac that protrudes through the skull, usually in the region of the posterior fontanelle, and there may be associated structural malformations of the mid-brain. Prognosis is variable and influenced by the presence or absence of neuronal tissue within the sac and associated anomalies.

The focus of this chapter is to outline the range of abnormalities that occur in spina bifida and to consider the management of the child with a myelomeningocele and the family. At the end of reading this chapter you will be able to:

Learning outcomes

- Outline the variable presentation of spina bifida and the pathophysiology changes that occur as a result of failure of the spinal cord to fuse
- Describe the nursing care of the child and family, where the child requires surgery to treat the myelomeningocele
- Discuss the long-term care needs of the child and family.

10.1 Spina bifida: incidence, aetiology, pathophysiology and diagnosis

Incidence and aetiology

Incidence

Spina bifida is the most frequent birth defect in children that results in long-term disability. The incidence of spina bifida has steadily declined over the last two decades and has probably stabilized to approximately 1 in 1,000 live births (Murphy *et al.* 1996).

Points to consider

The decline in spina bifida has been attributed to increased uptake of folic acid supplements by expectant mothers and improved antenatal diagnosis (Bell *et al.* 1996). Improved antenatal diagnosis has enabled parents to have a greater choice in relation to progressing with the pregnancy.

Aetiology

Spina bifida has no known cause but is thought to be multi-factorial in origin: a genetic susceptibility influenced by environmental factors (Botto *et al.* 1999). The genetic inference relates to the variations in the incidence of spina bifida between cultures, with the highest incidence occurring in Caucasian populations and an increased risk of the development of spina bifida if a sibling has the disorder (Feuchtbaum *et al.* 1999). An increased intake of folic acid, taken before and during pregnancy, can significantly reduce the risks of having a child with spina bifida (Medical Research Council 1991; Green 2002).

Essential care

The neural tube completely closes by the end of the fourth week of embryonic development. Many women will be unaware of being pregnant until after the neural tube has closed. Therefore, advising women to increase folic acid intake as a preventative measure needs to occur as part of pre-conception planning along with other measures to promote a healthy pregnancy, such as advice about not smoking and recommended alcohol intake.

The recommended daily intake of folic acid during pregnancy is 0.4mg but this may need to be increased to 5mg if women are identified as having a high risk of having a baby with spina bifida. This higher dose will need to be prescribed by a doctor. Drugs that lower folate levels in maternal red blood cells increase the risk of neural tube defects (Hernández-Díaz *et al.* 2001).

Points to consider

The range of drugs that are known to be folic acid antagonists include aminopterin, methotrexate, valproic acid, carbamazepine, phenobarbitone and trimethoprim.

Pathophysiology

Spina bifida occurs as a consequence of failure of the neural tube to close, which can manifest in a range of defects, usually classified as spina bifida occulta, meningocele and myelomeningocele (Figure 10.1a). Most defects occur in the sacral or lumbosacral region, but if arrest of the neural tube occurs early during embryonic development, high lesions such as thoracolumbar lesions may occur.

Normal spinal cord development:
the spinal cord is encased in the
meninges and the bones of the vertebra

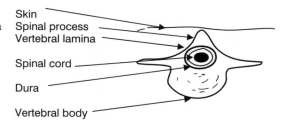

Spina bifida occulta:
failure of the posterior vertebral lamina
to fuse. The spinal cord and meninges
remain within the spinal column

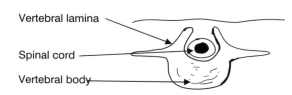

Meningocele:
failure of the posterior vertebral lamina,
muscle and skin to fuse. This results in
the meninges protruding through the
bony defect forming a sac that is filled
with cerebrospinal fluid. The nerve tract
remains within the spinal cord

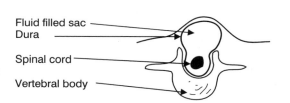

Myelomeningocele:
failure of the posterior vertebral lamina,
muscle and skin to fuse.
This results in the meninges and nerve
tract protruding through the bony defect
forming an open lesion that leaks
cerebrospinal fluid

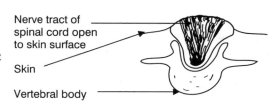

Figure 10.1a Normal spinal cord and the range of defects that occur if the spinal cord fails to close

Diagnosis

Neural tube defects are usually diagnosed in the prenatal period. Prenatal screening involves performing an ultrasound scan of the fetus and measuring alpha-fetoprotein levels. Routine fetal ultrasound scans may identify the presence of a membranous sac in the spinal region and, if hydrocephalus is present, distortion of the skull and ventricles. Alpha-fetoprotein is a glycoprotein produced by the fetal liver and is normally present in the amniotic fluid and maternal serum. Alpha-fetoprotein levels are routinely measured in maternal serum samples at about 12 weeks of gestation.

Points to consider

Abnormal alpha-fetoprotein levels can indicate the presence of gross chromosomal disorders or neural tube defects. However, there is a 30 per cent chance of a false-positive result, therefore a woman with an abnormal result will normally be offered an amniocentesis to confirm the presence of a neural tube defect.

Amniocentesis is a procedure that involves obtaining a sample of the amniotic fluid that bathes the fetus. To minimize any risk to the fetus, amniocentesis is offered at 16–18 weeks' gestation. In addition to measuring alpha-fetoprotein levels, a karyotype of fetal cells, found in the amniotic fluid, will identify the presence of any chromosomal abnormalities. Prenatal screening offers parents the opportunity to make decisions relating to the continuation or termination of the pregnancy. In addition to offering support to parents during this difficult period, it will be necessary to provide parents with information about spina bifida, such as the range of presentations and potential long-term sequelae. This information may assist parents when making a decision relating to the pregnancy.

10.2 Spina bifida occulta

Spina bifida occulta is considered the mildest form of spina bifida and may not always be obvious at birth because, other than a slight indentation over the lesion, the meninges and the spinal cord are not exposed (Figure 10.1a). Other indications that the child has spina bifida occulta include abnormal patches of hair in the skin surrounding the abnormality, or the presence of a telangiectasis, epidermoid cyst or lipoma at the site of the abnormality. Although spina bifida occulta requires no treatment at birth, recognition of the abnormality and long-term follow up of the child are important because there is a potential for the spinal cord to become fixed (tethered) at the site of the lesion (Chumas 2000). The consequence of a tethered cord is that the nerve tract can become stretched and distorted as the child grows. The management of a child with a tethered spinal cord is outlined in Section 5.

Points to consider

The child who presents with spina bifida occulta will require a full neurological examination, an MRI scan and a detailed urodynamic assessment to determine if the structural abnormality is likely to cause functional problems in the area of the body below the lesion.

10.3 Meningocele

A lesion is classified as a meningocele when the meninges protrude through the open vertebrae, muscle and skin, but the neural tissue is intact and remains within the spinal canal (Figure 10.1a). The sac-like lesion may be distended and filled with cerebrospinal fluid. Neurological function outcome is usually more favourable compared to myelomeningocele because there is potentially less damage to the spinal cord. A range of neurological deficits may occur in children who present with a meningocele, which will be influenced by the extent of nerve damage and location of the lesion. The infant will require surgery to close the lesion and appropriate management of any permanent neurological deficits. The surgical management of the infant with a meningocele will follow similar principles to those outlined for the child with a myelomeningocele (Section 4). Long-term needs will depend on the extent of neurological deficits and again will be similar to the principles outlined for the child with a myelomeningocele (Section 4).

10.4 Myelomeningocele

Pathophysiology

A lesion is classified as a myelomeningocele when the meninges and nerve tract protrudes through the open vertebrae, muscle and skin (Figure 10.1a). The myelomeningocele will be apparent at birth and presents as a visible raw tissue mass protruding above the skin. The lesion may be covered by a membrane of modified meninges which leaks cerebrospinal fluid. The exposed neuronal tissue appears disorganized. The degree of nerve damage at birth and location of the lesion will influence the range and extent of neurological deficits. Nerve damage causes paralysis, loss of sensation and loss of function in the body regions innervated below the lesion. The legs, bladder and bowel are usually affected. Hydrocephalus is usually present in children who present with a myelomeningocele because of associated malformations of the hindbrain.

An overview of the management of the child and family when the child has a myelomeningocele

Immediate care needs

A prenatal diagnosis of myelomeningocele will provide opportunity for healthcare professionals to ensure appropriate facilities are available to support the infant and parents following delivery. It will be necessary for the infant's care to be managed on a neonatal unit where there are healthcare professionals experienced in caring for the newborn with spina bifida and there are established links with a neurosurgical department (Sandler 1997). The initial aims of care are to prevent infection developing at the site of the lesion, and to minimize the risks of ascending meningitis, ventriculitis and urinary infections.

It may be necessary to cover the lesion with a dressing because the delicate neuronal tissue will be susceptible to infection, drying and traumatic damage. The choice of dressing will depend on the position of lesion and the likelihood of contamination with urine or faeces, and the amount of cerebrospinal fluid leakage. A clear film dressing allows inspection of the wound, is impermeable to water and microorganisms and may remain in place until surgery. If a woven dressing is indicated to absorb exudate it must be non-abrasive and non-adherent, for example a transparent, non-adherent hydrogel. The non-adherent dressing can be placed directly onto the lesion, which can be covered with gauze and secured with a light bandage. This will minimize trauma to the lesion during dressing changes. Meticulous nappy care is particularly essential in an infant with a low spinal lesion to prevent the lesion becoming contaminated with urine and excrement. The infant should be nursed prone with appropriate support to minimize the risk of nappy soiling.

In addition to meeting the infant's general care needs such as feeding, nappy care and maintaining comfort, the infant will require a thorough assessment of bladder and bowel functions, which will include regular renal ultrasound scans. This will ensure appropriate management strategies are implemented to minimize later complications and preserve urinary functioning from birth. Stagnation of urine in the bladder will increase the risk of urine infections and if combined with urinary reflux will predispose the child to kidney damage. The infant must be assessed for signs of continuous urine leakage or the bladder appearing full after voiding. Prophylactic antibiotics may be required to prevent urine infections. The infant may require intermittent catheterization to prevent urine stagnation and urine reflux from the bladder into the ureters. Expressing the bladder by applying pressure over the lower abdomen during nappy changes may increase the risk of urinary reflux into the ureters.

The infant will require a full assessment of neurological impairments including the range of sensory and motor deficits present at birth. The infant's care must include ensuring correct positioning of the limbs, observation of the skin for any signs of pressure damage, regular position changes and regular passive exercises to ensure the limbs are moved through a range of normal movements. The frequency of these routines will depend on the initial assessment but are usually performed with other care routines such as feeding and nappy care to minimize disturbances for the infant.

In addition to meeting the physical needs of the infant, healthcare professionals will need to offer support and counselling to the parents. Where possible, it is advantageous to provide parents with some indication of future predictions relating to the potential physical and cognitive long-term outcomes for their child (Kirpalani *et al.* 2000). This will assist parents when making decisions relating to the care of their child, in particular resuscitation if a life-threatening event occurs as a consequence of any early complications. In addition to predicting the potential long-term outcome for the child with spina bifida, it has been suggested that understanding parents' desires for their child, family functioning and support networks, and family coping strategies may assist with ethical decisions relating to the extent and nature of the treatments offered (Kirpalani *et al.* 2000).

Surgical closure of the myelomeningocele

If there are no coexisting conditions that result in cardiac or respiratory instability, surgery to close the lesion can usually be undertaken within 24 hours of birth (Sandler 1997). The aims of repairing the myelomeningocele early are to prevent continual leakage of cerebrospinal fluid, minimize the risk of the lesion becoming infected, prevent ascending cerebral infections, prevent traumatic injury to the lesion, preserve existing neurological function, and to facilitate normal handling of the infant and promote bonding between the infant and parents. Surgery consists of dissecting the neural tissue and covering the tissue with fibrous dura to prevent leakage of cerebrospinal fluid, correcting bone abnormalities and removing abnormal skin surrounding the lesion (Sandler 1997). If there is insufficient skin to cover the lesion a skin graft may be necessary. If hydrocephalus has been diagnosed a shunt may be inserted to manage the hydrocephalus.

If hydrocephalus occurs with the myelomeningocele it may be evident at birth. However, the ability of cerebrospinal fluid to drain through the open lesion may result in hydrocephalus not becoming evident until after the spinal lesion has been closed. Nursing staff will need to perform preoperative neurological observations because of the potential rise in intracranial pressure in infants with hydrocephalus. However, due to the infant's skull sutures not being fused, the infant may not present with the classic signs of RICP (Chapter 2, Section 3). Nursing staff must be alert to subtle changes in the infant such as irritability, poor feeding or vomiting, lethargy, pallor, large and tense anterior fontanelle and increased head circumference (Brett and Harding 1997).

Surgery undertaken in the neonatal period places additional demands on the infant compared to older infants and children. Neonates are physiologically immature and are less able to maintain body heat, respond differently to infectious agents, cannot maintain the circulatory system in response to even minor fluid losses and are less able to maintain their airway.

Points to consider

The principles of perioperative care for the neonate include:

- Maintaining the airway and providing adequate oxygenation
- Maintaining adequate circulatory fluid volumes and replacing blood loss
- Ensuring hypoprothrombinaemia is minimized by giving vitamin K preoperatively
- Ensuring the environment minimizes heat loss
- Monitoring and preventing metabolic abnormalities such as hypoglycaemia, hypocalcaemia or acidosis
- Maintaining strict precautions to minimize the risk of infections.

(Kelnar *et al.* 1995)

It will be necessary to nurse the infant prone and in a neutral position for 48 hours postoperatively. This will prevent cerebrospinal fluid pressure increasing at the wound site and any pressure being placed on the wound. The wound must be observed for cerebrospinal fluid leakage and signs of infection. The risk of wound infection can be minimized by ensuring meticulous skin care in the perianal region and frequent nappy care. A clear film dressing will allow inspection of the wound, and may help keep the wound free of urine and faeces. The wound will usually have been closed under tension, therefore nylon sutures are usually inserted and removed after 10–14 days.

Nursing staff will need to continue to perform neurological observations postoperatively. Infants with an associated hydrocephalus, not evident preoperatively, may develop an acute rise in intracranial pressure after closure of the spinal lesion. Hydrocephalus is likely to develop within 10 days postoperatively, as this is usually a sufficient time period to allow levels of cerebrospinal fluid to increase within the ventricles. Leakage of cerebrospinal fluid from the wound may be suggestive of the presence of hydrocephalus. In addition, the infant will require frequent measurement of head circumference and regular cranial ultrasound scans to detect development of hydrocephalus.

The infant can be discharged from hospital once the wound has healed, bladder and bowel functions have been assessed and are responding to initial management programmes, and the infant is feeding and gaining weight. Discharge from hospital must be planned effectively to ensure that parents feel confident to care for the infant and have sufficient community support networks. The discharge and subsequent care delivery will require a multidisciplinary team approach involving the family, specialist nurses, consultants, physiotherapists, community children's nurses, health visitor and the general practitioner. The number of individuals involved in the infant's care can be overwhelming and there are different models of care available to ensure the family receives appropriate support. Key workers are effective in facilitating relationships with the family. Care is probably best delivered at a child development or specialist centre, where there will be the range of specialist healthcare professionals with the skills necessary to meet the infant's and family's needs (Sandler 1997). The infant will require regular assessments through childhood to ensure care reflects changing needs as the infant grows and develops, and to ensure ongoing care needs are managed appropriately.

Ongoing care needs

The ongoing care needs of the child with a myelomeningocele relate to motor deficits, sensory deficits, urinary and bowel dysfunction, latex allergy and shunt malfunctions (McCarthy 1991). Hydrocephalus and its management are outlined in detail in Chapter 4.

Managing motor deficits and maximizing existing function

Leg movement is dependent on both upper and lower motor neuron activity. In children with myelomeningocele neuron damage results in weakness or paralysis of the muscles innervated by the nerves at the level of and below the lesion. Lack of movement in the limbs results in muscle wasting, poor growth, lack of mobility and poor circulation. The consequences are an increased likelihood of lower limb fractures, increased risk of pressure ulcers and obesity (Sandler 1997). Most centres, where possible, encourage early walking through a combination of extensive bracing, intensive physiotherapy and corrective orthopaedic surgery (Sandler 1997). Even a limited degree of mobility will offer the child increased independence.

Children with a myelomeningocele will require regular assessment of lower limb functions and formulation of an individualized care plan by a physiotherapist experienced in the care of the child with neurological problems. For treatments to be maintained on a regular basis, the child and family must be involved in the decision-making process and the formulation of care plans. Therapy must be incorporated into the child's everyday activities. Care will include passive and active exercise to maintain muscle tone, prevent muscle wasting, and prevent muscle and soft tissue contractures. Children with immobility problems must have their limbs maintained in good alignment at all times, which may require the use of splinting. Maintaining a regular exercise routine will improve blood circulation, relieve pressure, facilitate lung expansion, prevent urinary stasis and improve gut mobility.

In general, children with a myelomeningocele will require the use of mobility aids to achieve independent ambulation. Mobility aids range from walking aids such as braces to total dependence on a wheelchair. Most children will eventually require the use of the wheelchair. The child will require assessment of seating position and the degree of ability to support the spine to ensure the most appropriate wheelchair is selected. The child, parents and carers will require appropriate instructions about wheelchair safety and transferring to and from the wheelchair. Technological advances have resulted in techniques such as electrical stimulation of the spinal cord being developed to assist children in achieving independent ambulation; however, most developments are in their infancy (Karmel-Ross *et al.* 1992). As the child becomes older equipment to assist with moving and handling will be necessary and must be planned in advance. The child and family will require training with moving and handling and the use of equipment, to maintain safety and prevent injuries.

In addition to motor paralysis, children with myelomeningocele are likely to have a range of musculoskeletal deformities of the hips and feet, such as talipes equinovarus or calcaneovalgus, congenital dislocation of the hips, and fixed or hyper-flexed joints (Broughton *et al.* 1993; Frawley *et al.* 1998). Many children with spina bifida develop abnormal spinal curvature. Scoliosis may develop as a result of muscle weakness in the trunk and lower limbs. Associated problems linked to scoliosis such as respiratory difficulties do not appear common unless the spinal curvature becomes extreme. The child may undergo a range of orthopaedic procedures to correct any musculoskeletal deformities. This can result in additional periods of hospitalization for the child and treatments may interrupt usual therapy routines if immobilization is necessary.

Obesity is often associated with children with myelomeningocele and is partly attributed to immobility. The child and family must be provided with information relating to maintaining a well-balanced diet that reflects the child's calorific needs and provides the range of nutrients and vitamins needed to promote health.

Sensory deficits and preventing injury

Children with myelomeningocele have poor sensory perception due to peripheral nerve impairment. Poor sensory perception places the child at risk of injury to the lower limbs because pressure, temperature changes or pain may not be detected. The child is particularly at risk of pressure ulcers in the lower limbs and sacral region. Pressure ulcers are difficult to treat because of lack of mobility and long periods in the same position and may become infected if there are associated continence problems. The child and family must be encouraged to take active measures to prevent skin breakdown including: maintaining the limbs in a correct alignment, avoiding exposure to extremes of temperature, ensuring frequent position changes, maintaining exercise routines, ensuring meticulous skin care, maintaining a well-balanced diet and seeking prompt treatment if there are any signs of a pressure sore developing.

Managing urinary and bowel dysfunctions

A) URINARY INCONTINENCE

Urinary problems occur in children with a myelomeningocele if the normal neurophysiological interactions between the sacral spinal nerves and the cerebral cortex are disrupted. A range of symptoms, such as increased urgency when needing to void, increased frequency in voiding, retention of urine and incontinence, indicate disruption to normal urinary function. The child may be unable to completely empty the bladder and is at risk of urinary tract infections. Poor bladder wall compliance or detrusor muscle hyperreflexia can result in high intra-bladder pressures (Johnston and Borzyskowski 1998). High bladder pressures can result in urine reflux into the ureters, and may lead to kidney damage. Effective management and prevention of urinary problems requires accurate assessment of the child's renal function which may include renal and bladder ultrasound scans, urodynamic tests that measure bladder pressure and micturating cystograms which can image urine flow (Johnston and Borzyskowski 1998).

> **Points to consider**
>
> Children with spina bifida will require ongoing surveillance of renal and urinary function because of the potential for bladder function to deteriorate during the course of the child's life.

Points to consider

The aims of managing urinary problems are to preserve normal renal function and prevent kidney damage, achieve continence and allow the child to be independent in relation to their elimination needs (Johnston and Borzyskowski 1998).

Achieving continence is a major social achievement and will promote self-esteem in the child with spina bifida. Conservative management of incontinence includes toileting programmes. Continence nurse specialists provide the child and family with continence advice and support. An occupational therapist will provide positioning guidance and the need for supportive toilet seating. Children with cognition and memory difficulties may have additional learning needs which need to be considered when initiating toileting programmes.

The primary treatment of the child with a neurogenic bladder is anticholinergic therapy (bladder muscle relaxants) and clean intermittent catheterization (Geraniotis *et al.* 1988; Van Savage and Yepuri 2001). Clean intermittent catheterization is a technique used to empty the bladder at regular intervals, usually 5–6 times day. The technique considerably reduces the risk of developing upper renal tract dysfunction in children where the bladder does not empty completely (Geraniotis *et al.* 1988). In addition, children who are able to self-catheterize will have greater independence.

Essential care

The child and family will require input from a specialist children's continence nurse advisor who will provide support and guidance to the child and family including: teaching catheterization procedures, providing advice on the type of catheters and frequency of catheterization, providing advice relating to obtaining supplies of catheters, liaising between hospital and community services, advising schools about the procedures and facilities required, and monitoring for signs of urinary tract infections.

Although the usual treatment for incontinence in children with a myelomeningocele is intermittent catheterization, some children – because of neurological impairments, fixed lower extremities, obesity and urethral strictures – may not be able to perform the procedure (Van Savage and Yepuri 2001). Surgical procedures, where a catheterizable conduit is created, have been developed to enable clean catheterization for children who otherwise would not be able to perform the procedure (Van Savage and Yepuri 2001). The Mitrofanoff appendicovesicostomy is a urinary diversion procedure that involves mobilizing the appendix and using it as a conduit from the bladder to the abdominal wall. A stoma is formed on the abdomen, which can be used to catheterize the bladder. Bladder augmentation may be carried out at the same time as a Mitrofanoff procedure and involves using a piece of bowel inserted into the bladder wall. This procedure increases the capacity of the bladder, and is performed in children with high bladder pressure as a result of a small and overactive bladder to prevent urinary reflux.

More recently alternatives to the Mitrofanoff procedure, such as transverse retubularized sigmoidovesicostomy, have been developed in response to the increasing use of the appendix in antegrade continence enema procedures in children with faecal incontinence (Van Savage and

Yepuri 2001). Whichever urinary diversion is used the family will require input from a specialist children's continence nurse advisor who will provide support and guidance to the child and family on care of the stoma and catheterization procedures.

B) BOWEL DYSFUNCTION

In common with urinary functioning, normal bowel function in the child with a myelomeningocele will not be possible if the neurophysiological interactions between the sacral spinal nerves and the cerebral cortex are disrupted. Disruption to the nerve pathways can result in little or no awareness when the bowel is full because voluntary control that initiates or inhibits defecation is lost. Most children with spina bifida retain stool and develop constipation (Sandler 1997). Lack of sphincter control and faecal overflow as a consequence of constipation will result in faecal incontinence. This is extremely distressing for the child and family and limits many aspects of the child's life, including social and educational opportunities. The management of faecal incontinence must start with a detailed assessment of the child's bowel function. This will necessitate the child to keep a bowel diary to identify the nature of the problem. A systematic individualized approach to bowel management, negotiated with the child and family, and evaluation of the effectiveness of any interventions introduced is required.

Essential care

Bowel management has many interrelated components which include:

- Ensuring diet and fluid intake are appropriate to achieve appropriate stool consistency. This may be trial and error and will be individual to each child. A dietician will be able to provide dietary advice. Dehydration will increase consistency of the stool and should be avoided
- Abdominal massage may assist in maintaining gut motility and increase gut transit times
- Laxatives may be used as an adjunct to other treatments, with the type of laxative prescribed depending on the consistency of the stool. Laxatives are broadly divided into those which stimulate gut motility, for example bisacodyl, those which have an osmotic effect and prevent the stool becoming hard, for example lactulose and bulking agents, for example Fybogel
- The regular use of suppositories and enemas may be sufficient to maintain continence in some children
- Bowel training programmes that promote regular bowel habits may be beneficial but depend on the child having a degree of sphincter control and may not be suitable for children with memory or cognitive difficulties. An occupational therapist will be able to provide positional guidance and the need for supportive toilet seating.

The introduction of surgical procedures based on the principles of the antegrade continence enema (ACE procedure) – where the appendix is mobilized and used to form a stoma on the abdominal wall – have offered opportunity for children to achieve acceptable levels of continence. The stoma is used as a catheterizable conduit to allow the child or parents to perform bowel washouts, usually on alternate days, to achieve continence. A caecostomy button is a similar procedure but the caecum is brought to the surface of the abdominal wall to form a stoma, which is used as a conduit through which bowel washouts can be performed.

Latex allergy

Latex allergy is a common problem for children with a myelomeningocele (Barker *et al.* 2002). Although the specific cause of latex allergy is unknown, it is thought to be the result of the child becoming sensitized to rubber products through repeated contact during surgical procedures, diagnostic examinations, and bladder and bowel treatment programmes. Latex can be found in a range of healthcare products, such as surgical gloves, catheters, elastic bandages and elastic plasters. Allergic reactions to latex result in a range of symptoms: mild symptoms include eye irritations, sneezing, coughing and rashes; a severe reaction will result in anaphylactic shock due to the initiation of a major cell-mediated response causing acute vasoconstriction of the airways resulting in breathing difficulties, acute vasodilatation and increased permeability of the capillaries resulting in loss of fluid from the circulatory system and an inability to maintain the blood pressure. A latex-free environment can dramatically reduce latex sensitization in children (Nieto *et al.* 2002).

Essential care

The Task Force for Allergic Reactions to Latex (1993) provides information relating to maintaining a latex-free environment, which includes:

- Avoiding contact with latex products and using products with alternative components such as silicone, plastic or vinyl
- Healthcare professionals advocating for a latex-free environment for the child
- Providing parents with information relating to everyday products that contain latex; these include feeding bottle teats, pacifying dummies, disposable nappies, elastic in clothing and toys made of rubber
- Advising on contraceptive products that do not contain latex.

Enabling the child to develop to their maximum potential

The child and family will require support so that the child can reach their full potential and, where possible, achieve independent living.

Points to consider

The child will have a range of health and social care needs, which are best met by:

- Working in partnership with the child and family
- The child and family having a named key worker
- Having specialist centres where all aspects of care can be coordinated
- Ensuring effective transition strategies from child to adult service.

(Association for Spina Bifida and Hydrocephalus 2002)

Health, social and educational services need to ensure the child and young person with a disability are provided with opportunities that promote independence (Minchom *et al.* 1995). The child should be encouraged to take an active role in maintaining their health needs and preventing complications associated with a myelomeningocele. Healthcare professionals need to encourage the family and child to participate in decision-making processes. Parental overprotection, where paternal protection does not take into account a child's developmental stage or ability, is likely to be greater in children with myelomeningocele compared to able-bodied children (Holmbeck *et al.* 2002). This may be attributed to the child with myelomeningocele usually requiring an extensive range of healthcare interventions that can place physical, psychological and social demands on parents. Parental overprotection may be a consequence of psychosocial adaptation, and is used as a coping mechanism when tensions arise between the parent's desire to keep the child healthy, and the child's need for autonomy (Holmbeck *et al.* 2002).

Children with a myelomeningocele without hydrocephalus do not appear to have significant cognitive impairments (Iddon *et al.* 2004). Children will be able to attend mainstream nursery and school but will require detailed assessment to ensure educational settings can accommodate the child's physical limitations. This will require assessing the child's educational needs to comply with the current government codes of practice relating to children with special education needs (DfES 2001).

Support networks can be valuable for the child and their parents. Support groups can provide practical and emotional support and healthcare professionals should provide information about the availability of local support groups.

Adolescence is the time when young people are developing the skills necessary for independent living and life choices are being made. Young people with spina bifida will benefit from additional personal skills development support. This is particularly important for young people with communication difficulties and poor decision-making skills. The inclusion of children and young people with spina bifida into mainstream education has increased the need to ensure young people have a needs assessment which includes personal skills and access to appropriate advisors to help with the young person's future choices (Association for Spina Bifida and Hydrocephalus 2002).

The young person with a myelomeningocele will require specific information relating to potential sexual dysfunction in addition to routine sexual health information. Discussions relating to sexual health should be undertaken by a suitably qualified healthcare practitioner and must be handled sensitively. The young person will need advice relating to contraception, including ensuring products such as condoms and diaphragms are latex free. Sexual functions may be altered due to disruption of the neurophysiological interactions between the sacral spinal nerves and the cerebral cortex. This can result in altered sensations and may affect sexual function, including erection difficulties in men and altered vaginal secretions in women. Women may need to take extra precautions to prevent recurring urinary tract infections, such as emptying the bladder before and after sexual intercourse.

Points to consider

The young person planning a family may wish to have genetic counselling to enable them to discuss the likely risks of conceiving a child with spina bifida.

Transition to adulthood and to adult services can be an extremely anxious and difficult time for the child and family. This is compounded by the fact that health and social services that are available for children may not necessarily be available or funded once the child in no longer in full-time education (Association for Spina Bifida and Hydrocephalus 2002). Transition from child to adult services needs to be well planned, with a clear programme of care established before complete transition occurs (Tuffrey and Pearce 2003). Transition planning is discussed in Chapter 2, Section 8.

10.5 Tethered spinal cord

There is potential for the spinal cord to become fixed, known as a tethered cord, in children with spina bifida occulta or following surgical repair of meningocele or myelomeningocele as a result of anatomical abnormalities at the site of the lesion. A tethered spinal cord results in progressive neurological deficits such as decreased motor strength and increased spasticity in the lower limbs, lumbar pain, decreased mobility and incontinence (Barker *et al.* 2002). Children may not present with signs and symptoms of a tethered spinal cord until adulthood (Barker *et al.* 2002). The mechanisms for this late presentation are unclear but may be a consequence of mechanical and ischaemic damage at the site of the tethered cord. The cord becomes stretched during periods of rapid growth spurts such as adolescence (Yamada *et al.* 1995). The diagnosis is more difficult in children with myelomeningocele because neurological symptoms may already be present as a result of previous nerve damage (Fone *et al.* 1997; Jeelani *et al.* 1999). Consequently the signs and symptoms of a tethered cord in these children may only produce subtle changes in function.

Essential care

Children with spina bifida who present with progressive neurological deficits will require MRI and full neurological examination of spine and lower extremities to diagnose the presence of a tethered spinal cord (Fone *et al.* 1997; Jeelani *et al.* 1999). The child will require a detailed assessment of renal function as described in Section 4.

Surgery to release the spinal cord may be required in an attempt to restore function to previous levels and prevent further deterioration of neurological function (Jeelani *et al.* 1999). A laminectomy will be necessary to expose the tethered spinal cord, enabling the surgeon to release the adhesions and, where possible, correct any malformations. The care of the child post-laminectomy usually includes; bed rest for five days, followed by physiotherapy to assist the child in achieving previous levels of mobility. Wound drains are usually present for the first 24–48 hours following surgery; sutures are removed after 7 to 10 days. Usually the child is mobile and ready for discharge at about seven days following surgery. Children who are not suitable for surgery, or for whom surgery has been unsuccessful, will require appropriate care and management of permanent neurological deficits, outlined in Section 4.

Functionality following release of a tethered spinal cord is variable, and appears to depend on the level of the lesion, degree of neurological changes and the presence of a scoliosis (Fone *et al.* 1997). Estimates suggest that improvement in presenting symptoms occur in 70 per cent of children who undergo surgery (Herman *et al.* 1993; Fone *et al.* 1997). Improvements are more likely in children with spina bifida occulta. There is less evidence to support a benefit for children who have had previous surgery to repair a meningocele or myelomeningocele (Fone *et al.* 1997). There is the potential for the spinal cord to become tethered again as a result of scar tissue following surgery or additional growth, and repeat procedures may be necessary (Archibeck *et al.* 1997); however, a re-tethered cord may not always produce symptoms (Fone *et al.* 1997).

10.6 Long-term outcomes of spina bifida and effects on the child and family

The survival of infants born with spina bifida has increased four-fold since the 1960s as a consequence of improved neonatal care and improved operative procedures, particularly the development of shunts to manage hydrocephalus (Laurence 1974). However, spina bifida remains one of the leading causes of disability in children. This section will briefly discuss the long-term physical and psychological consequences of spina bifida for the child, family functioning and quality of life.

Long-term physical and psychological effects of spina bifida

The long-term outcomes for children with spina bifida appear to be related to the extent of neurological deficits, the presence of associated conditions and low birth weight. The-long term sequelae are variable and include reduced mobility, obesity, neurosensory deficits, and bladder and bowel incontinence (Hunt and Oakeshott 2003). The ability of children to gain independence on reaching adulthood is variable, ranging from independent living or minimal support within sheltered housing, to being highly dependent and requiring assistance to maintain activities of daily living (Hunt and Oakeshott 2003). Children with spina bifida can be socially disadvantaged because of a lack of community acceptance of disabilities and lack of peer support. In addition, young people with disabilities potentially have fewer employment possibilities and therefore reduced financial opportunities compared to able-bodied peers.

The impact of spina bifida is not dependent solely on neurological dysfunction and physical disability but also on psychosocial functioning (Minchom *et al.* 1995). It has been suggested that some young people with spina bifida have poor self-esteem, which is not necessarily linked to the severity of the disability (Minchom *et al.* 1995). Children with higher intelligence quotients and greater academic ability appear to have lower self-worth (Minchom *et al.* 1995). Unless associated with hydrocephalus, children with spina bifida can be expected to have normal intelligence and cognitive abilities (Iddon *et al.* 2004).

Effects of spina bifida on family functioning

Spina bifida is a permanent condition that can have significant effects on family functioning (Friedman *et al.* 2004). The effects will be similar to those experienced by families where a child has a long-term condition and include: maintaining normality, gaining skills in meeting the physical and emotional needs of the child, being alert to changes in the child's condition, providing adequate social opportunities for the child and being able to effectively orchestrate services for the child (Knafl *et al.* 1996; Gravelle 1997; Fisher 2001; Ray 2002). The ability of parents to respond to these issues are influenced by the family's health beliefs, their perception and understanding of the illness, adapting family routines to incorporate the child's routines, forming partnership with healthcare professionals and mastering technical aspects of care.

Maintaining normality

Making sense of the illness is a key component for parents caring for a child with a chronic illness. Parent's beliefs can impact, positively and negatively, on the expectations parents have for the child and the decisions they make to manage the child's condition. Parents of children with long-term conditions will make adjustments to accommodate the illness into family life, and evidence suggests that the unremitting nature of these adjustments is particularly challenging (Gravelle 1997; Fisher 2001). Families who work together appear to be more positive and less likely to focus on the child with a long-term condition (Knafl *et al.* 1996). In contrast are families who struggle to make adjustments to the situation do not appear to function as a family unit with the child becoming the main focus within the family and the source of conflicts (Knafl *et al.* 1996). Healthcare professionals need to support those families who are struggling to adapt to having a child with a disability within the family.

Physical and emotional overburden can be a direct result of providing care for the child to maintain the child's functions of daily living (Ray 2002). Care-giving usually falls to mothers (Gravelle 1997), and can place significant stress on partner relationships (Eddy and Walker 1999). Often families with a child with a long-term condition do not spend time together. Achieving normality can be difficult for some families because caring routines can become burdensome and everyday events can take an extraordinary amount of organizing (Knafl *et al.* 1996; Gravelle 1997; Fisher 2001).

Gaining skills to meet the physical and emotional needs of the child

Gaining the skills necessary to meet the physical needs of the child is a major aspect of parenting a child with a long-term condition (Knafl *et al.* 1996; Gravelle 1997; Fisher 2001; Ray 2002). Difficulties can be related to becoming confident with technical aspects of the child's care and obtaining appropriate equipment. Parents and the child will need clear, accurate and timely information in all aspects of care delivery including the use of equipment.

Essential care

Evidence suggests that equipment is not always specific to the individual child and therefore not suitable, the time taken for equipment to arrive is excessive, training and the timing of training is not always appropriate, written instructions are not clear, and parents perceive that there seems to be an inordinate amount of bureaucracy in funding and ordering equipment (Gravelle 1997; Ray 2002). Healthcare professionals must be proactive in ensuring the child is appropriately assessed and equipment recommended is not only appropriate for the child's needs but considers the home and school/nursery environment.

Provision of services for the child

Decisions about the needs of the child and family and type of care provision required should be negotiated between healthcare professionals and the child and family. Government policy has begun to recognize the importance of embedding the needs of the individual with chronic illness into models of healthcare delivery (DH 2001, 2004; Modernisation Agency 2002). However, parents have indicated that there is a lack of information about available services and they have to fit the child's requirements into the existing system rather than organizing services around the child's needs (Gravelle 1997; Ray 2002). Parents of a child with a long-term condition spend an excessive amount of time orchestrating services for their child (Ray 2002; Gravelle 1997). This is particularly problematic for parents of children who require complex care. A key worker can be effective in supporting the child and family and ensuring their individual needs are met.

Quality of life

The quality of life for children with spina bifida appears to be poor compared to children with other physical disabilities (Cate *et al.* 2002). This could be attributed to associations between quality of life and severity of the condition. Children with spina bifida who have associated medical problems, such as hydrocephalus and epilepsy, have a poorer quality of life compared to children with spina bifida in isolation (Cate *et al.* 2002). However, perceptions of quality of life in children with spina bifida vary between parents, physicians and the child (Kirpalani *et al.* 2000). It has been suggested that positive parent attitudes have a significant impact on the perceived quality of life for the child (Kirpalani *et al.* 2000). An additional factor that appears to influence the quality of life of children with spina bifida relates to the family's resourcefulness, namely care-giving efficiency and the ability to meet the whole family's needs (Cate *et al.* 2002). Detailed assessment of family functioning may help healthcare professionals identify those families who are struggling and prioritize service input accordingly.

Key messages from this chapter

- Spina bifida is the most frequent birth defect in children that results in long-term disability
- Spina bifida occurs as a consequence of failure of the neural tube to close, usually classified as spina bifida occulta, meningocele and myelomeningocele
- In children with a myelomeningocele the meninges and nerve tract protrude through the open bones of the spinal vertebrae forming an open lesion with the spinal cord nerve tract open to skin surface, allowing leakage of cerebrospinal fluid
- The child with a myelomeningocele will have motor deficits and sensory deficits, urinary and bowel dysfunction
- The long-term outcomes for children with spina bifida are variable and include reduced mobility, obesity, neurosensory deficits and bladder and bowel incontinence.
- Children with myelomeningocele may not achieve independent living and will require assistance to maintain activities of daily living
- Spina bifida is a permanent condition that can have significant effects on family functioning.

Web resources

Association for Spina Bifida and Hydrocephalus (ASBAH)
is the leading UK-registered charity providing information and advice about spina bifida and hydrocephalus to individuals, families and carers.
www.asbah.org.uk
Scope
provides support for people with disabilities.
www.scope.org.uk

References

Archibeck MJ, Smith JT, Carroll KL, Davitt JS, Stevens PM (1997) Surgical release of tethered spinal cord: survivorship analysis and orthopedic outcome. *Journal of Pediatric Orthopedics* **17** (6): 773–6.

Association for Spina Bifida and Hydrocephalus (2002) *A Constant Fight.* Association for Spina Bifida and Hydrocephalus, Peterborough.

Barker E, Saulino M, Caristro A (2002) Spina bifida. *RN* **65** (12): 33–9.

Bell WO, Nelson LH, Block SM, Rhoney JC (1996) Prenatal diagnosis and pediatric neurosurgery. *Pediatric Neurosurgery* **24** (3): 134–7.

Botto LD, Moore CA, Khoury MJ, Erickson JD (1999) Neural-tube defects. *New England Journal of Medicine* **341** (20): 1509–10.

Brett EM, Harding BN (1997) Hydrocephalus and congenital anomalies of the nervous system other than myelomeningocele. In Brett EM (Ed) *Paediatric Neurology*, 3rd edn. Churchill Livingstone, London.

Broughton NS, Menelaus MB, Cole WG, Shurtleff DB (1993) The natural history of hip deformity myelomeningocele. *Journal of Bone and Joint Surgery* **75** (5): 760–3.

Chumas PD (2000) The role of surgery in asymptomatic lumbosacral spinal lipomas. *British Journal of Neurosurgery* **14** (4): 301–4

Department of Health (2004) *The NHS Improvement Plan: Putting People at the Heart of Public Services.* DH, London.

Department for Skills and Education (2001) *Special Educational Needs: Code of Practice.* The Stationery Office, London.

Department of Health (2001) *The Expert Patient.* The Stationery Office, London.

Eddy L, Walker AJ (1999) The impact of children with chronic health problems on marriage. *Journal of Family Nursing* **5** (1): 10–32.

Feuchtbaum LB, Currier RJ, Riggle S *et al.* (1999) Neural tube defect prevalence in California (1990–1994): eliciting patterns by type of defect and maternal race/ethnicity. *Genetic Testing* **3** (3): 265–72

Fisher HR (2001) The needs of parents with chronically sick children: a literature review. *Journal of Advanced Nursing* **34** (4): 600–7.

Fone PD, Vapnek JM, Litwiller SE *et al.* (1997) Urodynamic findings in the tethered spinal cord syndrome: does surgical release improve bladder function? *The Journal of Urology* **157** (2): 604–9.

Frawley PA, Broughton NS, Menelaus MB (1998) Incidence of hindfoot deformities in patients with low-level spina bifida. *Journal of Pediatric Orthopedics* **18** (3): 312–13.

Friedman D, Holmbeck GN, Jandasek B, Zukerman J, Abad M (2004) Parental functioning in families of preadolescents with spina bifida: longitudinal implications for child adjustment. *Journal of Family Psychology* **18** (4): 609–19.

Geraniotis E, Koff SA, Enrile B (1988) The prophylactic use of clean intermittent catheterization in the treatment of infants and young children with myelomeningocele and neurogenic bladder dysfunction. *Journal of Urology* **139** (1): 85–6.

Gravelle AM (1997) Caring for a child with a progressive illness during the complex chronic phase: parents' experience of facing adversity. *Journal of Advanced Nursing* **25** (4): 738–45.

Green NS (2002) Folic acid supplementation and prevention of birth defects. *Journal of Nutrition* **132** (8 Suppl): 2356–60.

Herman JM, McLone DG, Storrs BB, Dauser RC (1993) Analysis of 153 patients with myelomeningocele or spinal lipoma reoperated upon for a tethered spinal cord. Presentation, management and outcome. *Pediatric Neurosurgery* **19** (5): 243–9.

Hernández-Díaz S, Werler MM, Walker AM, Mitchell AA (2001) Neural tube defects in relation to use of folic acid antagonists during pregnancy. *American Journal of Epidemiology* **153** (10): 961–8.

Holmbeck GN, Johnson SZ, Wills KE *et al.* (2002) Observed and perceived parental overprotection in relation to psychosocial adjustment in preadolescents with physical disability: the mediational role of behavioral autonomy. *Journal of Consulting and Clinical Psychology* **70** (1): 96–110.

Hunt GM, Oakeshott P (2003) Outcome in people with spina bifida at age 35: prospective community based cohort study. *British Medical Journal* **326** (7403): 1365–6.

Iddon JL, Morgan DJ, Loveday C, Sahakian BJ, Pickard JD (2004) Neuropsychological profile of young adults with spina bifida with or without hydrocephalus. *Journal Neurology, Neurosurgery, and Psychiatry* **75** (8): 1112–18.

Jeelani N, Jaspan T, Punt JA (1999) Lesson of the week: tethered spinal cord syndrome after myelomeningocele repair. *British Medical Journal* **318** (7182): 516–17.

Johnston LB, Borzyskowski M (1998) Bladder dysfunction and neurological disability at presentation in closed spina bifida. *Archives of Disease in Childhood* **79** (1): 33–8.

Karmel-Ross K, Cooperman DR, Van Doren CL (1992) The effect of electrical stimulation on quadriceps fermoris muscle torque in children with spina bifida. *Physical Therapy* **72** (10): 723–30.

Kelnar JH, Harvey D, Simpson C (1995) *The Sick Newborn Baby*. Baillière Tindall, London.

Kirpalani HM, Parkin PC, Willan AR *et al.* (2000) Quality of life in spina bifida: importance of parental hope. *Archives of Disease in Childhood* **83** (4): 293–7.

Knafl K, Bretmayer B, Gallo A *et al.* (1996) Family responses to childhood chronic illness: descriptions of management styles. *Journal of Pediatric Nursing* **11**: 315–26.

Laurence K (1974) Effect of early surgery for spina bifida cystica on survival and quality of life. *Lancet* **1** (7852): 301–4.

Medical Research Council Vitamin Study Research Group (1991) Prevention of neural tube defects: results of Medical Research Council Vitamin Study. *Lancet* **338** (8760): 131–7.

Minchom PE, Ellis NC, Appleton PL *et al.* (1995) Impact of functional severity on self concept in young people with spina bifida. *Archives of Disease in Childhood* **73** (1): 48–52.

Modernisation Agency (2002) *Involving Patients and Carers*. The Stationery Office, London.

McCarthy GT (1991) Treating children with spina bifida. *British Medical Journal* **302** (6768): 65–6.

Murphy M, Seagroatt V, Hey K *et al.* (1996) Neural tube defects 1974–1996 – down but not out. *Archive of Disease in Childhood* **75** (2): F133–4.

Nieto A, Mazón A, Pamies R *et al.* (2002) Efficacy of latex avoidance for primary prevention of latex sensitization in children with spina bifida. *Journal of Pediatrics* **140** (3): 370–2.

Cate IM, Kennedy C, Stevenson J (2002) Disability and quality of life in spina bifida and hydrocephalus. *Developmental Medicine and Child Neurology* **44**: 317–22.

Ray LD (2002) Parenting and childhood chronicity: making visible the invisible work. *Journal of Pediatric Nursing* **17** (6): 424–37.

Sandler A (1997) *Living with Spina Bifida: A Guide for Families and Professionals*. University of North Carolina Press, Chapel Hill, NC.

Task Force for Allergic Reactions to Latex (1993) American Academy of Allergy and Immunology. Committee report. *Journal of Allergy and Clinical Immunology* **92** (1): 16–18.

Tuffrey C, Pearce A (2003) Transition from paediatric to adult medical services for young people with chronic neurological problems. *Journal of Neurology, Neurosurgery, and Psychiatry* **74** (8): 1101–13.

Van Savage JG, Yepuri JN (2001) Transverse retubularized sigmoidovesicostomy continent urinary diversion to the umbilicus. *The Journal of Urology* **166** (2): 644–7.

Yamada S, Iacono RP, Andrade T *et al.* (1995) Pathophysiology of tethered cord syndrome. *Neurosurgery Clinics of North America* **6** (2): 311–23.

Appendix I

Terminology relating to neurosurgical procedures (adapted from Hickey 2003)

Burr hole   a hole made by a surgical drill into the skull which can be used to insert an endoscope, a catheter (such as a pressure monitoring device) or intracranial electrodes, and can be used to evacuate a haematoma

Craniotomy   an opening made into the skull that provides access to the intracranial contents for surgery. It usually involves creating a series of burr holes, using a specialized surgical saw, the holes are joined together to create a flap of bone which can be removed to allow access to the brain. The flap is replaced at the end of the procedure

Craniectomy   is the excision of a section of the skull, as in craniotomy, but the section is not replaced. It may be used after cerebral debulking procedure, such as tumour resection where there is anticipated to be excessive swelling or to relieve cerebral pressure

Laminectomy   excision of the posterior arch of a vertebra, sometimes performed to relieve pressure on the spinal cord or nerves or to allow access to the spinal cord for surgery

Linear craniectomy   excision of a fused suture

Stereotaxis   refers to a three-dimensional system that precisely locates the site for the surgical procedure. The principle is based on using a frame that is attached to the child's head and, with the aid of CT scanning probes, the area for surgery can be located.

Reference

Hickey JV (2003) Management of patients undergoing neurosurgical procedures. In Hickey JV (ed.) *The Clinical Practice of Neurological and Neurosurgical Nursing*, 5th edn. Lippincott, Williams & Wilkins, Philadelphia, PA.

Appendix II

Glossary

Acidosis   increased acidity and, if not specified, usually refers to the acidity of the blood plasma. It occurs as a result of an increase in hydrogen ion concentration resulting in a low blood pH

Adhesions   union between two surfaces that are normally separated

Amniocentesis   is a procedure where a small sample of amniotic fluid, the fluid that surrounds the **fetus** in the **womb,** is taken for testing in a laboratory.

Anencephaly   congenital absence of the cranial vault. The cerebral hemispheres are completely missing or reduced in size

Aneurysm   dilation of a blood vessel, usually an artery

Angiography   radiological examination of the blood vessels using an opaque contrast medium

Angioplasty   surgery of the blood vessels

Anosmia   impairment of the sense of smell

Antegrade continence enema (ACE)   a procedure that enables enemas to be administered through a stoma to empty the colon as a way of achieving continence

Anticholinergic therapy   bladder muscle relaxants

Arteriovenous   pertaining to both arteries and veins

Ataxia   poor muscle coordination resulting in irregular jerky movements or staggered walking

Atelectasis   collapse of the lung tissues, particularly bronchioles and alveoli

Atherosclerotic disease (atherosclerosis)   a condition in which fatty degenerative plaques cause narrowing and hardening of the blood vessels

Bacteraemia   presence of live bacteria in the bloodstream

Biparietal pinching   indentation of the parietal bones

Calcaneovalgus   is the term used to describe the position of the foot when it is pointing upwards and outwards, nearly always as a result of a congenital malformation

Canthoplasty   surgery to strengthen the lateral canthus, the tendon at the outer corner of the eyelids, which helps correct a drooping eye

Cardiac tamponade   life-threatening situation in which there is a large amount of fluid (usually blood) inside the pericardial sac around the heart, which affects normal heart functioning

Caudal   lower, for example the lower end of the spine

Central venous pressure   the pressure in the right atrium. Recorded by a central venous pressure monitor introduced via a catheter placed in the right atrium

Cerebral infarction   an area of necrosis in the brain produced by the blockage of a blood vessel

Cerebral anoxia   insufficient oxygen to the brain and if severe can cause irreversible brain damage

Cerebral perfusion pressure the difference between the mean arterial pressure and the intracranial pressure

Cerebrovascular pertaining to the arteries and veins of the brain

Cerebrovascular accident (stroke) a disorder arising from an embolus, thrombus or haemorrhage of the blood vessels of the cerebrum

Choanal atresia a congenital abnormality of the membranes of the nasal passages, resulting in blockage of the airways

Colloid solution a colloid is a **mixture** with **properties** between those of a **solution** and **fine suspension**, they are widely used in the replacement of fluid volume in resuscitation situations because they remain in the circulatory system longer than non-colloid solutions

Cortical relates to the cortex or outer portion of an organ

Cytogenetics the study of **chromosomes**, the visible carriers of **DNA**, the hereditary material

Dermatome collective name for regions of the body that graphically represent specific areas from which sensory spinal nerves carry information from the body to the central nervous system

Diabetes insipidus a condition of increased urine output and thirst caused by a lack of vasopressin, a hormone produced by the pituitary gland that regulates water reabsorption in the kidneys

Dysostosis defective ossification of fetal cartilage

Dysphasia difficulty in speaking due to brain damage that effects the ability to arrange words in the correct order

Effusion the escape of blood, serum or other fluid into surrounding tissues cavities

Encephalocele herniation of the brain through a congenital defect in the skull

Endocrinopathy disorder of the endocrine glands or their secretions

Endothelium the membranous lining of serous, synovial and other internal surfaces

Epidermoid cysts a **benign** lump of **squamous epithelium** cells

Equinovarus is the term used to describe the position the foot turns inward and downward, nearly always as a result of a congenital malformation

External ventricular drain (EVD) a system that uses a catheter which is placed in the ventricle of the brain and is connected to a drainage system as a temporary means of draining cerebrospinal fluid

Exophthalamus bulging of the eyes

Frontal bossing protrusion of the forehead

Fibrinolysis the process of breaking clots down and reabsorption of the clot

Fibrinolytic agent endogenous or exogenous chemicals that convert plasminogen to fibrinolysin, examples include urokinase, streptokinase and recombinant tissue plasminogen

Fistula an abnormal connection or passageway between two epithelium-lined organs or vessels that are not usually connected

Guillain-Barré syndrome a condition characterized by progressive symmetrical **paralysis** and loss of reflexes, usually beginning in the legs and usually proceeds towards the torso

Haemangioma benign tumours of the endothelial cells

Haematoma a swelling containing clotted blood

Hemiparesis weakness on one side of the body

Hemiplegia paralysis of one half of the body

Heterogeneous dissimilar elements; not uniform

Histology the study of the form of structures under the microscope.

Hypercalcaemia high levels of calcium in the blood

Hypercarbia/ hypercapnia   high levels of carbon dioxide in the blood

Hyperflexia   over-bending of a limb

Hyperlipidaemia   high levels of fat or lipids in the blood

Hyperpyrexia   an extremely elevated body temperature

Hypertelorism   abnormally wide spacing between the eyes

Hyperthyroidism   excessive circulation of thyroxin due to an overactive thyroid gland

Hypocalcaemia   low levels of calcium in the blood

Hypogonadism   a condition in which decreased production of gonadal hormones leads to below-normal function of the gonads and to retardation of sexual growth and development

Hypophosphatasia   an inherited absence of alkaline phosphatase, an enzyme essential in bone formation

Hypotelorism   abnormally narrow space between the eyes

Hypothalamic   refers to the hypothalamus; hypothalamic disorders affect many body functions and disrupt the function of the autonomic nervous system, metabolism and the endocrine system

Hypothrombinaemia   abnormally low thrombin in the circulating blood resulting in a tendency to bleed

Hypovolaemia   excessive loss of blood volume

Hypoxaemia   excessive reduction of oxygen levels in the blood

Hypoxia   reduction of the **oxygen** levels in tissues

Immunosuppression   decreased ability to form antibodies that may result in difficulty to respond to infectious agents

Incidence   the rate of new cases of a disease which occur in a population during a specified time period

Infarct   an area of necrosis as a result of tissue anoxia as a result of interruption to the blood flow

Infratentorial herniation   the infratentorial contents of the brain are displaced through the foramen magnum

Inotrope   a drug agent which alters the force of heart muscle contractions

Intracranial   within the skull

Intracranial pressure monitoring   the recording of pressure exerted by the cerebrospinal fluid within the subarachnoid space and ventricles of the brain

Ischaemia   deficiency in the blood supply to a part of the body

Lipoma   a benign tumour composed of fatty tissue that develops in the connective tissue and can arise in any part of the body

Mean arterial pressure   is the difference between the systolic and diastolic blood pressure

Meningocele   a protrusion of the meninges through the skull or spinal column, appearing as a cyst filled with cerebrospinal fluid

Microencephaly/

microcephaly   a small head and usually reflects an underlying reduction in the size of the brain

Mitrofanoff appendicovesicostomy   urinary diversion procedure to enable catheterization of the bladder through a stoma in the abdomen

Moyamoya disease   a rare progressive cerebrovascular disorder caused by blocked arteries where the basal ganglia are situated at the base of the brain

Morbidity   a specific incidence rate that relates to the effects of the condition in a defined population

Mortality   a specific incidence rate; death from a disease in a defined population

Mutism   an inability to speak

Myelomeningocele   a protrusion of the spinal cord and meninges through a defect in the vertebral column

Myelosuppression   decreased bone marrow activity as a consequence of chemotherapy resulting in a reduction of blood cells

Myotome   collective name for regions of the body that graphically represent specific muscles innervated by nerves from a particular spinal nerve

Necrosis   the death of living cells

Nephritis   **inflammation** of the **kidney**

Nephrotoxicity   substances that can potentially damage the cells of the kidneys

Neurofibromatosis   a genetic disorder of the nervous system that causes tumours to grow on nerves, affecting the development and growth of neural cell tissues

Neutropaenia   low **white blood cell**, specifically **granulocytes**, that are responsible for killing and digesting microorganisms

Nystagmus   rapid rhythmic repetitious involuntary eye movements

Occipital protuberance   prominence of the outer surface of the of the occipital bone

Oedema   an excessive amount of fluid in the body tissue

Oesteotomy   a surgical operation whereby a bone is cut to shorten, lengthen, or change its alignment

Oncogenesis   the causation and formation of tumours at cellular level

Optic atrophy   wasting of the optic disc

Ototoxicity   substances that can potentially damage the eighth cranial nerve or structures related to hearing

Pappilloedema   swelling of the optic disc

Peripheral neuropathy   numbness and/or tingling of the hands and feet

Phonetic   refers to sound

Polydactyly   more than usual number of fingers and toes

Porencephaly   cysts or cavities in the cerebral hemisphere of the brain

Positron emission tomography (PET)   diagnostic examination that involves obtaining body images based on the detection of radiation from the emission of positrons. Positrons are tiny particles emitted from a radioactive substance administered to the patient.

Prevalence   the proportion of the population that have a named condition, usually at a single period in time

Prognathism   the positional relationship of the mandible and/or maxilla to the skeletal base where either of the jaws protrudes

Ptosis   drooping of one or both upper eyelids

Rostral   Uppermost, for example the upper end of the spine

Septicaemia   a blood infection causes by multiplication of bacteria within the blood

Sclerotherapy   a procedure where blood vessels are injected with a sclerosing solution which causes them to collapse

Scoliosis   lateral curvature of the spine

Serum osmolarity/osmolality   the osmotic concentration of blood serum solution expressed as osmoles of solute per litre of solution. Osmolarity is the osmoles of solute per litre of solution. Osmolality is the osmoles of solute per kilogram of solvent

Single positron emission computerized tomography (SPECT)   a **nuclear medicine tomographic** imaging technique using gamma rays

Somatic   refers to the body as distinct from some other entity such as the mind

Spherocytosis   diseased red blood cells where the surface membrane of the cell is defective and the blood cells become spherical in shape

Strabismus   muscle failure or nerve defects in the eyes causing them to move in separate directions

Subcortical   below the cortex

Subdural haemorrhage   a bleed between the arachnoid and dura mater

Supratentorial   the area of brain above the tentorium

Syndactyly   a condition in which two or more of the fingers or toes are joined together

Talipes   a deformity caused by a congenital or acquired contraction of the muscles or tendons of the foot

Telangiectasis   a group of dilated capillary blood vessels, web-like or radiating in form

Tentorium   a fold of dura mater that covers the cerebellum and supports the occipital lobes of the cerebrum

Thrombocytopaenia   decreased number of platelets that may result in bruising and tendency to bleed

Thrombolytic agent   a chemical that is able to dissolve a clot (**thrombus**) and reopen an artery or vein

Thrombosis   the formation of a clot inside a blood vessel, obstructing the flow of blood through the circulatory system.

Tinnitus   ringing in the ears

Tissue plasminogen activator   an enzyme that helps dissolve clots

Transverse retubularized sigmoidovesicostomy   urinary diversion procedure

Tuberous sclerosis   a genetic disorder characterized by abnormalities of the skin, brain, kidney and heart. The brain abnormalities are mainly benign cortical tumours (tubers) which cause seizures, developmental delay, and mental retardation

Ventriculitis   inflammation and/or infection of the ventricles

Visceral   the internal organs of the body, specifically those within the chest such as the heart, lungs and abdomen

Index